MEDICINE THAT WALKS

Disease, Medicine, and Canadian Plains Native People, 1880–1940

In this seminal work, Maureen Lux takes issue with the 'biological invasion' theory of the impact of disease on plains Aboriginal people. She challenges the view that Aboriginal medicine was helpless to deal with the diseases brought by European newcomers and that Aboriginal people therefore surrendered their spirituality to Christianity. Biological invasion, Lux argues, was accompanied by military, cultural, and economic invasions, which, combined with both the loss of the bison herds and forced settlement on reserves, led to population decline. The diseases killing the plains Aboriginal people were not contagious epidemics but the grinding diseases of poverty, malnutrition, and overcrowding.

Medicine That Walks provides a grim social history of medicine from the end of the nineteenth to the middle of the twentieth century. It traces the relationship between the ill and the well, from the 1880s, when Aboriginal people were perceived as a vanishing race doomed to extinction, to the 1940s, when they came to be seen as a disease menace to the Canadian public. Drawing on archival material, ethnography, archaeology, epidemiology, ethnobotany, and oral histories, Lux describes how bureaucrats, missionaries, and particularly physicians explained the high death rates and continued ill health of the plains people in the quasi-scientific language of racial evolution that inferred the survival of the fittest. The plains people's poverty and ill health were seen as both an inevitable stage in the struggle for 'civilization' and as further evidence that assimilation was the only path to good health.

The Native people lived and coped with a cruel set of circumstances, but they survived, in large part because they consistently demanded a role in their own health and recovery. Painstakingly researched and convincingly argued, this work will change our understanding of a significant era in western Canadian history.

MAUREEN K. LUX is a post-doctoral fellow at the Hannah Institute for the History of Medicine.

Infectious Ideas

Infectious Ideas

Contagion in Premodern Islamic and Christian Thought in the Western Mediterranean

Justin K. Stearns

The Johns Hopkins University Press
Baltimore

This book has been brought to publication with the generous support of the Program for Cultural Cooperation between Spain's Ministry of Culture and United States Universities.

Printed in the United States of America on acid-free paper
2 4 6 8 9 7 5 3 1

The Johns Hopkins University Press
2715 North Charles Street
Baltimore, Maryland 21218-4363
www.press.jhu.edu

Library of Congress Cataloging-in-Publication Data

Stearns, Justin K., 1974–
Infectious ideas : contagion in premodern Islamic and Christian thought in the Western Mediterranean / Justin K. Stearns.
p. ; cm.
Includes bibliographical references and index.
ISBN-13: 978-0-8018-9873-0 (hardcover : alk. paper)
ISBN-10: 0-8018-9873-0 (hardcover : alk. paper)
1. Diseases—Causes and theories of causation—History—To 1500. 2. Medicine, Medieval—Western Mediterranean. 3. Epidemiology—History—To 1500. 4. Medicine—Religious aspects—Islam—History—To 1500. 5. Medicine—Religious aspects—Christianity—History—To 1500. I. Title.
[DNLM: 1. Medicine in Literature—Africa, Northern. 2. Medicine in Literature—Portugal. 3. Medicine in Literature—Spain. 4. Christianity—history—Africa, Northern. 5. Christianity—history—Portugal. 6. Christianity—history—Spain. 7. Communicable Diseases—Africa, Northern. 8. Communicable Diseases—Portugal. 9. Communicable Diseases—Spain. 10. Cross-Cultural Comparison—Africa, Northern. 11. Cross-Cultural Comparison—Portugal. 12. Cross-Cultural Comparison—Spain. 13. Islam—history—Africa, Northern. 14. Islam—history—Portugal. 15. Islam—history—Spain. 16. Leprosy—history—Africa, Northern. 17. Leprosy—history—Portugal. 18. Leprosy—history—Spain. 19. Plague—history—Africa, Northern. 20. Plague—history—Portugal. 21. Plague—history—Spain. WZ 330 S7995i 2011]
RB152.S74 2011
362.196′9—dc22 2010019679

A catalog record for this book is available from the British Library.

To Mataio
for everything you have given us
and
for everything that will come

Contents

Preface

Disease, and especially epidemic disease, has played an influential or even central role in human history. Not too long ago, when the focus of historians was largely political, and disease made at best an anecdotal appearance in standard historical narratives, such a statement would have needed justification. But in the past half century, historians and scholars have argued convincingly that disease has been a factor in nearly every aspect of the human experience.[1] Few would now dispute that epidemic disease influenced (and continues to influence) political, social, and economic developments; a classic example is the role played by smallpox in the Spanish conquest of the New World. How has humankind responded to this influence? What were the cultural and intellectual responses to epidemics? How have societies made sense of these terrible and traumatic natural disasters that they could neither fully control nor understand? This book examines one aspect of the human experience of epidemics, the transmission of disease—commonly known as contagion—in the context of Christian and Muslim societies in Iberia and North Africa. Much of the attention is focused on the example of the Black Death of the fourteenth century, but in order to fully contextualize the variety and richness of the meanings given to the concept of contagion, the book considers examples from the ninth to the nineteenth centuries.

Epidemic disease disrupts societies and threatens the established social and ethical order. As is true of both the plague and leprosy, the two diseases that figure most prominently in this work, epidemics commonly arouse fear, disgust, helplessness, and incomprehension. How and why epidemics occur have always been closely associated if not interwoven questions, and any discussion of contagion in medieval Iberia involves an at least implicit discussion of how Christians and Muslims responded to these epidemics themselves. Yet the focus here is on the many significances of contagion itself, and specifically on how Christian and Muslim scholars presented understandings of contagion that drew productively and creatively on medical knowledge, empirical observation, religious sources, and previous scholarship. This is a comparative study, in that the worlds of Christian and Muslim scholarship here examined were largely distinct, though they both drew on Greek sources and Abrahamic scriptures. Simultaneously, it strives to avoid the comparativist tendency to reduce a given religion, culture, or society's response to a narrow set of characteristics that can be easily juxtaposed with those of another. Instead, the study aims to identify the different parameters within which these two groups of scholars debated the notion of contagion and to clarify why each found it to be of such interest.

Christian Scholarship in Iberia

The Iberian peninsula was at least tentatively united under Roman rule by the end of the third century BCE, following Rome's defeat of Carthage in the Second Punic Wars, and it was through Rome that Christianity came to Iberia in the first century CE.[2] Although Christians of the time were persecuted for their faith, shortly before 313 CE, when the emperor Constantine issued the Edict of Milan, declaring a policy of religious toleration, the first public council of the Church in Spain boasted nineteen bishops. In the beginning of the fifth century, as the Roman Empire's control over Iberia weakened, Visigothic tribes crossed the Pyrenees, bringing with them Arianism, a Christian heresy that they continued to profess for another century and a half.[3] The Visigoths were not able to consolidate their hold over Iberia until the end of the sixth century, at roughly the same time that they abandoned their adherence to Arianism and officially adopted Catholicism, removing a barrier between them and their Hispano-Roman subjects. The following century witnessed a rapid growth of Christianity in the peninsula. While it is impossible to know what percentage of Iberia's population was Christian by the time of the Muslim invasion in 711, archaeological evidence strongly suggests that by then the majority of Iberians had adopted Christianity. This Christian population was tended to by an affluent and powerful church, which had become one of the largest landowners in Iberia, second only to the Visigothic royalty.

The authors considered in chapters 2 and 4 of this book largely belonged to the ecclesiastical classes of this church. Beginning with the bishop Isidore of Seville (d. 636), they were concerned with policing the purity of the faith of their flock and with maintaining their own social importance. These anxieties were initially reflected in their worry over the survival of remnants of Arianism, a theme that continued to be manifested, if only rhetorically, until the fifteenth century in the sermons of Saint Vincent Ferrer (d. 1419). After the arrival of Islam in the eighth century, however, the Catholic clergy were faced with a new heresy, Islam. It continued to be considered a heresy for much of the Middle Ages.

From the eighth to the end of the fifteenth century—significantly longer than Europeans have been in the New World—Muslims ruled substantial parts of Iberia. In both the Alphonsine corpus of the thirteenth century and the sermons of

Saint Vincent Ferrer of the fifteenth, we find contagion being marshaled as a metaphor to describe first the danger of Muslims as an external threat and then, later, an internal one. Of course, Christian scholars also discussed contagion as a medical problem, as did Isidore in the seventh century and the Catholic humanists Enrique de Villena and Alonso Fernández de Madrigal of the fifteenth century, discussed in chapter 4. Their discussions of leprosy and contagion, however, were at least nominally directed to clarifying biblical passages, but they also served as explications of contemporary understandings of the natural world. The writings on contagion examined in these chapters were produced by a body of scholars who were innocent of the modern preoccupation with distinguishing between religious and scientific knowledge; moreover, they accepted without question the proposition that revealed scripture and the natural world were the works of the same Creator and could inform each other. The problem was how to elucidate most accurately the relationship between the two.[4] A similar challenge was faced by Muslim scholars of the time.

Muslim Scholarship in al-Andalus and the Maghrib

As part of the extraordinary Muslim military and political expansion of the first/seventh–second/eighth centuries, a mostly Berber army led by Arab Muslims invaded Iberia in 711, putting an end to Christian Visigothic rule. Despite this early political prominence of Muslim elites in what they soon came to call al-Andalus, Muslim scholarship in this region depended a great deal initially on intellectual ties to Egypt, Arabia, and Iraq.[5] Islamic law and theology were still very much in the process of being articulated during the very centuries when Muslim political control expanded so quickly. Next to the Qur'an, Muslims have generally considered the sayings of the Prophet Muḥammad—the hadith—to represent the greatest scriptural authority. Following the compilation of these sayings into collections in the third/ninth century that later became canonical, knowledge of the hadith and of how to interpret them became central to Sunnī Muslim scholarship. Although, as briefly discussed in chapter 3, acknowledgment of the authority of the hadith took a little longer with the Mālikī law school, which came to be dominant in al-Andalus and North Africa, by the fifth/eleventh century any substantive legal or theological debate involved a discussion of the relevant sayings of the Prophet. Chapter 1 takes up the place of contagion in the collections of the hadith and the commentaries on these collections. These sources, even those not written in the western Mediterranean (often referred to simply as "the West," or al-Maghrib), carried considerable authority there and, second to the Qur'an, formed the heart of what many Muslims considered knowledge (*ʿilm*) to be. The hadith was itself, however, only a body of texts. How to read these texts, how to relate them to each other and to elucidate their significance, demanded a body of interpretive principles, and this need was met in two different ways in the fields of law (how one should act, and why) and theology (what one should believe, and why). Muslim jurists and theologians were not necessarily specialists in the hadith, although they often were, but they knew at least which books to consult to find pertinent information. The legal and theological status of contagion for Muslim scholars is discussed in chapter 5, and the reader will note how both there and in the other chapters on Muslim scholarship, the Muslim West is considered as a unit, within which scholars wrote, read, and debated with each other regardless of the political divides that may have separated them.

The lines between the scholarly disciplines of hadith studies, law, and theology were often blurred, and similarly, Muslim authors of medical works had often distinguished themselves in other fields. While some of the scholars introduced in chapter 3 are known only for their writings on medicine, many others also wrote with authority in the fields of law, theology, and mysticism and were, in addition, accomplished poets. It is precisely this ability of scholars in the premodern period—both Muslim and Christian—to master multiple fields of knowledge that frustrates any attempt to easily characterize them as a group, particularly when considering their views on contagion over more than a thousand years.

Medicine, Theology, and the State

When we think of responses to the threat of epidemic disease today, as in the case of the H1N1 swine flu virus, we commonly turn to the state for broad, sweeping solutions when it comes to developing vaccines and possibly implementing quarantines. The state, in turn, sees itself as responsible for protecting its population against health risks, its economy from potential disruption, and its armed forces from potential strategic disadvantages. The state response to the threat of an epidemic involves attempting to manage it through the organization of a coherent, coordinated effort of physicians and health care specialists. During the premodern period, because state power was comparatively weak and decentralized, the situation was considerably different (with some notable exceptions, such as the city-states of late-medieval Italy). Scholars who wrote on contagion or epidemic disease did so primarily as spiritual, legal, or medical authorities; they may have expressed a clear preference for a specific response, but they seldom had the authority to put their recommendations into effect. Even in the case of Ibn al-Khaṭīb, vizier of the emirate of Granada in the eighth/fourteenth century, when the Black Death struck, it is unclear whether his staunch defense of the phenomenon of contagion had any effect on the official responses of the Granadan state to the disaster. Instead, the scholars whose opinions are presented in the following chapters were, almost without exception, presenting the results of their own individual research and thought. The degree to which their opinions were considered definitive by fellow scholars was directly correlated to how much authority they possessed. It is, in any event, difficult to know to what degree these opinions represent the views on contagion held by the nonliterate classes, although in the case of the sermons, legal opinions, and plague treatises considered here, we know at least that they were intended to reach the broader Christian or Muslim public.

In Iberia, as the political fortunes of the Muslim community waned from the eleventh century onward and Christian kingdoms gradually became ascendant, a large number of medical, philosophical, and scientific works were translated from Arabic into Latin and later into Castilian. In part reflecting the high degree of scholarly interconnectedness of the two religiously defined political and social spheres, a great deal has been written in recent years on the creation of a "tolerant" multireligious society in medieval Iberia.[6] Yet, although Muslim and Christian scholars drew on some of the same medical authorities and at times were reminded of similar scriptural precedents, they differed starkly in how they made sense of epidemic disease and in how they determined the significance of contagion. How and why this was so, as well as why it would be dangerous to exaggerate these differences, is the subject of this book.

The Structure of the Book

Comparative history is difficult, in part because it implies equivalences where they often do not exist. More treacherously, characterized by the desire to better understand cultural, social, and religious differences, comparative history can encourage us to simplify complex traditions and create generalizations based on a series of striking examples. Resisting this tendency toward reductionism, *Infectious Ideas* aims to elucidate the complexity within Christian and Muslim discussions of contagion as much as to offer a comparison of the two traditions. This goal is reflected in the book's structure. The introduction discusses some of the broader and perhaps unexpected historiographical and theoretical issues raised by the study of contagion in the premodern Mediterranean world. The chapters that follow alternate between Muslim and Christian scholarship. Chapter 1 examines contagion in the collections of sayings and actions (the hadith) of the Prophet

Muhammad, which purport to date back to the first half of the seventh century—the very same period when Isidore of Seville wrote—when the Muslim community first encountered the plague and leprosy. The chapter then traces the discussion of contagion in commentaries on these sayings that were written down to the eighteenth century. The sayings and the commentaries on them both provide the basis for and reflect the premodern legal and theological debates of Muslim scholars in al-Andalus and North Africa. Chapter 2 turns to the metaphoric uses of contagion in Christian Iberian writings, taking a similarly longitudinal approach by beginning with the work of the seventh-century bishop Isidore of Seville and continuing through to the copious sermons of the fifteenth-century Valencian preacher Vincent Ferrer. Chapter 3 is devoted to contagion in the Muslim medical tradition, focusing specifically on the plague treatises written in the aftermath of the Black Death. Chapter 4 offers initially a summary discussion of the plague treatises written by Christian authors in Iberia but then takes up more extensively the phenomenon of visual contagion that was debated by Christian humanists in the fifteenth century. Chapter 5, drawing on material introduced in chapters 1 and 3, explores the ways in which contagion was discussed within Islamic law and theology. Chapter 6, following on chapters 3 and 5, examines Muslim treatments of contagion in North Africa from the sixteenth to the nineteenth century. In the conclusion, I return to the broader subject of Muslim and Christian communities' responses to the Black Death in the fourteenth century and to how previous comparisons of their respective conceptions of contagion have largely missed the mark.

Although the chapters are organized in roughly chronological order, their structure is primarily thematic. I have privileged tracing the development of a particular discussion or rhetorical trope—the permissibility of fleeing the plague in Islamic law, for example, or the contagiousness of heretics—over a purely temporal order. In taking this approach, I have been influenced by the conviction that although the various medical, legal, literary, and theological discourses in which contagion featured influenced each other, they also possessed their own coherence, which deserves attention in its own right. I recognize that moving back and forth chronologically within two different scholarly traditions may be challenging for the reader, and so, for reference, on pages xvii–xx I have supplied an annotated list of the main Muslim and Christian authors discussed in the book.

Acknowledgments

My thanks go first and foremost to my advisers Michael Cook and William Jordan, with whom I had the good fortune to study at Princeton. Graduate school was for me a challenging, rewarding, frustrating, and often humbling experience, but both of my advisers not only gave me the tools to begin to ask the questions in which I was interested, but also, through their examples, impressed upon me the full potential of being a scholar. In two separate seminars that they offered, I caught the first glimpses of what led me to this rather peculiar topic. I am especially grateful to Michael Cook for his patience and his exceedingly generous comments, suggestions, and corrections. I would also like to thank Andras Hamori and Abraham Udovitch for their scholarship and counsel.

Conceived in Princeton, this project came into the world in Madrid, in the Department of Arabic Studies at the Consejo Superior de Investigaciónes Científicas. During an initial visit in the summer 2002 and then again for a year in 2003–4, I benefited from the warm and collegial atmosphere I found there and from conversations with Elena de Felipe, Maribel Fierro, Mercedes García-Arenal, Rashid Hour, Manuela Marín, Fernando Mediano, Cristina de la Puente, and Delfina Serrano. I am indebted to Maribel Fierro for her ongoing support, her numerous references, her comments, her time, and in general for helping a clueless American graduate student find his way through the scholarship on al-Andalus. In addition, I am grateful to Cristina Álvarez Millán for her advice and support during my initial attempts to understand plague treatises. Finally, during my first summer in Spain, I was blessed by the hospitality of Sofía Torallas-Tovar and by her friendship during both that summer and the year I returned to Spain.

This project was improved by the feedback of numerous friends and colleagues, including Najam Haider, Toby Jones, Ben Lerner, Judith Loebenstein, and Nathalie Peutz. I also profited from the comments, generosity, and advice of Jocelyn Hendrickson, Sayeed Rahman and (again!) Nathalie Peutz. I would like to profoundly thank the first anonymous reader for the Johns Hopkins University Press, who took the time to offer corrections and improvements on every page of the manuscript. I have tried to resolve the issues raised by the second anonymous reader, for whose careful reading of the manuscript I am similarly grateful. I wish to express as well my deep gratitude to Jacqueline Wehmueller of the Johns Hopkins University Press for her support, her patience, and her guidance through the process of turning manuscript pages into a book. Finally, I am indebted to Lois Crum for her detailed and patient copyediting of the manuscript. She improved the text immensely.

During the past five years, my academic home has been the Religion Department at Middlebury College, and I am truly grateful to have been part of such a warm and collegial environment. During this time, I not only have begun to learn how to teach but have also been stimulated by conversation with my colleagues and, most of all, with my students.

Since I began work on the subject of contagion, it has followed me from Egypt, Yemen, New Zealand, Spain, and Morocco to Vermont. My constant companion has been my wife, Nathalie Peutz, to whom I am grateful for so much more than academic support. Without her presence, little in these years would have made much sense at all. In the past three years our son Mataio has had many opportunities to turn and run out of his father's office when faced with perilously teetering piles of books related to this project, or to ask me "Why?" when I say that I am going to work now. I can only hope that he will continue to remind me of what Gary Snyder has called "the real work."

Chronological List of Relevant Muslim and Christian Scholars Who Wrote on Contagion in the Premodern Period

Ibn Sahl b. Rabbān al-Ṭabarī (d. after 240/855), Christian doctor who converted to Islam; lived in Sāmarrā'.

Ibn Qutayba (d. 276 / 889), theologian, traditionist, and jurist; lived much of his life in Baghdad.

Thābit b. Qurra (d. 288/901), doctor, mathematician, and astronomer from Ḥarrān; flourished and died in Baghdad.

Muḥammad b. Zakariyyā al-Rāzī (d. 311/923), doctor and student of the natural sciences in general; born and died in Rayy, spent many years in Baghdad.

Al-Khaṭṭābī (d. 338/998), traditionist, hadith commentator, and poet from Bust (in southern Afghanistan).

Ibn Sīnā (d. 428/1037), philosopher and doctor from Bukhara; died in Hamadan.

Ibn Baṭṭāl (d. 449/1057), traditionist and hadith commentator from Cordoba.

Ibn ᶜAbd al-Barr (d. 463/1070), traditionist and jurist from Cordoba.

Al-Bājī (d. 474/1081), theologian and jurist from Badajoz; died in Almería.

Ibn Rushd al-Jadd (d. 520/1126), jurist and judge from Cordoba; grandfather of the philosopher.

Al-Māzarī (d. 536/1141), jurist and hadith commentator from al-Mahdiyya in Ifrīqiya.

Ibn al-ᶜArabī (d. 543/1148), traditionist and jurist from Seville; buried in Fez.

ᶜIyāḍ b. Mūsā (d. 544/1149), jurist from Ceuta; died in Marrakesh.

Ibn al-Ṣalāḥ (d. 643/1245), traditionist and jurist from Shahrazūr (on the border of Iraq and Iran); died in Damascus.

Abū ᶜAbbās Aḥmad b. ᶜUmar al-Qurṭūbī (d. 656/1258), jurist, traditionist, and hadith commentator from Cordoba; died in Alexandria.

Abū ᶜAbdāllah Muḥammad b. Aḥmad al-Qurṭūbī (d. 671/1273), traditionist and Qur'anic exegete from Cordoba; died in Upper Egypt.

Al-Nawawī (d. 676/1277), jurist, traditionist, and hadith commentator from Nawā, near Damascus.

Ibn Abī Jamra al-Andalusī (d. 699/1300), traditionist and ascetic; place of birth and death unknown.

ᶜUmar al-Sakūnī al-Ishbīlī (d. 717/1317), theologian and jurist; lived and died in Tunis.

Shams al-Dīn al-Dhahabī (d. 748/1348), traditionist and jurist; lived and died in Damascus.

Ibn al-Wardī (d. 749/1349), jurist and poet from Ma^{c}arrat al-Nu^{c}man; died in Aleppo.

Ibn Qayyim al-Jawziyya (d. 751/1350), theologian and jurist; lived and died in Damascus.

Ibn Mufliḥ al-Maqdisī (d. 763/1362), jurist and legal theorist; lived and died in Damascus.

Ibn Khātima (d. 770/1369), jurist and physician from Almería.

Ibn al-Khaṭīb (d. 776/1374), jurist, physician, and Sufi; flourished in Granada and died in Fez.

Ibn Abī Ḥajalah (d. 776/1375), poet, prose writer, and Sufi from Tilimsān; died near Cairo.

Ibn Lubb (d. 782/1381), jurist and judge; lived and taught in Granada.

Al-Manbijī (d. 785/1383), jurist and traditionist from Syria.

Al-Kirmānī (d. 786/1384), jurist, theologian, and hadith commentator; died on pilgrimage and was buried in Baghdad.

Al-Shāṭibī (d. 790/1388), jurist and legal theorist; was born and died in Granada.

Al-Ubbī (d. 827/1425), traditionist, jurist, and hadith commentator; lived in Algeria.

Ibn Ḥajar al-^{c}Asqalānī (d. 852/1448), traditionist, jurist, and judge; born and died in Cairo.

Al-^{c}Aynī (d. 855/1451), jurist, hadith commentator, and judge from ^{c}Ayntāb in Syria; flourished and died in Cairo.

Al-Raṣṣā^{c} (d. 894/1489), jurist, doctor, and judge from Tlemcen; died in Tunis.

Al-Sanūsī (d. 895/1490), theologian, Sufi, and doctor; was born and died in Tlemcen.

Al-Mawwāq (d. 897/1492), jurist and judge; died in Granada.

Al-Qasṭallānī (d. 923/1517), traditionist, hadith commentator, and theologian; was born and died in Cairo.

Al-Yūsī (d. 1102/1691), jurist, Sufi, and theologian from near Sefrou; died in Fez.

Al-Zurqānī (d. 1122/1710), jurist and traditionist; was born and died in Cairo.

Muḥammad b. Aḥmad al-Ḥājj (d. 1128/1715), jurist and traditionist; was born and died in Fez.

Aḥmad b. Mubārak al-Sijilmāsī al-Lamṭī (d. 1156/1743), Sufi and jurist; lived in Fez.

Abū ^{c}Abd Allāh Muḥammad al-Shabbī al-Ḥāmidī al-Sūsī (d. 1163/1749), doctor.

Muḥammad b. al-Ḥasan al-Banānī (d. 1194/1780), jurist and preacher; died in Fez.

Aḥmad Ibn ᶜAjība (d. 1224/1809), Sufi and jurist from al-Khamīs, near Tangiers; died in Zammīdj (also near Tangiers).

Muḥammad b. Aḥmad al-Rahūnī (d. 1230/1814), Moroccan jurist.

Muḥammad b. Abī al-Qāsim al-Fīlālī (al-Filālī) (d. after 1252/1836), jurist from Sijilmāsa; died in Rabat.

Ḥamdān b. ᶜUthmān Khoja (d. ca. 1258/1842), Algerian jurist; died in Istanbul.

Muḥammad b. al-Madanī b. ᶜAlī Junūn (d. 1302/1884), Moroccan Sufi and jurist.

Al-Gharisī (d. 1313/1895), jurist and poet from Tlemcen; died in Morocco.

Cyprian (d. 258), bishop of Carthage; lived and died in Carthage.

Ambrosiaster (fourth century), name given to an anonymous author, previously thought to be Ambrose (d. 397).

Jerome (d. 420), biblical translator and theologian from Stridon in Dalmatia; died near Bethlehem.

Isidore of Seville (d. 636), bishop and historian; flourished in Seville.

Beato of Liebana (d. 798), Cantabrian monk; wrote a commentary on the book of Revelation.

Qusṭā ibn Lūqā (d. 297/910 or 308/920), doctor; lived in Baghdad and died in Armenia.

Haymo Halberstatensis (d. 850), Benedictine monk and bishop of Halberstadt.

Rupert of Deutz (d. ca. 1130–35), monk and theologian from Liège; became abbot of Deutz and served there until his death.

Hervé de Bourg Dieu (d. 1150), Benedictine monk and biblical exegete; died near Tours.

Richard of Saint Victor (d. 1173), theologian and mystic of the abbey of Saint Victor in Paris; lived and died in Paris.

Thomas Aquinas (d. 1274), theologian from Roccasecca in Italy; died in Fossanova, near Rome.

Alfonso X (d. 1284), king of Castile and León; born in Toledo, died in Seville.

Alfonso of Cordoba (fl. 1348), physician from Cordoba.

Jacme d'Agramont (d. 1348), physician and professor of medicine at Lleida (in Catalonia); died in Lleida.

Anonymous Practitioner of Montpellier (fl. 1349).

Gui de Chauliac (d. 1368), physician; died in Avignon.

Vincent Ferrer (d. 1419), Dominican preacher from Valencia; died in Brittany.

Alonso de Chirino (d. between 1429 and 1431), converso Castilian physician.
Enrique de Villena (d. 1434), Castilian noble and humanist.
Alfonso Fernández de Madrigal (El Tostado) (d. 1455), professor of theology and bishop of Avilá; died in Avilá.

Infectious Ideas

Contagion and Causality in the Study of Premodern Muslim and Christian Societies

> Now if a deadly epidemic strikes, we should stay where we are, make our preparations, and take courage in the fact that we are mutually bound together . . . so that we cannot desert one another or flee from one another. First, we can be sure that God's punishment has come upon us, not only to chastise us for our sins but also to test our faith and love—our faith in that we may see and experience how we should act toward God; our love in that we may recognize how we should act toward our neighbor. I am of the opinion that all the epidemics, like any plague, are spread among the people by evil spirits who poison the air or exhale a pestilential breath, which puts a deadly poison into the flesh. Nevertheless, this is God's decree and punishment to which we must patiently submit and serve our neighbor, risking our lives in this manner as St. John teaches, "If Christ laid down his life for us, we ought to lay down our lives for the brethren" [1 John 3:16].
>
> Martin Luther, 1527

> Surely, it were to be wished that one would not see the hearts of many who term themselves reformed Christians, confused with the mad error of the Turks.
>
> Antoni Duizing, Dutch doctor, 1664

THIS BOOK DEALS with how Muslims and Christians in the premodern world conceived of contagion and what meaning they gave to it in their theological, medical, and literary writings. Within this vast subject, I have focused my study on contagion as discussed by authors living in Iberia and North Africa during the premodern period. This project began as a study of the effects of the second bubonic plague pandemic (fourteenth–eighteenth centuries CE) on the Muslim and Christian societies of late medieval Iberia and early modern Spain, and texts that were written in the initial aftermath of the Black Death of the late 740s/1340s figure prominently in the book. Yet to situate these texts and their authors, I found it necessary to deal with the scholarly traditions that determined how Muslim and Christian scholars understood the nature of the challenge they faced in the eighth/fourteenth century and what significance they attributed to the concept of contagion. Similarly, in order to clarify the subsequent development of the reactions to the Black Death of the eighth/fourteenth century, I also address how Muslim scholars of North Africa continued to debate the nature of contagion well into the fourteenth/nineteenth century, when, in the context of colonialism, they were exposed to broad European support for the imposition of quarantine in times of epidemic disease.

My book's aim, therefore, is to provide a longitudinal treatment of the concept of contagion in Iberian Muslim and Christian circles from the end of late antiquity to the beginning of early modernity. This investigation occurs chiefly in the context of two diseases, known today as the plague and leprosy. Although Muslim and Christian treatments of contagion can be compared, neither one is easily reduced to a single position or characterization. I have therefore attempted to approach scholars' discussions of contagion in terms of the way they embedded it within broader theological, medical, and legal discourses.

The reason for choosing contagion as the subject of a comparative historical study might not be immediately apparent. However, the ways in which societies conceive of and cope with transmissible diseases offer valuable insights into their social and intellectual practices. In the past decade, scholars have grown increasingly interested in tracing the history of contagion through a variety of cultural and political contexts.[1] As natural disasters of horrendous proportions, contagious diseases such as the plague posed complicated problems for both Muslim and Christian scholars: What is the plague's larger significance? What is the appropriate response? Can one flee from it, or does one have an obligation to stay and look after the sick? Could the plague be transmitted from one victim to another, or is it also possible that it is the product of corruption of the air? These were the more general quandaries that arose. More subtle ones soon followed, and those offer insights into how Muslim and Christian scholars approached the concept of contagion: What is the proper metaphoric significance of the plague, and how is it similar to other transmissible diseases, such as leprosy? Does the plague have the ability to transmit itself, or is God directly involved in its transmission? To what degree is the manner of the plague's transmission similar to the evil eye or even the effects of pornography? As I explore some of scholars' answers to these questions, my most substantive contribution may well be insight into the criteria scholars considered both relevant and authoritative when constructing the significance of the diseases, more than clarifying their individual positions on the nature of the diseases.

Contagion before the Laboratory

Although entering the worlds of premodern Christian and Muslim theology and law in search of depictions of contagion is not without its difficulties, the chief obstacle for the reader is more general. It is characterized by the widespread acceptance of modern understandings of disease. In the second half of the nineteenth century, following what Andrew Cunningham has called the "laboratory revolution" and what K. Codell Carter has characterized as the emergence of an etiological research program, the conception of disease, and with it contagion, changed profoundly.[2] This change was so significant, and today is so widely held to be normative and natural, that without taking it into account, it will be difficult to approach the worldview of the premodern scholars with any understanding or sympathy.

Historians of medicine have devoted a great deal of attention to developments in European medical thought in the nineteenth century, and my brief discussion of aspects of the work of Cunningham and Carter does these rich and nuanced contributions a disservice.[3] In addition, I should stress that these authors differed in their approach to the history of disease: Cunningham examined the effect of the laboratory revolution on our understanding of the transmission of plague, and Carter focused on theories of the causes of diseases. While it is certainly true that disease transmission and disease etiology are separate subjects with their own histories, for the purposes of this book, which is devoted to premodern constructions and interpretations of contagion, I am primarily concerned with how nineteenth-century developments collectively changed the ways in which people currently understand diseases, the origins, and their natures. The following observations, though mundane for historians of medicine, may be of value for students of Islamic history and nonspecialists.

Today, both medical practitioners and the wider public generally believe that diseases have distinct causes that define them and without which they would not exist. As Susan Sontag has noted—with only mild hyperbole—regarding cancer, it is only in the case of diseases for which we have no cure, diseases we do not fully understand, that we accept the possibility of multiple causal factors.[4] This understanding, which is of particular salience in the case of contagious diseases, emerged gradually during the nineteenth century within the debates surrounding a bacterial theory of disease.[5] As Carter has argued eloquently, the success of the bacterial theory—perhaps most famously employed by Louis Pasteur (d. 1895) and Robert Koch (d. 1910)—was not solely or even principally the result of technological advancements or empirical discoveries. Instead, it rested upon a theoretical reformulation of the nature of disease, which, once correctly understood, could be applied to diseases caused not only by bacteria but also by viruses or deficiencies. Quoting Koch, Carter describes this shift in the understanding of disease as the result of the adoption of an "etiological standpoint," which he defines as follows:

> The etiological standpoint can be characterized as the belief that diseases are best controlled and understood by means of causes and, in particular, by causes that are *natural* (that is, they depend on forces of nature as opposed to the willful transgression of moral or social norms), *universal* (that is, the same cause is common to every instance of a given disease), and *necessary* (that is, a disease does not occur in the absence of its cause). This way of conceiving disease has dominated medical thought for the last century. . . . At the same time it is clear from historical and anthropological literature that an interest in universal causes is unique to modern western medicine. There is no such interest in non-western medicine or in medicine prior to the middle of the nineteenth century. This concept is a defining characteristic of modern western thinking about disease.[6]

The etiological standpoint did not arrive at its contemporary dominant status without resistance. Although today it might be assumed that its opponents were blindly subservient to the authority of tradition, or that they rejected empirical evidence, it would be more accurate to argue that they were simply more aware than we are today of the limitations of the evidence presented by Pasteur, Koch, and others.[7] For the work of bacteriologists to be convincing, its premises had to be accepted beforehand, and this required something akin to an act of faith:

> In their work on anthrax, both Koch and Pasteur accumulated empirical evidence of causality and their evidence was of different kinds. However, it is impossible to prove causation by empirical evidence alone. This is reflected in the standard objection—which continued to be raised throughout the century—that, no matter how carefully organisms were isolated, it was always possible that an unknown virus or some totally different entity in the blood was the true cause of the disease. Proving bacteria cause a particular disease, such as anthrax, was impossible in the absence of a theory within which bacteria were recognized as possible causes—one needed an assumption like the Bacterial Hypothesis. . . . Where rational persuasion fails, the only alternative is *conversion,*

> and converting opponents to the bacterial theory required successes that were "supernatural" in the sense of being outside what could reasonably have been expected within the framework of traditional medicine. To achieve conversion, bacteriologists required, not mere evidence, but something akin to *miracles*.[8]

The susceptibility of empirical evidence to alternate interpretations is also relevant to the bitter debates between contagionists and anticontagionists that raged throughout much of the nineteenth century in England and were often characterized by invocations of the primary importance of contagion and miasma. Here again it may be assumed that the anticontagionist position, in its rejection of the etiological standpoint, is characterized by a radical anti-empiricism. Yet as Hamlin and Worboys have argued, not only did the medical profession at the time often make no clear distinction between contagion and miasma, but both contagionists and anticontagionists often accepted similar premises while advocating for different policies.[9]

The excellent recent scholarship on the changing medical paradigms of the nineteenth century, with its close readings of the importance of theoretical frameworks and the contingency of interpretations of empirical evidence, is of paramount importance for the discussion of contagion in the premodern period. It cautions against a too-Whiggish attitude regarding the "natural" status of the etiological standpoint and strongly undermines any easy equivalence between modern Western medicine and notions of rationality. The need for this distinction may not yet be apparent, but in the course of this study we will encounter numerous occasions when Western scholarship has privileged certain premodern Muslim understandings of contagion and disease over others because they resembled (in some manner) the etiological standpoint. To be blunt—and I recognize that this point may not be granted by scholars in the natural sciences, though it is a commonplace among historians of medicine—if we recognize that diseases are social constructions at least as much as they are biological entities, then we need to maintain constant vigilance against the temptation of finding today's diseases and their means of transmission in the past. This point has been made admirably by Arrizabalaga, Henderson, and French in their study of the Great Pox, especially with regard to their reading of the theory of "seeds of disease," suggested by the Italian scholar Fracastoro (d. 1553).[10] Regardless of how easily one can read Fracastoro's writings today as prescient of germ theory, he situated disease transmission within a conceptual framework completely distinct from the etiological standpoint. The works of far too many other scholars—the Andalusī polymath Ibn al-Khaṭīb

(d. 776/1374) is a prominent example—have not been as carefully approached.[11] In this book, I situate discussions of contagion within broader theological, legal, mystical, and literary discourses in order to elucidate its contemporaneous significances. The connection between contagion and causality, alluded to earlier by Carter, demands to be addressed in this context, for it plays an important role.

The Challenge of Causality, the Purpose of Occasionalism

In travel literature of the early modern period, European visitors to the Middle East, observing the behavior of local residents in times of epidemic disease, often remarked on the "fatalistic" behavior of Muslims, linking it to their belief in predestination or, more appropriately, in occasionalism.[12] The virulence of the European rejection of the behavior of those Muslims who refused to flee from the plague may have had as much to do with intra-Christian debates as it did with Orientalist bias, and I will return to this point later in the introduction. Here it is worth considering the theological basis, which for some Muslim scholars linked a denial of secondary causation with a rejection of contagion. In the Muslim world, occasionalism, the belief that events have no necessary causal connection and that God creates everything anew at every moment, has its roots in theological debates going back to the third/ninth century on the implications of the omnipotence of God. Most recently, Dominik Perler and Ulrich Rudolph have treated the history of occasionalism in a nuanced and perceptive manner, tracing its development in the Muslim world and its transfer to Western Christendom through the writings of Moses Maimonides in the thirteenth century. Perler and Rudolph show how occasionalism, a theory supported by influential European Christian thinkers down to the time of David Hume (d. 1776), was an answer to two very different problems.[13]

In the Muslim world, we find causality to be a central concern of the early and influential Muᶜtazilī school of theology, which originated in Basra and Baghdad in the second/eighth century.[14] Beginning with a few prominent Muᶜtaziī scholars, and continuing in a fully expanded form with the founder of the Ashᶜarī school, Abū al-Ḥasan al-Ashᶜarī (d. 323/936) himself, Muslim theologians attempted to systematically elucidate the consequences of God's omnipotence.[15] To understand this issue, they considered it necessary to clarify the nature of physical reality and to determine whether created entities (implicitly including diseases) had "natures" of their own that could act upon other beings. For these scholars, the question of causality was directly tied to the nature of human action and the freedom of will, as well as to whether there is a natural order and how miracles are to be understood. The variety of positions taken on the subject by Muᶜtazilī thinkers speaks to the difficulty of the issue: while affirming the possibility of human action, Abū Hudhayl (d. 227/842) described the material world as composed of atoms without natures of their own, though they possessed attributes (often termed "accidents"). Although Abū Hudhayl emphasized the ability of God to intervene in the natural order at any time, he also implicitly affirmed the existence of such an order and thus the possibility of secondary causes.[16] Abū Hudhayl's famous student al-Naẓẓām (d. 232/847), however, constrained the potential for human action in order to stress the existence of objects possessing independent natures. Al-Naẓẓām's understanding was in turn rejected by one of his own students, Ṣāliḥ Qubba (d. 246/860), who seems to have been the first of the Muᶜtazila to argue that God was the agent behind each action and occurrence. Ṣāliḥ Qubba faced substantial opposition from other Muᶜtazliī thinkers, in part certainly because by denying the possibility of a natural order and affirming God's role in creating each and every action, he failed to offer any explanation for the appearance of regularity in material reality (stones falling when dropped, wool burning when brought into contact with flame, etc.) or any assurance that people's sensory impressions are reliable.[17] A solution to this problem was offered by Jubbā'ī (d. 302/915), the first Muᶜtazilī to clearly articulate the notion that one may rely on God's regularly causing actions to occur in the same fashion according to his habit (*ᶜāda*).[18] The individual components of occasionalism were first fully assembled and explored, however, by Jubbā'ī's student, the aforementioned al-Ashᶜarī, who clearly stated that neither people nor any other created entity has the ability to cause anything, that God creates reality anew at every moment according to his habit. Although he began as an adherent to Muᶜtazilism himself, al-Ashᶜarī ultimately parted ways with the Muᶜtazilī school and came to be seen as the founder of his own school of thought. As a comprehensive theory, occasionalism flourished only under al-Ashᶜarī's followers and was never fully accepted by later Muᶜtazilīs, Maturidis (a school of theology that emerged in the fourteenth century), or those Muslims who rejected the legitimacy of speculative theology (*kalām*).[19] As a school of theology, Ashᶜarism was largely accepted by the Mālikī law school, and by the fifth/eleventh century it had spread throughout North Africa and al-Andalus.[20]

It should not be thought, however, that Ashᶜarīs' support of occasionalism implies any sort of fatalism or, more specifically, an opposition to the possibility that diseases are transmitted between people. For all practical purposes, the concept of God's habit had a predictive value similar to an acceptance of secondary causation: claiming that wool burns when brought into contact with fire not because of any property of fire, but because God habitually causes this to happen, protects against a polytheistic belief in multiple causality as much as it offers a description of reality. In addition, not all Ashᶜarī theologians necessarily understood occasionalism in the same way. Doubtless the most prominent example of an Ashᶜarī who argued for secondary causes is al-Ghazālī (d. 505/1111), but later examples such as al-Yūsī (d. 1102/1691) can be found; those are discussed in chapters 5 and 6.[21]

The danger that a belief in secondary causation—in which God gives his creations a degree of causative power—could lead to polytheism might not be immediately clear. How Muslim scholars debated this issue in the context of Prophetic Tradition is discussed in detail in chapter 1. In general, however, it should be remembered that the coalescing Islamic legal and theological tradition of the second/eighth–third/ninth centuries depicts Islam as emerging into an intellectual environment characterized by a strong belief in polytheism and thus in the causative power of multiple gods.[22] In this context, many scholars—though by no means all, as the Muᶜtazilī examples cited above demonstrate—were wary of countenancing any hint of a belief in secondary causality, which they depicted as characteristic of the bedouin of pre-Islamic Arabia. While sophisticated scholars such as al-Ghazālī and al-Yūsī might be able to reconcile secondary causation with a strict monotheism within an Ashᶜarī framework, their views were not shared by the majority of their colleagues, who may well have felt that such sophistication would have confused the average believer.[23]

Occasionalism was of interest to European Christian theologians in a decidedly different context. When Thomas Aquinas (d. 1274) refuted occasionalism as presented in the Latin translation of the *Guide to the Perplexed,* by Moses Maimonides (d. 1204), he understood it as an attempt to address the relationship of form and matter in the Aristotelian concept of hylomorphism—the theory that all things are composed of a permanent aspect, matter, and a current aspect, form, that can change.[24] Later European thinkers invoked occasionalism to explain the interaction between the spiritual and physical worlds: God was responsible for using the occasion of someone's seeing a flower to create the concept of flower within a human mind, just as he was responsible for using the occasion of a mental decision to move one's body into actual physical motion.[25] Despite the exceptional case of philosophers such as the French thinker Nicholas Malebranche (d. 1715), who developed a theory of occasionalism that would have been familiar to Ashᶜarī theologians, in which he described secondary causes as minor deities, occasionalism in Christian European thought played little if any role in discussions of contagion. Nonetheless, Christian authors, especially Protestant ones, did make statements similar to Muslim scholars' conclusion that it was impermissible to flee from the plague.

Fleeing Essentialist Interpretations

In the following chapters, I examine Muslim and Christian writings on contagion from Iberia and North Africa and show that while Muslim scholars generally denied the phenomenon of contagion and Christian scholars tended to invoke it favorably, the meanings they attributed to it varied widely. I recognize, however, that the reader who is otherwise unfamiliar with Muslim and Christian views on the plague may generalize from my examples to the respective religious traditions as a whole. Although certain lines of thought may well be representative of scholars of either religion from various regions and time periods, other elements of the materials discussed here represent only one of many positions taken. This is the case with the Iberian Christian plague treatises discussed in chapter 4. Contagion is discussed there in detail, but the reader may deduce that, contrary to Muslim precedent, no Christian author advocated remaining in a plague-struck area. Yet in sixteenth- to seventeenth-century Protestant northern Europe, numerous Christian authors argued, as had many Muslim authors farther south, that one has a duty to remain in plague-afflicted areas and take care of fellow believers.[26] To be sure, Luther, who affirmed the concept of contagion in a general fashion, argued that persons not in an immediate position of spiritual or temporal authority, as well as those whose faith was not strong, were free to flee.[27] Simultaneously, he chided those Christians who overzealously refused to seek medical attention, thereby placing themselves in the way of harm; Luther equated this with suicide.[28] In his attempt to find an ethical decision that would balance the spiritual and physical needs of the community and would address a variety of believers, Luther was acting much like the Muslim jurists discussed in chapter 5, who struggled with the implications of affirming or denying contagion.[29] Luther's epistle should not be taken as representative of all Protestant thought, however; later authors of plague tracts in the Protestant Netherlands noted the mistaken belief of Christians who held that because the plague originates with God, it cannot be contagious.[30] Nevertheless, as Ole Grell has argued, by the end of the sixteenth century, the early Protestant emphasis on community and neighborly love, so well displayed in Luther's treatise, had been replaced by a focus on self-preservation and communal good in the influential tract of the Calvinist Theodore Beza (d. 1605).[31] Of particular interest here are the sixteenth- to seventeenth-century debates between Protestant theologians, physicians, and scholars, in which a fatalistic Muslim denial of contagion was introduced as a foil that could be used to criticize persons who opposed fleeing from the plague.[32] A belief in God's omnipotence and predestination and a denial of the contagious nature of the plague were by no means necessary bedfellows, but the connection between them seems to have been sufficiently widespread that the invocation of Muslim fatalism was considered a viable refutation of them throughout the seventeenth century, as exemplified in the work of Gottfried Leibniz (d. 1716) (see chapter 6). Although I have mentioned only Protestant authors here, sixteenth-century Catholic authors in France also addressed the responsibility of taking care of one's fellow believers, although they struggled less extensively with the implications of predestination.[33]

These few examples indicate the difficulty of attempting to assign to religious traditions single, even majority, positions on the subject of contagion, but they also suggest the benefits of using contagion as a lens through which to approach disparate bodies of scholarship within premodern Islam and Christianity.

Cultures of Scholarship

This book is structured comparatively, with chapters alternating between Christian and Muslim discussions of contagion, and it is the comparative nature of the study that offers some of the most useful insights into how humankind has come to terms with the effects of disease. By adopting this approach I am placing this book in direct conversation with an influential article by Michael Dols, published in 1974, which compared Muslim and Christian responses to the Black Death. Dols, whose work on the plague in the Middle East was foundational, argued that the responses of the two religious communities were entirely different, particularly regarding the issue of contagion, with Christians affirming and Muslims denying its existence. I will return in greater detail to Dols's article in the conclusion, but I should note here that I differ not only with Dols's conclusions, but also with the way in which he framed his comparison, including his belief that the respective positions of Muslims and Christians on the issue of contagion could productively be reduced to a series of contrasting characteristics. Generally speaking, Muslim and Christian discussions of contagion were qualitatively distinct to the degree that they reflected awarenesses of different problems that needed to be addressed and resolved. Admittedly, by the High Middle Ages, Muslim and Christian scholarship shared a common medical heritage, one in which the concept of contagion can easily be found. Yet, what contagion *signified* for Muslims and Christians was determined by their respective cultural and religious traditions, and these differed substantially. By offering the reader a close examination of how Christian and Muslim scholars discussed the concept of contagion, I argue for the importance of a nuanced and detailed approach to comparative intellectual history. Instead of reducing Muslim and Christian understandings of contagion to a clear opposition between two approaches characterized by religious or civilizational labels, I attempt to delineate the parameters that directed these two groups of intellectuals toward qualitatively distinct constructions of contagion. Because the subject of contagion came to present both a legal and a theological problem in Islamic thought, and the resulting debate produced its own defined body of work, more space has been devoted here to Muslim thinkers.[34] Tracing the concept of contagion in the writing of Christian Iberian scholars involved, on the one hand, observing how they employed it metaphorically—a practice rarely employed by the Muslim writers examined here—and, on the other, paying close attention to how they defined the concept medically.

The broader contribution of this book—not novel but, I hope, usefully incremental—lies in its emphasis on the creativity and richness of both Muslim and Christian scholarship in the premodern period. I have deliberately chosen the binary premodern-modern when referring to Christian and Muslim scholarship, instead of using the term *Middle Ages,* because that term has little relevance for the Muslim world and because thinking on the subject of contagion in both European and Muslim scholarship changed qualitatively in the nineteenth century with the laboratory revolution and the expansion of European colonialism into the Middle East. In addition, while students of the history of Islamdom and Christendom are seldom unaware of the ability of individual scholars to reinterpret authoritative materials to reflect their own contexts and needs, many scholars continue to see the "Middle Ages" and Christian or Muslim "orthodoxies" as anathema to rational inquiry, reasoned reflection on the importance of empirical evidence, and vigorous engagement with established precedent. The chapters that follow challenge this depiction and show the extent to which premodern Muslim and Christian scholars engaged in thoughtful and rational attempts, using both textual authority and empirical evidence, to best define the significance of contagion. While emphasizing the flexible nature of individual discourses, I also argue that the work of the scholars discussed in this book reflects an ethical engagement on their part, at the heart of which is a desire to protect the physical and spiritual health of their respective communities. Their changing conceptions of this health, and the factors that influenced them in their investigations into the nature of contagion, frame the following discussions.

Contagion in the Commentaries on Prophetic Tradition

> Moslem response to plague was (or became) passive. Epidemic disease had been known in Arabia in Muhammad's time, and among the traditions that Islamic men of learning treasured as guides to life were various injunctions from the Prophet's own mouth about how to react to pestilential outbreaks. . . . The effect of such traditions was to inhibit organized efforts to cope with plague.
>
> William McNeill, *Plagues and Peoples*

IN THE MIDDLE of the eighth/fourteenth century, after the Black Death had swept through the Mediterranean region and Europe, the Granadan vizier Ibn al-Khaṭīb (d. 776/1374) composed a medical treatise on the epidemic entitled *That Which Satisfies the Questioner regarding the Appalling Illness* (*Muqniᶜat al-sā'il ᶜan al-maraḍ al-hā'il*). Toward the end of the work, the author observes that several traditions related from the Prophet deny the existence of contagion but that these traditions should be ignored in light of clear empirical evidence to the contrary: "One principle that cannot be ignored is that if the senses and observation oppose a revealed indication [i.e., Prophetic Tradition] the latter needs to be interpreted, and the correct course in this case is to interpret it according to the position of a group of those who affirm contagion."[1] Recent scholarship has seen Ibn al-Khaṭīb's attitude toward contagion as exceptional, at odds with both the accumulated scholarship of preceding centuries and the views of such respected scholars as Ibn Ḥajar al-ᶜAsqalānī (d. 852/1448), who succeeded him.[2] At times he has been portrayed as a member of a small group of seventh–eighth/fourteenth–fifteenth-century Muslim rationalists, expounding views that were rejected by the religious establishment.[3] In his remarks directed against those who deny contagion, Ibn al-Khaṭīb cites a Prophetic tradition that supports his own views. By contrast, he merely alludes to those traditions of the Prophet that deny contagion, stressing that they must be interpreted to confirm its existence. Before reevaluating Ibn al-Khaṭīb's place in the debate regarding the nature of contagion, a task that is taken up in a later chapter, it is worth looking more closely at the body of traditions to which he referred.

Defending the Integrity of Prophetic Tradition

The Prophetic traditions relating to contagion were discussed, and their apparent contradictions reconciled, in a series of exegetical commentaries. Such reconciliation should be understood as part of a larger enterprise on the part of a group of Muslim scholars to defend the integrity of Prophetic Tradition, a project that is well documented by the third/ninth century. Conceivably, contradictions in the Prophetic Tradition could have been dealt with by simply denying the validity of all problematic material. However, for those scholars who believed that Prophetic Tradition was, after the Qur'an, the most trustworthy guide to correct conduct, such a general rejection of seemingly contradictory traditions would have meant the end of the authority of Prophetic Tradition as a whole. It would have conceded too much ground to those Muslims who privileged reason or experience over the reported words and acts of the Prophet. Instead, it was necessary, on the one hand, to refute those who saw Prophetic Tradition as contradictory and, on the other, to explain how that tradition was to be correctly understood. A first step in this direction was the compilation in the third–fourth/ninth–tenth centuries of what became the six canonical collections of Prophetic traditions.[4] This process effectively separated the thousands of traditions that were not thought to be reliable from those that were. In the commentaries written in the following centuries, the scholars who supported the status of Prophetic Tradition attempted to reconcile most—if not all—remaining inconsistencies. Their project had a precedent in the earlier writings of scholars such as Ibn Qutayba (d. 276/889), who had vigorously defended the reliability of Prophetic Tradition.[5]

In this chapter, two examples are given, evil omens and contagion, in which apparent contradictions in Prophetic Tradition are reconciled. I have chosen to consider the case of evil omens along with that of contagion in order to show that the analytical method applied by the commentators on Prophetic Tradition to the subject of contagion is representative of a broader interpretive approach. In both cases I show how the hadith folk (*ahl al-ḥadīth*)—the supporters of Prophetic Tradition—resolved apparent contradictions by arguing that the Prophet had anticipated the tendency of many Muslims to fall into doubt and fear in the face of evil omens and transmissible diseases.[6] Far from being contradictions, these traditions are revealed, at least implicitly, to be proofs of the Prophet's understanding of the weaknesses of human nature. To accomplish this goal, the hadith folk interpreted some of the Prophet's statements as being metaphoric and limited the scope of others.[7] The phenomenon of contagion was in the end conditionally acknowledged in the cases of leprosy and mange but denied in the case of the plague. In conclusion, I argue that previous discussions that differentiated between scholarly and administrative conceptions of contagion are flawed and that the response of premodern Muslim administrations to transmissible diseases was in fact in accord with, if not based on, the writings of the hadith folk.

In what follows, I examine the Prophetic traditions that relate to the subject of contagion in the six canonical hadith collections, along with those in the earlier *Muwaṭṭa'* of Mālik (d. 179/796), the *Muṣannaf* of ᶜAbd al-Razzāq al-Ṣanᶜānī (d. 211/827), and the *Musnad* of Aḥmad b. Ḥanbal (d. 241/855). In the centuries after the compilation of these works, some of them were frequently commented upon, with each commentator attempting to summarize and reconcile earlier views. The commentators contributed, in part, to an ongoing conversation on the topic of contagion. Instead of proceeding in a linear fashion, for example, from a rejection to an acceptance of contagion, this literature tacks back and forth, each scholar taking up certain past arguments but not always giving others the same consideration. Often the actual question of the existence or nonexistence of contagion seems to fade into the background as the debate focuses more on *how* exactly and by whose will the transmission of disease occurs. This occurs in large part because the subject of contagion was drawn into two of the central theological debates of early Islam: the question of the unity of God and that of God's decree (*qadar*) and free will. The role of contagion in theological arguments on the nature of causation is discussed in a later chapter, but the potential for contagion to become a point of contention for the Muᶜtazila, the hadith folk, and the Ashᶜarites should be emphasized at the outset.[8]

Contagion was not discussed in a vacuum. At least by the time the hadith collections were assembled, it was one of a group of pre-Islamic beliefs that the Prophet was held to have denied. Foremost among these, and given at least as much attention as contagion, was the topic of evil omens, sometimes seen in the flight of birds and in other forms of augury. In order to better understand the interpretive choices made by the *ᶜulamā'* in their discussion of contagion, it is of comparative interest to examine how they treated evil omens.[9]

Before entering into a discussion of the traditions in question, I should note that my approach to the material differs from that of some recent scholarship. Instead of attempting to outline the progressive development of individual traditions through analysis of their chains of transmission (*isnād*) and comparison of alternative versions of similar material, I have chosen to give a composite overview of traditions as they could have been perceived by the later commentators themselves. Thus, I do not attempt to untangle the complex web of the beliefs of the early Muslim community, but rather to establish how later scholars approached their tradition once it had somewhat solidified.[10]

Evil Omens and Augury: The Prophetic Traditions

In Prophetic Tradition, *ṭiyara,* while at times referring to augury in general, most often carries the sense of "evil omen." The word seems to have originally referred to seeing omens in the flight of birds, and the fifth form of the verb, *taṭayyara,* is more generally understood as carrying out any type of augury.[11] Yet the way in which *ṭiyara* is used in the body of traditions in question shows that it referred exclusively to an omen of evil import, and the Prophet contrasted it with the good omen (*fa'l*).[12]

The Prophet clearly denied the existence of both contagion and the evil omen, saying, "[There is] no contagion, no evil omen, no death bird [*hāma*], no tapeworm [*ṣafar*], no ghoul, and no malignant star."[13] Much more frequently found in the canonical collections of traditions, however, are formulations in which, even as the evil omen is denied, the existence of the good omen (*al-fa'l*) is affirmed.[14] Lest it be thought that this leaves the door ajar for the possibility of augury, the Prophet is held to have defined the good omen as a felicitous phrase or word.[15] In the hadith collections and, presumably, in the minds of those who compiled and read these collections, these traditions were closely associated with the denial of other types of augury as well: the Prophet is held to have similarly forbidden having recourse to soothsayers,[16] and seeking to know the future from the flight of birds (*al-ᶜiyāfa*) or through the use of pebbles (*al-ṭarq*) is described as a type of polytheism.[17] Though not of immediate pertinence to this study, it is interesting to note that the Prophet did not deny that soothsayers had access to secret knowledge through their association with jinn, but he affirmed that the jinn corrupted what they heard from the inhabitants of the higher spheres.[18] To avoid underestimating the danger of believing in augury, there is an additional tradition in which belief in evil omens is openly declared to be polytheism.[19]

At the same time that evil omens are repudiated, and often in the same tradition in which their general existence is denied, their presence in a small number of things is acknowledged. This group is frequently composed of houses, horses, and women.[20] In addition, the Prophet is portrayed as considering names of people and places to bode well or ill.[21] Here, as opposed to the good omens that may be found in well-chosen speech, there is the possibility that a person or place might also be seen as having an ill-fated name.[22] In addition to omens in houses, horses, and women, the existence of the evil eye is also confirmed.[23] The tension between the denial of evil omens in general and the admission of certain exceptions to this rule is addressed in the traditions themselves. At least one incident is reported in which people come either to Mālik b. Anas (the founder of one of the four Sunnī law schools) or the Prophet, complaining that their fortunes have declined since they moved into their current house. The responses vary in emphasis, but the questioners are left in no doubt that they should leave the house.[24] This reply may be seen as already forming the beginning of a later attempt to explain the exceptional status of horses, houses, and women by offering practical reasons for considering them ill-omened (e.g., a woman's inability to bear children). In addition, it is implied that these three have the potential to damage the faith of believers by making them doubt the unity of God. Similarly, a line of argument taken by later commentators, and one present in some of the traditions themselves, is that far more important and dangerous than evil omens is the power people emotionally and mentally confer upon omens.[25] This has a parallel in associating the evil omen with thinking poorly of others or feeling envy.[26] The Prophet addressed the danger of believing in evil omens by stating that one should avoid giving credence to evil omens by placing one's trust in God.[27] Dwelling on the beliefs and convictions of Muslims was similarly important for the commentators on the traditions surrounding contagion, and this shift of emphasis from what people did to what they thought can be seen as part of a continuing desire on the part of the *ʿulamāʾ* to address internal attitudes and not just external actions.

Evil Omens and Augury: The Commentators

Following the Qur'an, the canonical collections of traditions—and first and foremost those of al-Bukhārī and Muslim—form the source of law and correct conduct for the vast majority of the Muslim community. And just as the desire to understand the Qur'an produced a body of exegetical material—the *tafsīr* literature—many commentaries were written on the collections of Prophetic traditions. The commentators attempted to explain to the faithful the significance of individual traditions and their relation to other Prophetic traditions and the Qur'an itself. Since the number of accepted traditions, after the initial selections made by the compilers of the canonical collections, remained beyond the ability of the average believer to master, an authoritative point of reference was necessary.[28] And although certain commentaries attained greater respect than others, the process of commentary itself never ended, and it continues today.[29]

There is little doubt that the intended audience of the commentaries was the scholarly community, not the average believer.[30] The commentaries are most often written in a tight, allusive style that would be obscure to one who had not received formal training in the religious sciences. The layman was far more likely to take his questions regarding Prophetic traditions to a *muftī* or an *imām* than to consult a commentary. If he took the former course, the *fatwā,* in accordance with its form, would likely contain a precise and usually conclusive answer to a specific question, whereas the commentaries on Prophetic traditions, like Qur'anic commentaries, often present several interpretations of a given tradition without necessarily giving preference to one over the others. Since many doubts and misunderstandings, as well as differences of opinion regarding the interpretation of traditions, could come about even among scholars, different strategies and tools had to be used to reconcile them and offer convincing explanations.

Addressed to a community of scholars, the commentaries reflect this community's preoccupations along with a certain conservatism. While earlier opinions were weighed and valued, each commentator, relying to a large degree upon his predecessors and the framework within which they worked, was representative of the outlook of the hadith folk. That is, commentaries on Prophetic Tradition are not a site where one expects to find the views of philosophers, Muᶜtazilites, physicians, or natural scientists treated sympathetically on a regular basis. These views could be, and at times were, introduced to be refuted or shown to be in accordance with Tradition, but seldom did they, in the fashion of Ibn al-Khaṭīb's plague treatise, provide the basis of understanding with which the traditions had to be reconciled. In addition, the commentaries themselves should not be seen as progressing linearly, each scholar summarizing previous work and then adding new material. It was often the case that commenting on a tradition entailed choosing and affirming one of the previously stated opinions.[31] Because there were thousands of traditions to cover, one may have some sympathy with commentators who contented themselves with summarizing previous opinions.

In addition to the content of the traditions, the commentators had to deal with the many thorny issues raised by the question of the reliability of their transmitters, a subject that had grown into a entire field of knowledge in itself long before the Black Death: the science of men, or *ᶜilm al-rijāl.* Masters of this field, such as Ibn Ḥajar, were able to invoke extensive amounts of biographical knowledge in their discussion of traditions, while lesser exegetes contented themselves with quoting the opinions of earlier commentaries or those of the compilers of the collections of traditions.[32] Still, it was seldom the *isnād* alone that decided the importance that was placed on a tradition. The weight given to the *isnād* depended in part on the relative strength and number of other traditions that agreed or disagreed with a given tradition, and the final opinion on a tradition's significance certainly depended in part on the theological presuppositions of the exegete. Looking back from the time of Ibn Ḥajar in the ninth/fifteenth century, one could see that the *ahl al-ḥadīth* had made a decision relatively early on to attempt to reconcile as many of the seemingly contradictory traditions as possible. The motive behind this was most likely to ward off the criticisms of those, such as the Muᶜtazilites, who cast doubt upon the reliability of Prophetic Tradition in general.[33] The decision to reconcile apparent contradictions in Prophetic Tradition was defended at length by Ibn Qutayba in his appropriately titled *Ta'wīl Mukhtalif al-Ḥadīth* (*The Interpretation of Contradictory Ḥadīths*) and was later taken up in the commentaries.[34] Ibn al-Ṣalāḥ (d. 643/1245) addressed the same topic in his introduction to the science of traditions.[35] The commentators saw Prophetic Tradition as a crucial and essential source for understanding the nature not only of Islam as a series of ritual obligations, but also of the world itself. It is, to be sure, a complicated source that requires study and dedication to comprehend, but once mastered it is a reliable guide to correct action and belief. The great value ascribed to these commentaries in the Muslim world today speaks to the authority the vision of the hadith folk achieved in the formative period of Islam, a vision that has since rested in a comfortable position of dominance alongside competing philosophical and mystical lines of thought. That Prophetic Tradition can be read in various ways by jurists, theologians, doctors, and mystics goes without saying; in subsequent chapters, some of these ways that are relevant to contagion are examined. First, however, the commentators' opinions on the issues of the evil omen are considered.

The Commentaries

I have drawn chiefly upon the following commentaries on Mālik's *Muwaṭṭa'* and the *Ṣaḥīḥayn* of al-Bukhārī and Muslim (arranged chronologically with respect to the work commented upon):

Ibn ᶜAbd al-Barr (d. 463/1070): *Al-Tamhīd li-mā fī-l-Muwaṭṭa'*
al-Bājī (d. 474/1081): *Al-Muntaqā: Sharḥ Muwaṭṭa' Mālik*

Ibn al-ᶜArabī (d. 543/1148): *Al-Qabas fī Sharḥ Muwaṭṭa' Mālik b. Anas*
al-Zurqānī (d. 1122/1710): *Sharḥ al-Zurqānī ᶜalā Muwaṭṭa' li-l-Imām Mālik*
al-Khaṭṭābī (d. 338/998): *Aᶜlām al-Sunan fī Sharḥ Ṣaḥīḥ al-Bukhārī*[36]
Ibn Baṭṭāl (d. 449/1057): *Sharḥ Ṣaḥīḥ al-Bukhārī*
Ibn Abī Jamra al-Andalusī: (d. 699/1300): *Bahjat al-Nufūs*
al-Kirmānī (d. 786/1384): *Al-Kawākib al-Darārī fī Sharḥ Ṣaḥīḥ al-Bukhārī*
Ibn Ḥajar al-ᶜAsqalānī (d. 852/1449): *Fatḥ al-Bārī bi-Sharḥ Ṣaḥīḥ al-Bukhārī*
al-ᶜAynī (d. 855/1451): *ᶜUmdat al-Qārī fī Sharḥ al-Bukhārī*
al-Qasṭallānī (d. 923/1517): *Irshād al-Sārī li-Sharḥ Ṣaḥīḥ al-Bukhārī*
al-Māzarī (d. 536/1141): *Al-Muᶜlim bi-Fawā'id Muslim*
ᶜIyāḍ b. Mūsā (d. 544/1149): *Ikmāl al-Muᶜlim bi-Fawā'id Muslim*
al-Qurṭubī (d. 656/1258): *Al-Mufhim li-mā Ashkala min Talkhīṣ Kitāb Muslim*
al-Nawawī (d. 676/1277): *Sharḥ Ṣaḥīḥ Muslim*
al-Ubbī (d. 827/1425): *Ikmāl Ikmāl al-Muᶜlim*
al-Sanūsī (d. 895/1490): *Mukammal Ikmāl al-Ikmāl*[37]

I have also included the *Ta'wīl mukhtalif al-ḥadīth* of Ibn Qutayba and Ibn al-Ṣalāḥ's *'Ulūm al-ḥadīth,* because the first book is often quoted in the commentaries, and Ibn al-Ṣalāḥ, whose work attained a considerable reputation, presented himself as Ibn Qutayba's successor in matters of Tradition.[38] Spanning, for the most part, the fifth/eleventh to the ninth/fifteenth centuries, these sources offer representative, though not exhaustive, material pertaining to the exegetical world of the commentaries on Prophetic traditions. The interpretative choices made and the conclusions reached during this period remain authoritative for many Muslims today and are seen as representative of the apogee of the science of Tradition. Instead of summarizing each commentator's opinion in a chronological fashion, I have chosen to present the views thematically, drawing attention to points of disagreement.

The Historical and Qur'anic Background

The evil omen and contagion are closely bound together by the Prophetic tradition "No contagion, no evil omen, no death bird [*hāma*], no tapeworm [*ṣafar*]," and the commentators frequently note that belief in all of these goes back to pre-Islamic times, a period when, however, belief in evil omens was far from universal.[39] Passages of Jāhilī poetry are cited to show that the practice of divination was rejected by some, though hardly all.[40] At that early time, an augury was carried out by observing the movement of animals, most frequently birds, but gazelles are also mentioned. With the coming of Islam and the Prophet's denial of the legitimacy of divination, belief in evil omens was forbidden. Giving up this belief entirely proved difficult for many people, though, and they continued to hold that evil omens could exist in women, horses, and houses.[41] What is the nature of these omens? Do they have any actual power? An initial attempt to define the limited influence of omens involved the citation of verses 18 and 19 of Sūrat Yā-Sīn: " 'We [a people to whom prophets were sent] think you [i.e., the prophets] are an evil omen (*innā taṭayyarnā bi-kum*). If you do not stop, we shall stone you, and inflict a painful punishment on you.' The messengers said, 'The evil omen (*ṭā'iru-kum*) is within yourselves.' "[42] This exchange is set in the greater context of verses 13–27 of the same Sūra, where the story is given of three messengers who in pre-Islamic times were sent to a sinning people in order to convert them.[43] Here, an ill augury seems to function as a thinly veiled threat, carried out when the obstinate community imprisons the first two people sent to it, but ultimately the threat rebounds upon those who issue it.[44] The commentators cite this story to show that although thinking ill of someone has no power in itself, such ill will can harm the one who bears it.[45] This interpretation finds a parallel in the tradition that auguring ill comes true for the one who engages in it.[46] Yet the parallel is only approximate: in the Qur'an, augury is clearly used as a metaphoric threat (i.e., we foresee bad things for you because we are going to stone you), as opposed to the actual practice of seeing omens in the behavior of animals, and perhaps because of this, this Qur'anic verse is not cited in later commentaries.[47]

The other reference to the Qur'an arose in the context of a debate about to whom the Prophet was referring when he said that the evil omen remains in women, houses, and horses.[48] The Prophet's wife ᶜĀ'isha was reported to have become enraged upon hearing that the Prophetic Companion Abū Hurayra (d. 58/678) was relating this tradition from the Prophet, and she stated that the Prophet, when he said this, had been speaking of the beliefs of the Jāhiliyya. To support her claim, she cited Sūrat al-Ḥadīd, 22: "No misfortune can happen on earth or in your souls but is recorded in a decree before we bring it into existence."[49] Earlier exegetes tended to side with ᶜĀ'isha in this matter, whereas later ones, notably Ibn al-ᶜArabī and Ibn Ḥajar al-ᶜAsqalānī, argued that it was possible to reconcile this tradition with that of the Prophet's saying "No evil omen."[50] Ibn al-ᶜArabī argued that the Prophet had been sent to inform people of what they should believe, not to describe what they had believed previously, and Ibn Ḥajar stated that if one can reconcile two traditions, one should not press the case for abrogation.[51] Later scholars seem to have accepted Ibn Ḥajar's rationale, although, as we will see in the next section, if the existence of evil omens was to be admitted, the nature of their existence would have to be differentiated from that of the omens of pre-Islamic times.[52]

Causation and the Nature of Evil Omens

The belief in evil omens was not merely a historical issue for the commentators. It was common in their day and was by no means confined to the three cases mentioned by the Prophet.[53] For most commentators, both evil omens and contagion are inextricably caught up in the mechanics of causation. As Conrad has indicated, denying the possibility that contagion occurred *by its own nature* (as opposed to being caused by God) was far more important than denying its existence absolutely.[54] Similarly, if, swayed by the abundance of Prophetic traditions supporting the presence of a small number of evil omens, one advocated their limited existence, there was then the danger that doing so would acknowledge some power other than God. The Prophet, after all, had equated believing in evil omens with idolatry.[55] Although it was noted that Mālik had interpreted this tradition literally and that the evil omens actually existed in these three cases, care was taken to see that the tradition was interpreted correctly.[56] Commentators showed that Mālik's observation that many people had experienced a change of fortune for the worse when moving from one house to another did not mean that the new house itself had any power but that the move between houses had coincided with God's decreeing a change in the fate of their inhabitants.[57] This coincidence was further explained to mean that one should leave a house if many bad things happened in it, not because it was ill-omened but because it might be tempting to think it was.[58] The case is similar to one in which the Prophet said, when he was asked his opinion about a particular house, that it should be abandoned because it was at fault (*dhamīmatan*).[59] The Prophet's statement did not refer to some power of the house but to God's having created in human nature a fear of what humans associate with ill fortune. The Prophet's order to leave the house reflected his understanding of man and his own (i.e., the Prophet's) mercy but by no means a belief in any power belonging to the house.[60] It follows that one is similarly allowed to divorce a woman whom one considers to be ill-fortuned and to sell a servant who brings bad luck.[61]

For some commentators, the topic moved them to address the subject of causation in more general terms. As mentioned above, it was important to emphasize that nothing but God has the power to cause anything to happen. It was possible, however, that God would give something else the power to do something, not through *its own* nature, but through God's.[62] I emphasize the possible existence for the exegetes of such a complex web of causation, one in which God endows objects and processes with causative power on a regular basis, precisely because such a vision ultimately did not win broad acceptance.[63] The view was refuted at least once in the commentaries themselves, most likely because of the danger posed by the heresy of the natural philosophers, who believed in the inherent power of the nature of things:[64] al-Māzarī, in a critique of astrologers' belief that planets had an effect on happenings on earth, cites their own criteria for the nature of causative agents in arguing against them.[65] However, for the majority of the commentators, the principles of causation are less important than giving concrete justifications for the application of the term *evil omen* to women, houses, and horses. After all, if the term can be shown to be purely metaphoric, many of its potentially problematical aspects would no longer have to be explained. Thus, ill-omened women are those who are barren, sharp of tongue, pining for a former husband, or possessed of an unpleasant disposition; or they may be simply women whose company one does not like. Ill-omened houses have bad neighbors, are small, or are so far from the mosque that the call to prayer cannot be heard in them. Ill-omened horses are those that are hurt or cannot be used for raiding. And ill-omened slaves, a category not present in most of the traditions, are those who are lazy and do not carry out the tasks entrusted to them.[66]

Despite these explanations, or perhaps in part because of them, it was stated that everyone believes in evil omens.[67] Later traditions of the Prophet maintain that no Muslim is free of three things—a belief in evil omens, doubt, and envy—and that one must ignore all of these, although it is hard to remove a belief in them from one's soul.[68] One is able to accomplish such a removal by placing one's trust in God and by repeating an invocation that credits him as the only cause of anything.[69]

Good Omens, Human Nature, and the Parallels with Contagion

Once the nature of evil omens had been elucidated, along with the way one might protect oneself against them, there was still the question of how it was possible for the Prophet to affirm the existence of good omens while denying that of evil omens.[70] Following the indications already present in the Prophetic traditions, the commentators met this challenge by defining the good omen as a fortuitous word or phrase coming at an opportune moment.[71] This explanation was substantiated in the many accounts of how the Prophet saw good omens in the names of places and people.[72] Yet the Prophet's phrasing of his acceptance of the good omen required additional grammatical explanation, since it appeared that he described the good omen as a subcategory of the evil omen.[73] The good omen is presented as a clarification, or as an exceptional type of evil omen that is influential whereas the evil omen itself is not.[74] Perhaps because this explanation was not considered entirely satisfactory, the commentators additionally defined the good omen as trusting in God, whereas the evil omen, being the opposite—not trusting in God—was clearly false.[75] That the Prophet had seen good omens in certain things was further justified by the argument that God created in human nature a favorable impression of natural phenomena such as pretty views, clear flowing water, and gardens in bloom.[76]

The notion that God places in human nature attractions and aversions to certain phenomena is important, for it causes the commentators to compare explicitly how humans react to what they perceive as evil omens with how they deal with the perceived danger of contagion. Ibn Ḥajar observes that Mālik's saying that one should leave a house that one thinks is ill-omened is similar to fleeing from the leper. In both cases one's heart is tormented by being close to the feared object, and one should leave it because if God's decree does coincide with proximity to the house or leper, one might sin in thinking that the house had caused one's fortunes to decline or that the leper had transmitted his sickness.[77] Creatively confused sinners might even conflate both forbidden phenomena and describe evil omens as being contagious.[78]

The Prophet forbade people to leave a plague-stricken country but allowed them to leave an ill-omened house, a stance scholars were aware could be misconstrued as contradictory.[79] Al-Māzarī relates from an unidentified source that one can differentiate between the two pronouncements because the first, the epidemic, is a general affliction, and the latter is a specific one. In the first case, harm can come about from people fleeing the area, while in the second case, people could alleviate their situation by leaving the house.[80]

In explaining the Prophetic traditions on the subject of the evil omen, the commentators moved far beyond simply glossing the traditions themselves. In order to show how the majority of the traditions can be reconciled, they had to offer a richer conception of human nature and behavior than was to be found in the hadith. To do so, they showed that humans generally are endowed with instinctive reactions, both positive and negative, to pleasing and repulsive phenomena. It was the challenge of the exegete to keep these reactions from interfering with correct belief, especially with faith in the unity of God. Far from being contradictory, Prophetic Tradition was shown to have taken into account human nature with all its foibles and to have been accommodating to human needs. Needless to say, the commentators do not agree about every issue, but if anything, the lack of agreement only ensures the need for further commentaries and the production of more scholarship on the commentators' differences.[81]

The arguments developed to deal with the problems raised by the evil omen are also employed in the case of contagion. Here too, the commentators pay close attention to how the believer's internal world is affected by the temptation to suspect that something besides God—in this case a disease—is endowed with agency. And the logic that allows al-Māzarī to distinguish between the plague and the ill-omened house is similarly used, if not as explicitly, to differentiate the contagion of leprosy from that of the plague.

Contagion: The Traditions

The presentation of contagion falls into four general subtopics in the collections of traditions. It is initially referred to implicitly in traditions concerned with not fleeing from the plague if one is in a land that is struck by it and not approaching such an area if one is outside it. The development of this tradition has been discussed at length by both Conrad and van Ess.[82] Yet this tradition, while tangentially present in later discussions of contagion, is usually addressed in terms of the debate surrounding fate and trusting in God.[83] Contagion itself, as noted above, is introduced by the Prophet and then denied, along with the evil omen: "[There is] no contagion, no evil omen, tapeworm, no death bird, no ghoul, and no malignant star."[84] The other pre-Islamic beliefs denied in this tradition are defined in other Prophetic traditions or in the commentaries.[85]

Like the evil omen, contagion is no sooner denied than certain apparent contradictions are introduced, thanks to other traditions from the Prophet: one should not water healthy animals with sick animals,[86] and lepers are to be treated with the same degree of caution as lions; that is, one should flee from them.[87] The subject of lepers is a particularly thorny one, for the Prophet and the first caliphs are said to have avoided their proximity and yet also to have welcomed them, even shared meals with them.[88] The tension between the denial of contagion and the injunction to avoid sick animals and people is most dramatically displayed when Abū

Hurayra is confronted with having related both the Prophet's denial of contagion and his admonition not to water sick with healthy animals:

> Abū Salama b. ᶜAbd al-Raḥmān b. ᶜAwf[89] related that the Prophet of God, Peace be Upon Him, said "No contagion," and he related that the Prophet said "Don't water the sick with the healthy." Abū Salama said: Abū Hurayra related both of these from the Prophet of God, Peace be Upon Him. Subsequently, Abū Hurayra was silent regarding the saying "No contagion" and emphasized (*aqāma 'alā*) [the tradition] "Don't water the sick with the healthy." He [Abū Salama] said, so al-Ḥārith b. Abī Dhubāb, the paternal nephew of Abū Hurayra, said: I have heard you, oh Abū Hurayra, relate to us along with this tradition another tradition. You have been silent regarding it. You used to say the Prophet of God, Peace be Upon Him, said: "No contagion." Abū Hurayra denied knowing this and said, "Don't water the sick with the healthy." Al-Ḥārith did not leave off about this until Abū Hurayra grew angry and blathered in Ethiopic (*raṭana bi-l-ḥabashiyya*). And he said to al-Ḥārith: "Do you know what I said?" He said: "No." Abū Hurayra said: "I said, I denied [it]."[90] Abū Salama said: "By my life! Abū Hurayra has been relating to us that the Prophet of God, Peace be Upon Him, said "No contagion," and I don't know if Abū Hurayra forgot or if one of the two sayings abrogated the other."[91]

Whether or not the traditions are contradictory in their essence, this episode suggests that Abū Hurayra perceived them to be so and chose to resolve the conflict by relating only the tradition that implies the existence of contagion.[92] In another confrontation, played out between the Prophet and an unnamed bedouin, Muḥammad is asked explicitly about the cases that had been observed in which one sick animal mingles with others and they then become sick.[93] The Prophet explains the phenomenon of diseases spreading with a rhetorical question as to who caused the first incidence of the disease:[94] implicit is that God, who caused the first occurrence, caused the second as well. In some traditions, the Prophet adds that contagion does not exist and that God has written out the fate of everyone and their afflictions beforehand.[95] The explicitness of these last traditions on the subject of fate (*qadar*) suggests that, as Conrad has argued, contagion was drawn into the theological debates of the second and third centuries of the Muslim calendar when the nature of man's fate and the limits of his free will were hotly debated.[96] These debates, which resulted in part in the development of Ashᶜarī theology, had a continued influence on the hadith folk's approach to contagion.[97] Other themes that shaped the hadith folk's discussion of contagion are referred to in the following discussion of the commentaries. One of them, the duty of every Muslim to take care of the sick and to sit with them, bears mentioning here, because it recurs in later arguments against acting on the basis of the existence of contagion.[98] In addition, we already find in the traditions a hint of what later commentators focused on when they interpreted the traditions in a manner that addressed the doubts, fears, and weaknesses of individual Muslims. Following his exhortation not to water the sick with the healthy animals, the Prophet was asked to specify what he meant: "They said: 'And what is that oh Prophet of God?' The Prophet of God said: 'It is a harm (*adhan*)!' "[99] It is unclear what exactly the Prophet was referring to. It could be the disease, or it could also, with some exegetical license, refer to the harm that would come through believing that the disease is the reason for the transmission of the sickness. In their desire to reconcile the various traditions and to preserve a belief in God as the immediate cause of all events, the commentators on Prophetic Tradition tended toward the latter interpretation.

Contagion: The Commentaries

The hadith commentators scrutinized the actions of the Prophet and his Companions in order to understand the correct reaction to epidemics and diseases that the pre-Islamic Arabian tribes had considered transmissible. One of the episodes that attracted a great deal of attention in the commentaries, and to which Ibn al-Khaṭīb later alluded, involved the second caliph ᶜUmar and a foray led by him from Medina toward Syria.[100] At Sargh, on the road between the Hijaz and Syria, ᶜUmar was informed that the plague had broken out in Syria, and after consulting with his companions, he decided to return to Medina. In what Conrad has convincingly argued to be a later development of the tradition, one of ᶜUmar's companions, Abū ᶜUbayda (d. 18/638), challenged the caliph's decision to return, asking him if it was right to flee the will of God. ᶜUmar retorted that he was fleeing *from* the will of God *to* the will of God, and in the final form of the episode, he was supported by ᶜAbd al-Raḥmān b. ᶜAwf (d. 32/652), who arrived at the critical moment, saying that he heard the Prophet say that one should neither leave nor approach a plague-stricken area.[101] In Conrad's view, this episode most likely had a historical kernel—ᶜUmar fleeing the plague that had broken out in Syria—around which a polished narrative developed in accordance with the theological demands of later generations. He suggested that the narrative was fashioned by al-Zuhrī (d. 124/742) out of earlier, regional traditions.[102] Relevant to our discussion of contagion is this: the caliph ᶜUmar's statement that he was fleeing to the will of God provides an eloquent rebuttal to anyone arguing for a fatalistic attitude toward epidemic disease, while the tradition related by ᶜAbd al-Raḥmān b. ᶜAwf provides what later generations could easily see as a justification for quarantine procedures.[103] Yet these two statements were not generally interpreted in this fashion, either in the premodern or the modern period.[104] Instead, the commentaries emphasize the impossibility of success in fleeing from the plague, cite the tradition of not entering or leaving a plague-stricken country, and omit ᶜUmar's remarks on fleeing from the will of God to the will of God.[105] Such a line of argumentation could be pursued by noting that on his deathbed ᶜUmar regretted fleeing the plague,[106] and by citing *Sūrat al-Baqara,* 243: "[Prophet], consider those people who abandoned their homeland in fear of death, even though there were thousands of them. God said to them, 'Die!' and then brought them back to life again."[107] This verse, along with being interpreted as an admonition against fleeing epidemics, served to explain the pre-Islamic history and origins of the plague.[108] Yet the plague itself and the episode of ᶜUmar at Sargh played only a minor role in the commentators' treatment of the issue. Of greater importance were the issues raised in the traditions on contagion discussed above.

The Prophet, the Bedouin, and Mangy Camels

Upon being told that there was no contagion, one of the bedouin, drawing on what would have been common experience, challenged the Prophet Muhammad with the example of a mangy camel that mingles among other camels that then become mangy themselves.[109] The commentators were unanimous in seeing the Prophet's response—"Who infected the first?"—as a rejection of the idea that the disease could transmit itself and an indication of God's agency in the origin of the disease.[110] Still, it was allowed that God could have created proximity to a sick animal to be a reason for the transmission of the disease.[111] The tradition, according to which Ibn ᶜUmar was sold camels sick with what previously had been thought to be a contagious disease, was given perfunctory treatment in comparison to the energy expended on interacting with lepers.[112] A possible reason for this is that the social reality of the commentators included lepers, but they, unlike the Prophet and the bedouin, may not have had much experience with camels. With careful scholarship, however, the empirical realities of the situation can be reconstructed: the thirsting sickness *hiyām* may be transmitted by smelling the urine of a camel afflicted with the disease.[113] This conclusion begs the question, however, of why

Ibn ᶜUmar would have been content with the sick camels he had bought if their sickness could be transmitted, whether through their urine or whether God had made proximity to them a cause for the transmission of illness. While this question is neither explicitly posed nor addressed in any other way, the danger of relying too much on sensory perception is taken up directly by Abū ᶜAbbās al-Qurṭūbī in a passage later quoted by Ibn Ḥajar:

> The meaning of this [i.e., Muḥammad's saying, Who infected the first?] is, where did the mange come from with the mangy camel that, as they claim, gave mange to the healthy ones? From another camel? That would necessitate a sequence [of transmissions]. Or from a cause other than a camel? And this is what created the mange in the first and the second: God, the Most High, the creator of everything, capable of everything. The doubt that appeared in them is that which occurred in the natural philosophers (*al-tabā'iᶜyyīn*) first and the Muᶜtazila second. The natural philosophers argued for (*qālū bi*) the mutual influence of things upon each other and their production (*ījād*) of each other. And they called that which influences (*al-mu'aththir*) "nature." The Muᶜtazila argued similarly regarding the acts of animals and acts (*mutawalladāt*). They said that their powers influence them through production. They are creators of their actions independently and by their own device (*bi-ikhtirāᶜihim*). They base all of the described on sensory perception (*al-mushāhada al-ḥissiyya*) and perhaps they consider the denial of this a denial of the obvious. This is a grave error and its cause is that they have confused sensory perception with perception through reason. What they have witnessed is the influence of one thing on another thing, and this is that which pertains to the senses (*ḥaẓẓ al-ḥiss*). Yet the influence of one thing upon another is not perceived by the senses, but by reason. For the senses perceive the presence of something with something else, and its ceasing (*irtifāᶜu-hu*) with its ceasing, but the senses have no access to its production. Concerning successive events being of the same state (*fa-ammā al-mutaqāribāt fī-l-wujūd ᶜalā ḥālatin wāḥidin*), it is reason that discerns and decides according to their being attached to each other, by means of reason and by their habitual association with each other, with its being permissible to do so rationally (*maᶜ jawāz al-tabaddul ᶜaqlan*). One of the wise and honored theorists did well when he said: You are deceived in the matter of existence and nonexistence [i.e., if you think you can rely solely on your senses in this matter, you are wrong]. The exhaustive treatment of this subject is in theology (*ᶜilm al-kalām*). In it is the indication that it is permissible to speak with one who doubts due to a belief in a rational proof if

> the questioner is of the people of understanding. Concerning the people of limited ability (*ahl al-quṣūr*), they speak according to what their minds grasp of the matters of conviction (*min al-umūr al-iqnāᶜiyyāt*).[114]

Perhaps most striking in this passage is the use of reason to refute the impressions of sensory perception. Al-Qurṭubī, like al-Māzarī in his discussion of astrologers, uses arguments drawn from Ashᶜārī theology to refute the claims of the rationalist natural philosophers and Muᶜtazila. After stating that the observation of a succession of events does not prove they are causally linked, he is able to establish an equivalence between reason and the commentator's interpretation of the Prophet's words.[115] It may be argued that in this understanding Muḥammad is portrayed as a theologian par excellence, showing weaker minds the intrinsic link between reason and revelation.[116]

Watering Sick Animals with Abū Hurayra

The question of abrogation was raised by commentators who saw a contradiction between the Prophet's answer to the bedouin and his exhortation not to water sick with healthy animals.[117] Far more attention, however, was given to the Abū Hurayra incident, in which he had denied relating the "There is no contagion" tradition after beginning to relate the "Do not water" tradition. Here, after all, was testimony that one of the Prophet's Companions and one of the most important relaters of traditions had seen these traditions as standing in tension. For the most part, the commentators simply repeat the words of Abū Salama, namely, that Abū Hurayra never erred save in this.[118] Even if this was so, however, the commentators still had to address the tension between the two traditions. Was the admonition not to water the animals together abrogated by the "no contagion" tradition? Are the two traditions irreconcilable? There was some difference on this issue, but the majority was clearly opposed to abrogation.[119] An easier way to reconcile the traditions is with the argument, already suggested above in the Prophet's answer to the bedouin, that God made proximity to the sick a cause for the occurrence of disease.[120] It needs to be emphasized that the commentators do not see here a transmission of any kind, but rather that proximity to the sick is related to God's direct creation of the mange as a casually, not causally, related phenomenon. The possibility that God might use transmission to create disease was a minority view among the hadith folk and was given a detailed physical form as early as Ibn Qutayba:

> The case is similar with the scab on a camel. It is a moist [form of] mange (*jarab raṭb*). If camels associate with it, rub against it (*ḥikka-hā*), and seek shelter in where it [a mangy camel] has lain down (*mubārakahā*), they are infected (*ūṣila ilayhā*) through the water that flows from it. The drops (*al-nuṭaf*) are similar to what is in it (*naḥwan mimmā bihi*) and this is the matter regarding which the Prophet, God bless Him and grant Him salvation, said: "Don't water one with a defect with a healthy one." It is hateful to associate a diseased one (*al-ma*ᶜ*yūh*) with a healthy one, for he obtains it [mange] from his drops and his itching (*ḥikkati-hi*), according to what he has (*naḥw mimmā bihi*).[121]

In the same section Ibn Qutayba denies a different interpretation, which later received greater prominence than his own views: the reason one should not mix sick and healthy animals is that if one of the healthy ones should then get sick, one might be tempted to believe in contagion and thus sin by associating another power with God, so falling into polytheism.[122] Such an interpretation has clear parallels with the commentators' explanation of the Prophet's advice to leave a house that is thought to be ill-omened. In both situations, the commentators see the principal danger to be to the beliefs of the community and not to their physical well-being. Parallels to this approach can also be found in explanations for why ᶜUmar turned back at Sargh or, more commonly, why one should avoid associating with lepers.[123]

Leprosy, the Other Contagion

It is in the context of leprosy that the commentators spend the most time discussing the subject of contagion. Here is a disease that had been present in the Muslim world from before the time of the Prophet and which continued to be relevant on a daily basis.[124] How should one interact with lepers? Could one share a source of water with them? Could one buy goods and food from them? Pray next to them? From the commentaries it is clear that many believers did not wish to interact with lepers, but how could this popular feeling be incorporated into a genre that tended to deny the transmission of disease? Two possibilities have already been discussed: The first is to emphasize the danger of being close to lepers because if one is struck down with leprosy, one may doubt the unity of God and believe in contagion.[125] The second—although this is a line of argument that in the long run may have caused more confusion than clarity—is the suggestion that the smell given off by lepers is dangerous in and of itself and that they should be avoided for that reason. This smell is described as being strong enough to cause the wife of a leper to miscarry and to make conjugal relations harmful in the extreme.[126] A third option is to argue, much as the evil omen was denied save in three things, that there is no contagion save in the cases of leprosy, mange, and a small number of other diseases (but not the plague).[127] These three tactics, despite being mutually contradictory, could be offered by the commentators with the tacit justification of comprehensiveness. The issue was further confused by several commentators who, drawing on the example of the Prophet and his Companions, strongly denied that leprosy is contagious.[128] This muddle could be cleared up in part by distinguishing between those believers whose strength of faith allowed them to remain in the proximity of lepers without any harm and the greater mass of common Muslims, who were mercifully exempted from such extreme demonstrations of trust in God.[129] It was also clarified by applying a logic similar to that used with the mangy camels, namely that proximity to a leper may be an occasion for the occurrence of the disease.[130]

The commentators also give opinions on a variety of practical issues that reveal a certain acceptance of popular apprehension regarding lepers: if an alternative water source can be provided for the use of lepers, then it should be;[131] lepers should be forbidden to attend any but the Friday mosque on Friday; and if their number grew large, they should be resettled.[132] These are topics that recurred in legal opinions (*fatāwā*) of the premodern period, reflecting a continued interest in the subject.[133] The trend toward allowing Muslims to avoid lepers was tempered by the reminder that it is both a sign and an act of piety to sit with the sick, a recommendation that was taken up in the context of the plague more than of leprosy.[134]

A Reconciliation of the Traditions?

Most of the commentators included or indicated their preference for only a selection of the preceding interpretations. Faced with such a wide range of opinions and approaches, what was the final judgment on the issue of contagion? Generally speaking, there is none; the process of commentary and interpretation continues both in the commentaries and in other genres, such as fatwas, plague treatises, and works on medicine. Many of the commentators express their positions by including only those views with which they agree or giving a brief statement at the end of each chapter. Yet some do offer a series of final positions on the subject along with an authorial preference. Contagion had no greater opponent than the esteemed Cairene scholar Ibn Ḥajar al-ᶜAsqalānī. Because of his influence on later scholarship, and because he wrote a book on the plague itself, his view is of special importance.[135] In his chapter on leprosy, he offers a list of the possible ways in which the relevant traditions may be reconciled, and all but one—the fifth—involved a denial of contagion:[136]

1. Completely deny contagion. In this understanding of the matter, one should stay away from lepers in order to avoid increasing their sense of loss by showing them a healthy body.
2. Assume that the two traditions have different addressees. The contagion hadith is directed to those who are strong in conviction and are able to reject belief in transmission of diseases, just as they are able to reject believing in evil omens. Ibn Ḥajar compares this case to the body's vitality in repelling an illness. The tradition on fleeing from lepers, in contrast, is directed to those who are weak in conviction and are not able to stop believing in contagion.
3. Take the "no contagion" statement as a general one to which there may be exceptions, such as leprosy and mange.
4. Consider that fleeing from a leper may have nothing to do with contagion at all, but rather reflects the unpleasantness of being around someone who smells bad and the possibility of becoming sick from the smell.
5. Understand the denial of contagion as meant to refute the pre-Islamic belief that it is the nature of sickness to be contagious and to show that everything depends on the will of God. For this reason the Prophet ate with lepers, to show people that it is God who causes sickness and heals. Yet he also advised against being in proximity to lepers in order to make it clear that proximity is one of the causes through which the will of God operates.
6. Completely reject contagion. Here Ibn Ḥajar explains that the issue of avoiding the leprous was used as an excuse to argue that interaction with the sick is a cause of the transmission of disease. This is the opinion of Abū ᶜUbayd (d. 224/838), whom Ibn Ḥajar proceeds to quote.[137] He then turns to the views of Ibn Khuzayma (d. 311/924), whom Ibn Ḥajar believes to have gone on at length (*aṭnaba ibn khuzayma*) in his exposition of the matter.[138] The former's style is rambling: after citing numerous accounts supporting the denial of contagion, he argues that the traditions that deal with fleeing from the leprous either have as their aim alleviat-

> ing the situation of Muslims who are afraid of coming to harm or were uttered by the Prophet out of compassion for the leprous, who would be pained by the sight of healthy bodies. It is clear in any case that affirming contagion goes against the sayings of the Prophet.

To some extent Ibn Ḥajar followed the division established by Ibn Qutayba between contagion in the cases of leprosy and of plague. Whereas the earlier author clearly had argued that leprosy could be transmitted by physical means, if not under the name of contagion, the evidence marshaled by Ibn Ḥajar suggested that this was not the case; nevertheless, there were other reasons to avoid lepers. Yet Ibn Qutayba and Ibn Ḥajar agreed that people could not escape from the plague and should not flee from it. The reason for this division of contagion into two types most likely has its origins in the Prophetic traditions themselves. With both the plague and leprosy, observers had problems establishing an airtight case for contagion. The plague occurs erratically, and some succumb to it while their neighbors escaped unscathed. With leprosy, transmission is related to the severity of affliction and the length of contact.[139] In neither disease was contagion constantly observable, although popular belief had long associated it with both. Another possible reason for the distinction between the two is that for the hadith folk, the plague was determined early on to be a gateway to martyrdom.[140] This view is the central argument of Ibn Ḥajar's book on the plague, in which he also argues that the plague is transmitted by jinn.[141] There is no room here for the doctrine of contagion: God affects victims individually by sending jinn to pierce them internally.[142] The case is different for lepers. Their affliction is in no way associated with martyrdom, and it has been shown that in the first century of Islam, leprosy may have been considered a curse.[143] Such explanations of the distinction between two types of contagion are, however, tentative at best. It is also possible that the difference had a great deal to do with the ways the two diseases differ, for as al-Māzarī noted, the plague is a collective disease, afflicting a large group of people at one time, whereas leprosy is an individual disease that is perceived to spread from one individual to another.[144] A final point regarding leprosy should be mentioned: neither Ibn Ḥajar nor any of the other commentators who emphasize the danger of the smell of lepers while also denying contagion could explain what may well strike the modern reader as a contradiction. For if the smell of leprosy, or the liquid resulting in the smell of mange, causes others to acquire the sickness, does that not mean that the disease is contagious? At best, the focus on the negative effects of leprosy's smell seems to have been a compromise between the demands of theological and medical discourses, allowing the hadith folk to insist that it is not the sickness itself that is transmitted—that this is not the contagion of the pre-Islamic period that the Prophet had denied. A similar compromise was not at hand in the case of plague, and it is this that Ibn al-Khaṭīb had occasion to lament in Granada in the eighth/fourteenth century.

Authoritative as Ibn Ḥajar's views may have been for later generations, other opinions were expressed during and after his lifetime. Al-Ubbī argues that proximity to disease was made by God to be a cause of disease transmission and that it is important not to deny medical principles. At the same time, he notes, one should interpret these principles so that they do not conflict with the unity of God (*tawḥīd*).[145] Al-Qastallānī, a compatriot of Ibn Ḥajar's who lived in the century after the latter's death, expresses a similar view, that God designated proximity as a cause for the transmission of disease, though he does not mention the importance of reconciling medicine and law.[146] Neither of these scholars refers to the views of Ibn al-Khaṭīb, with which I began this chapter, but if the Andalusian vizier had wished to, he could have cited earlier commentators who were closer to his own views, though he would have found none who supported him with respect to the plague.[147] In addition, the reliance on empirical evidence that is seen in Ibn al-Khaṭīb, so lauded by modern commentators, was examined a century before he wrote by a fellow Andalusian, Abū ᶜAbbās al-Qurṭūbī—and was found wanting. It would be dangerous, then, to see Ibn al-Khaṭīb as an isolated voice of reason in a wilderness of strict theological imitation. Within the realm of commentaries on traditions, there were many views, often set on the same page in tense juxtaposition, offering the reader the opportunity to make his own choice. While the ability of diseases to transmit themselves *by means of their own natures* was universally denied, many commentators, from the time of Ibn Qutayba to that of al-Qasṭallānī, supported the existence of disease transmission, if only under certain conditions and limited to a specific group of diseases.[148]

Conclusion

In order to explain apparent contradictions in the Prophetic traditions regarding both evil omens and contagion, the hadith folk employed a variety of techniques. Perhaps the most impressive of these was their focus on the inner world of the believer. In both the case of the ill-omened house and that of the leper, the commentators argued that prolonged contact with them could lead the believer into the temptation of thinking that something other than God possessed causative power.

This is not simply a makeshift solution to a difficult exegetical problem, though a skeptic might argue that it began that way, but rather a principle that commentators consciously use in differing cases for similar reasons.[149] Such a focus on a Muslim's internal belief system reflects the concerns of the second and third Islamic centuries more than those of the first. They are the result of what, from the perspective of Ibn al-Khaṭīb, was a relatively early episode in the venture of Islam: the attempt of Muslims to understand the nature of disease and to order society.

It is worthwhile to consider Conrad's evaluation of the hadith folk's understanding of contagion: "Medieval Islam provides a valuable case of a society in which public health measures against contagion were clearly being implemented, while at the same time contagion theory was quite controversial. . . . What this seems to indicate is that society was prepared to accommodate the subject in multiple contradictory registers, with contagion being critiqued and often denied in religious scholarship, while it was accepted as a matter of course in more practical secular spheres."[150] Instead of seeing a dichotomy between "religious scholarship" and "more practical secular spheres," I would suggest that the acceptance referred to by Conrad was actually based in, and not in tension with, the exegetical world of the hadith folk. By denying contagion and yet preserving the possibility of disease transmission in the case of lepers, Muslim legal scholars were, for example, able to give cogent reasons based on Prophetic Tradition for why the activities of lepers in the marketplace should be regulated.[151] The reasons they could not do so in the case of people afflicted with the plague, reasons examined in this chapter, were responsible well into the nineteenth century for the continued failure of the scholarly community and, in part, the government, to advocate measures for the containment of plague outbreaks.[152] This outcome was not due to a stale tradition rooted in imitation, but rather to continuously creative scholarship that evolved in a direction distinct from that chosen by natural scientists in the twentieth century. It is only when the scholarship of the hadith folk is seen in this light that it can be correctly understood as an ongoing dialogue between specialists attempting to explain the world and, to the best of their ability, legislate the will of God therein.

Contagion as Metaphor in Iberian Christian Scholarship

> For it was my doleful observation, repeated again and again, that the metaphoric trappings that deform the experience of having cancer have very real consequences: they inhibit people from seeking treatment early enough, or from making a greater effort to get competent treatment. The metaphors and myths, I was convinced, kill. I wanted to offer other people who were ill and those who care for them an instrument to dissolve these metaphors, these inhibitions. I hoped to persuade terrified people who were ill to . . . regard cancer as if it were just a disease—a very serious one, but just a disease. Not a curse, not a punishment, not an embarrassment. Without "meaning."
>
> Susan Sontag, *AIDS and Its Metaphors*

IN HER ESSAYS on epidemic disease, Susan Sontag argues powerfully against granting diseases metaphoric significance. She observes that by describing diseases with figurative language, we force upon the ill a host of associations that determine both the nature of their sickness and the significance of the state of those suffering. To help them confront their condition directly, it is vital to strip disease of its metaphors and allow the sick to understand their illness as nothing more than a clinical condition.[1] Diseases have no "meaning" for Sontag; they are nothing more than physical ailments. She advises us to calm our imaginations and to moderate our language on the subject of illness. It is possible that Sontag's arguments have so much power because the reader, while acknowledging their eloquence, also senses their futility. Disease, especially contagious disease, has shown a remarkable capability to repeatedly break through the narrow confines of literal language in order to accommodate the fears and fantasies of society.

Sontag's analysis gains authority from its reference to the effectiveness and legitimacy of modern medicine. In her writings, the division between premodern and modern medicine is a clear one.[2] Relying perhaps too easily on the clarity of the modern-premodern distinction, she directs an intense critique toward overly psychological paradigms of health, linking contemporary theories of psychosomatic causation to medieval miasma theory.[3] The references here and elsewhere to medieval notions of disease etiology occur when Sontag wishes to disparage views with which she disagrees. It was because people did not understand the diseases they observed, she argues, that they gave them so much meaning. The same is true for cancer and, now, AIDS. It is characteristic of diseases that are imperfectly understood, she claims, that we assign them complex and opaque etiologies with multiple causes.[4] Comparing cancer to leprosy, the disease often portrayed as characterizing the Middle Ages, Sontag writes: "Leprosy in its heyday aroused a similarly disproportionate sense of horror. In the Middle Ages, the leper was a social text in which corruption was made visible; an exemplum, an emblem of decay. Nothing is more punitive than to give disease a meaning—that meaning being invariably a moralistic one. Any important disease whose causality is murky, and for which treatment is ineffectual, tends to be awash in significance. First, the subjects of deepest dread (corruption, decay, pollution, anomie, weakness) are identified with the disease. The disease itself becomes a metaphor. . . . Feelings about evil are projected onto a disease. And the disease (so enriched with meanings) is projected onto the world."[5] Sontag asserts that despite the widespread presence of leprosy in many parts of the world today, it has lost the significance it possessed previously. This shift occurred principally after the nineteenth-century discovery of the relevant bacillus, a discovery that rendered the disease less mysterious.[6]

It is not my intention to dispute Sontag's use of the Middle Ages, although her polemic certainly leaves itself open to charges of ahistoricism and an overly optimistic faith in the powers of modern medicine.[7] The current chapter shows, on the contrary, to what degree Sontag's concerns can productively direct our attention to the metaphoric uses of the concept of contagion in Iberian Christian texts. Throughout the Middle Ages, disease figured prominently in biblical exegesis, popular sermons, and even chronicles, as a way of referring to people or beliefs thought to be dangerous. Yet, instead of flattening the premodern period into a continuum, as Sontag did, I will show how the meaning of certain diseases such as leprosy and the plague in Iberian Christian texts were contingent upon not only the immediate concerns of specific authors, but also medical developments in the understanding of contagion itself.

Characterizing "Christian Contagion": Tropes, Disease, and the Religious Other

As we saw in chapter 1, after the Black Death, the Muslim *ᶜulamāʾ* of the eighth/fourteenth century could look back and contemplate an extensive discussion of contagion centered on the words of the Prophet himself. Christian scholars had pursued no such debate. Jesus had said little about the existence or nonexistence of contagion, and his disciples had alluded to the subject only obliquely, in a metaphoric fashion. Similarly, one could consult the Old Testament without finding any explicit allusion to the subject of contagion, although, as in the New Testament in 1 Corinthians 5:6–8, there are several episodes there, notably Leviticus 13, that with exegetical help were found to be relevant.[8] The broader significance of the concept of contagion in the Christian world has its roots in the classical literature of Greece and Rome, especially in metaphors or tropes for beliefs and practices that were considered dangerous and unorthodox. From Thucydides in the fifth century BCE to Bede in the eighth century CE and Fracastoro in the sixteenth, contagion was employed to describe the transmission of heretical faiths or immorality.[9] Although Christian authors later used the metaphor of contagion in their writings against heresies, the image did not originate with them, and it had even at times been used against them: Pliny the Younger (d. 110), for example, once noted that there was yet hope to check the contagious superstition of Christianity.[10]

When used by Christian authors metaphorically to refer to the transmission of beliefs or moral values, contagion was significant in relation to several other tropes, principally those of sin as disease and Christ as physician (*Christus medicus*). Both of these tropes are present in the New Testament, and biblical exegetes argued for their presence in the Old Testament as well. They were so prevalent in the writings of Christian authors of the Middle Ages that the role of contagion as a metaphor seems comparatively minor if not largely determined by the other two. All three tropes were influenced by medical writings and the developing understandings of disease. Which diseases were associated with which sins, which diseases were thought to be contagious, and how the transmission of sin and disease took place all shaped the meaning of contagion. In addition, and of special relevance here, is how and when contagion was used to refer to the dangers of contact with religious minorities, specifically Muslims and Jews living under Christian rule in the Iberian peninsula.

Situating Biblical Exegesis and Allegorical Thinking

It is difficult to write the history of a metaphor. By laying out equivalences, a metaphor, even more than literal language, forces the reader to bring his own knowledge of the world into the text. In making sense of the statement "Christ is a doctor," for example, the reader draws on all of her or his associations with both terms.[11] Although I have used the word *metaphor* in the chapter's title, tropic language is notoriously difficult to define; in many of the cases discussed here, *allegory* may be the more accurate designation. As Joseph Lienhard has observed, however, the creative endeavor of biblical exegesis more often involved the commentator's use of a passage to elaborate on what it reminded him of, rather than setting up one-to-one correspondences between terms or figures.[12] Instead of focusing on the various tropological modes in which contagion is employed, therefore, I have attempted to elucidate its significance within its larger semantic context.

As social, cultural, and intellectual circumstances change, so do a reader's associations, whereupon a metaphor acquires new significance. This observation may seem commonplace, but acknowledging the importance of context encourages studies with a narrow temporal and geographic focus, which aim to acquire a clear understanding of a metaphor's significance at a particular point in time. A valuable example of this type of approach can be found in a recent essay by Abigail Firey, where she observes that Carolingian exegetes attempting metaphoric interpretations of leprosy in Leviticus 13 in the ninth century were directed by their interest in the "formulation of Christian identity in the midst of cultural diversity."[13] Firey shows, drawing in part on the work of the seventh-century Iberian polymath Isidore of Seville (d. 636), how Claudius of Turin (d. ca. 827) and Hrabanus Maurus (d. 856) both argued that the spiritual significance of leprosy discussed in Leviticus represented the danger of Judaism and heresy.[14]

The approach taken here differs from Firey's. Instead of discussing why Leviticus would have attracted exegetical attention in one period, I have chosen to follow the ways in which contagion was both defined and employed through four important bodies of text over an extended period of time: the work of Isidore of Seville (d. 636), the writings of Beato of Liebana (d. 798), the corpus of Alfonso X (thirteenth century), and the sermons of Saint Vincent Ferrer (d. 1419). These examples represent a broad selection of prominent examples of different genres—etymological dictionary, chronicle, biblical commentary, law code, and religious sermon. By grouping them together, the chapter offers a broad, necessarily impressionistic, account of the metaphoric uses of contagion in medieval Iberian Christian scholarship. Although none of the texts discussed here are explicitly medical, when they employ contagion, metaphorically and otherwise, they often slide seamlessly between the physical and the spiritual, the medical and the theological. The scope of this chapter provides the reader with an understanding of the origins and nature of the rhetoric used by Christian scholars to designate heretical beliefs, as well as emphasizing when and how this rhetoric shifted in accordance with medical advances and a changing political landscape.

The Case of Isidore

Standing on the threshold between late antiquity and the Middle Ages, Isidore of Seville was a prolific encyclopedist who drew extensively on the works of classical Latinity. His writings, especially the famed *Etymologiae,* enjoyed great influence throughout the Middle Ages, not only in the Iberian peninsula but also throughout Europe. Judging from the manuscript tradition, he was being read in Ireland, England, France, and Italy before the end of the eighth century.[15] Bischoff has argued that this popularity came about in part because he represented Christian Iberia's cultural prominence in the seventh century, a period of stagnation in much of the rest of Europe.[16] Possibly of equal importance was the exodus of Latin manuscripts from Iberia following the Arab invasion of 711.[17] That Isidore's work was considered especially precious, however, can be seen in the almost complete failure of any of his Christian Iberian contemporaries to have their works transmitted outside the peninsula.[18]

Isidore held the position of bishop in Seville from 599, when he succeeded his brother Leander in the office, to his death in 636. In 633 he presided over the fourth synodal council in Toledo and was able to implement reforms in clerical education, stressing the importance of the liberal arts.[19] Influenced by both classical and patristic sources, he deals with contagion in many of his works, where his treatment can be roughly divided into medical and metaphoric. This distinction, while at times useful, is admittedly forced, so instead of postponing discussion of his medical writings to a subsequent chapter, I have chosen to include them here. The influence of Isidore on posterity transcended disciplinary boundaries, and his encyclopedic *Etymologiae,* which includes his extensive definition of contagion, served as a general reference throughout the Middle Ages. Generally speaking, contagion carried a medical meaning when Isidore was discussing the plague or pestilence, but in his treatment of leprosy it fulfilled both a medical and a metaphoric purpose. It is therefore difficult and perhaps misguided to try to make a clear distinction between the two.[20]

Isidore discusses both the plague and leprosy in the fourth book of the *Etymologiae, De medicina.*[21] While the plague is equated with contagion, the question of whether leprosy can be transmitted is not addressed here. Isidore's remarks on the plague, influential throughout the Middle Ages, deserve to be quoted in full:

> Plague, *pestilential,* is a contagion which, when it takes hold of one person, quickly spreads to many. It arises from corrupt air, *corrupto aëre,* and by penetrating into the viscera settles there. Even though this disease often springs up from air-borne potencies, *per aërias potestates,* nevertheless it can never come about without the will of Almighty God. It is termed "pestilence" as though a "little pasture," *pastulentia,* or because it feeds like a fire, as Vergil [Aeneid 5, 683] : *Toto descendit corpore pestis,* "The plague fell upon the whole body." Likewise, it is called "contagion," *contagium,* from "touch," *contingere,* for whomsoever it touches, it infects. It is also called *inguina* because it attacks the groins, *inguen.* The same disease is also called *lues,* from "destruction" and "grief," *luctus,* since its course is so acute and rapid that one does not have enough time in which even to hope for life or for death, but a feeling of faintness comes on suddenly, bringing death at the same time.[22]

Perhaps only a modern reader would read two different etiologies of plague into Isidore's words, one in which plague is caused by a corruption of the air or miasma, and another in which it arises from physical contact with a transmissible disease. Strikingly, here the disease itself is referred to as "contagion," and not the mode of its transmission. This conflation helps explain how for Isidore's contemporaries there was no tension between miasma and contagion theories of causation, for one could understand the miasma itself to be contagious.[23] As Isidore notes, the corrupt air enters into the body and settles into the viscera, that is, anything under the skin.[24] In the accepted Galenic paradigm, in which a person's health depends on an equilibrium of the four humors, this corrupt air, by causing a severe imbalance between the humors, leads to death.[25] In another of his books, *De natura rerum,* Isidore discussed plague and, influenced by the Galenic phrase "seeds of disease," refined and complicated the notion of corrupted air:[26]

> Likewise, others say that many pest bearing seeds of things are carried into the air and borne up, then are transported either by winds or by clouds to the farthest parts of the heavens. Then, wherever they are carried, either they fall through our pores and joined together, encompass the beginnings of death for animals, or they remain suspended in the air, and when we breathe, we take in air, absorbing them at the same time into the body, then, falling ill, the body is extinguished either by foul ulcers or as though by a single blow. For just as bodies exposed to this unusual state of the heavens or unwholesomeness of the waters take the disease, so also corrupted air coming from other parts of the heavens snatch up the body with a sudden blow and quickly extinguish life.[27]

Again, a modern reader might deduce from this passage that Isidore was speaking of germs or bacilli that brought a disease into the body.[28] Certain similarities do exist: in both cases an external agent enters the body and causes a disruption of its internal harmony. But the similarities should not be overstated. The "seeds of disease" were for Isidore one factor among many, and in the end their possible effect was understood and treated within the Galenic framework of the humors, radically different from modern medicinal models.[29] It was clear, however, that plague was transmitted through the air and that it could be contagious, though how such contagion took place remained vague.

The case was different with Isidore's treatment of leprosy in *De medicina.* He differentiated between leprosy, elephantiasis, and scabies by drawing on Leviticus 13:1–6: leprosy is the skin disease in which patches of rough skin of a different color appear.[30] That leprosy of a moral kind is contagious becomes clear through a consideration of Isidore's exegetical writings. Isidore wrote two works that deal with the Old Testament, *Allegoriae quaedam sacrae scripturae* and *Questiones in Vetus Testamentum.* The first consists of a list of the allegorical meanings of people or events in the Old and New Testaments.[31] The glosses given here by Isidore employ leprosy as a sign of heretical beliefs or, in the case of the Jews, error. Miriam, Moses's sister, is said to prefigure the synagogue, sprinkled with the contagion of leprosy (*contagio leprae perfunditur*) because of its murmurings against Christ. Conversely, Moses's Ethiopian wife, against whom Miriam had railed, represents the multiethnic Church drawn together by Christ (*Ecclesiam ex gentibus Christo conjunctam*).[32]

These equivalences should not be seen as set in stone. As mentioned above, Joseph Lienhard has noted that "when one asks about the meaning of Scripture beyond the literal, 'allegory' is not a particularly helpful category. In many cases it may be better to speak simply of 'reminding.' Water reminded the Fathers of Baptism, bread or manna reminded them of the Eucharist, rock or stone reminded them of Christ."[33] Isidore had no compunction about being reminded of different things. In a letter to a Bishop Massona in which he discusses the punishment for a sinning member of the clergy, he writes that Miriam's punishment is that of the erring priest: "When, given to pride, she is stained with the most sordid contagion of corruption (*sordissimis corruptionum contagiis maculatur*), she is cast outside the camp for seven days, that is, outside the body of the Holy Church for seven years."[34] Here again, contagion is used as a synonym for disease and not as a description of how disease is transmitted. It refers to the corrupted state of an individual body, not the danger of being in close proximity to the sinner.

Isidore also contemplates leprosy in his *Quaestiones in Vetus Testamentum,* where he devotes a chapter to the subject. After citing Leviticus 13:1–3, he quickly turns to a symbolic exploration of the different types of leprosy. That "leprosy is false doctrine" is clear, but the disease is apt as an image of heresy because heretics have not one faith but many varied ones, which stain them as variously as leprosy does the healthy body.[35] Isidore then divides leprosy into six different types, according to the parts of the body in which the disease manifests itself, and assigns to each a different heresy. The technique of assigning various categories of the same disease to different sins or sinners was not uncommon; it was particularly popular with the plagues God had sent upon the Egyptians, upon which I will touch below. Needless to say, Isidore's division has little to do with true leprosy (Hansen's disease), but it corresponds with Isidore's own understanding of the disease's nature as defined in the *Etymologiae.*[36] Like Uzziah, the worst offenders were those who bore leprosy on their heads. This is the leprosy of those who sinned with regard to the divinity of the Father or that of Christ, who is his head. It was the leprosy of the Jews, the Arians, and the Manicheans, among others.[37] One could, of course, have several types of leprosy, as the Manicheans did, who were also afflicted with the leprosy of burning scars (*in cicatrice ustiones*).[38] Isidore's final use of leprosy regards the significance of Moses's hand, which God first made leprous and then cured (Exod. 4:6–7). This was one of the three signs with which Moses and Aaron were sent to the Jews to persuade them to depart from Egypt. For Isidore this episode stands for the current leprous nature of the Jews: they have been removed from the side of God, like Moses's leprous hand when he took it from his side, but one day they will be called back by God and will acknowledge Christ as their Savior, thus regaining their previous color.[39]

The ten plagues that God sent against the Egyptians, even more than leprosy, gave exegetes the opportunity to set up an equivalence of sin to disease and punishment. The nature of the groups identified might change, but the principle remained a constant.[40] There is no mention of contagion here, but it should be remembered that Isidore had declared *pestilentia* and *contagio* to be synonymous in the *Etymologiae.* That the meaning of one of these words could slip onto the other can be seen as far back as Leviticus 13:2–3, which in the Vulgate reads "plaga leprae" (plague of leprosy).[41] The slippage was aided by the explicit links of both plague and leprosy to sin.[42] How easy it was for Isidore to mix his use of the terms can be seen in his historical work, where the Arians, identified as lepers in his commentary on the Old Testament, are now described as both pestilence and contagion.[43] In all cases they and other heretics are referred to as dangerous and diseased. It is unclear, however, to what degree his choice of words reflects the possible transmissibility of their illness.[44]

Isidore wrote compilations of material collected from classical sources, and the brevity and exhaustive nature of these works is what earned him his lasting audience. This also may have been his contribution to the signification of contagion: he juxtaposed and collected its associations with illnesses and sin, transmitting them onward to his readers as largely interchangeable.

The Heresies of Iberia: Beato of Liebana and Elipando of Toledo

A little more than a century and a half after Isidore's death, and well over a half century after the Muslim invasion of Iberia, a Cantabrian monk by the name of Beato of Liebana (d. 798) wrote a long commentary on the Apocalypse of Saint John as well as a refutation of what he saw to be the heretical beliefs of the bishop of Toledo, Elipando (d. ca. 800).[45] Beato's works represent one of the first extensive bodies of writing set down in northern Iberia following the conquest. Writing in the mountainous north of the peninsula, Beato displays a surprising erudition, which suggests that he enjoyed access to a substantial number of books that must have reached him from the south, possessions of Christians who had fled north after the Muslim invasion.[46] Among these were the works of Isidore, which he acknowledges along with those of others in his introduction to *De Apocalipsis.*[47]

In recent scholarship, Beato's works have been discussed predominately in the context of the debate around adoptionism, the heresy Beato attributed to the bishop Elipando.[48] It is surprising that Beato never mentions the conquest or Islam, much less Muslim control over more than three-fourths of the peninsula at the time.[49] This absence is particularly intriguing when the nature of his two main works is considered: the first is the *Tractatus de Apocalipsis,* in which the plagues connected with the end of time are given due attention, and the second consists of a spirited criticism of a Christian heresy whose main proponent, Elipando, was living under Muslim rule. As a partial explanation, it may be argued that while Beato was not in a position to ignore the reality of Muslim rule, he may well have considered it of secondary in importance to the danger that Elipando presented to the Church from within.[50]

Beato seldom employs the image of contagion explicitly. In his commentary on Saint John, it is largely implicit within his discussion of the evils of Babylon and the many plagues sent down upon the sinning at the end of time. *De Apocalipsis* consists of two glosses, one less extensive than the other. In his initial comments on Revelation 16:21, Beato states that the plague of hail (*plaga gradinis*) represents the anger of God and that it is present in the Church of his time, for those who do not follow the laws of God are destroyed spiritually by hail. He returns to the dangers of heresy in his extended discussion of Revelation 9:17–19, describing the four horsemen of the Apocalypse. Here, he defines as follows the fire, smoke, and brimstone that, leaving the mouths of the horses, kill one-third of mankind:

> It is clear that these things do not leave its mouth, but that they are the words of those very men. Because of this he said fire, smoke, and brimstone. As he promises them in another text: those that worship the beast will be punished and for their torment he will raise up fires, smoke and brimstone for centuries upon centuries (Revelations 14, 9–10). *By these three was the third part of men killed, by the fire, and by the smoke, and by the brimstone, which issued out of their mouths.* By the words of their heads, that is to say, their princes, they rushed into these plagues for ever. *Because the power of the horses is in their mouths and in their tails,* that is, in the word, the act and in the office. We have already said that the tails were the prelates, that is, the bishops who are false prophets. *Their tails, like serpents, have heads.* We say regarding the heads that they are the princes of the world. *And with them they cause harm.* For without them the prelates couldn't cause harm within the Church.[51]

For Beato, the plagues said to have killed upward of one-third of mankind represent false belief, transmitted by the words of those who misuse their positions of authority. That the collusion of secular authorities ("princes") is said to be necessary for the bishops to cause harm is suggestive. Sánchez-Albornoz has argued that during Beato's time the Church in Christian Iberia was entirely dependent on the goodwill of the king. Conversely, for Beato, the fact that Elipando was writing from within Islamdom would have been at least suspect and possibly damning.[52]

Still, Beato admits that secular authorities might not recognize that they are misguided, even as they advance into sin. The ability to sin is itself a plague, sent down upon men: "To receive the power to sin and not to repent, is an incurable plague, and represents a great anger, especially against the saints. The cause of even greater anger of God is to help oneself, through an alleviation of sins, in order to please oneself for memory's sake. Each one believes that the holy thing he does is holy for him, saying in his heart, *What I do is just.* Many paths appear just for men, but in the end they lead to the depth of hell (Proverbs 14, 12)."[53] In passing,

Beato notes that the plagues God sent down on the Egyptians, similar to those of hail, sulfur, and fire mentioned in Revelation, are to be understood spiritually, though he does not assign the individual plagues specific meanings.

It is in his attack on Elipando that Beato is most creative in his use of imagery that evokes contagion. In his monograph on adoptionism, John Cavadini has convincingly argued that the debate between Beato and Elipando, which later expanded to include Alcuin (d. 804) and Felix of Urgel (d. 818), has been consistently misunderstood by scholars ever since Alcuin succeeded in portraying adoptionism as a regional heresy. Instead of seeing in it a replay of earlier Eastern Christological debates, Cavadini maintains that it should be considered a controversy with wholly Western Christian roots, in which both sides displayed creativity and originality.[54] For the purposes of this study, however, it is not the nature of the debate between Beato and Elipando that is of interest as much as the way in which they referred to each other and to heresy in general.

For Beato, heresy is that which is adulterated, the pure mixed with the false. Although there is no explicit reference to 1 Corinthians 5:6–8, the image of adulteration may remind the reader of it.[55] The word of God, Beato states, is like pure wine, but once water has been added to it in the form of the wisdom of heretics, the diluted wine is entirely infected.[56] The image of the first plague of Egypt, when part of the Nile was turned into blood, is an image of the spirit of error being mixed with Church doctrine. This is the spiritual danger of heresy. The blood is the dangerous and dark perversion of those philosophers—for heretics are necessarily philosophers—which will be corrected by the light of the cross of Christ.[57]

In the second book of the *Apologeticó,* entitled *De Christo et eius Corpore, quod est Ecclesia et de Diabolo et eius Corpore, quod est Antichristus* (*Of Christ and His Body, Which Is the Church, and of the Devil and His Body, Which Is the Antichrist*), Beato employs a series of images of the body in order to clarify the difference between correct and heretical belief. Taking up an image that goes back at least to Augustine, he describes Christ as the physician who in his blood and flesh provided us with the diet we need to preserve our health.[58] This description frames a clear dichotomy of the orthodox belonging to the spiritual body of Christ, while the heretics are the very body of the Devil.[59] The extent to which Beato took this analogy seriously is seen in his depiction of the heretics' devilish fertility, which is again linked to the corruptive power of language: "They [the heretics] are the testicles of the Antichrist, from whose semen perverse offspring are engendered that are united in the mouth of the Antichrist. Regarding the voice of the

Antichrist, it is said for Job: *The nerves of their testicles are entwined.* (Job 40:17). The Antichrist has as many testicles as he does preachers of his iniquity. Are they not his testicles, who with malicious persuasions corrupt men's hearts, pouring out the virulent seed (*semen*) of error?"[60] In his powerful representation of the words of heretics as the semen of the Devil, Beato was likely drawing upon Isidore, who in his gloss on Genesis 3:15 noted that "the seed of the Devil is perverse suggestion."[61] But the image of satanic offspring swirling in the mouth of the Antichrist is Beato's own, and the passage suggests that Beato saw the words of heretics as infectious seeds, planted in the hearts of those who listened to them. The allegory is continued in Beato's characterization of correct doctrine as a fetus, needing spiritual attention until it is fully formed: "As semen takes on form in the stomach bit by bit, and it is not considered murder until the confused elements have taken on their proper form and members, so also with the meaning of doctrine, conceived by reason. If it does not exit to the light through works, it will remain in the stomach. The aborted fetus perishes due to lack of nourishment, when it sees the abomination of the desolation setting itself up in the Church, and that Satan is transformed into the angel of light, that is, the heretic." The seeds of true faith, if preachers do not care for them, will die in childbirth due to the sermons of the heretics.[62] The figure of seeds, then, is not here linked inherently to sickness but to fertility and a reproductive process that, depending on the nature of the seeds, can lead either to the body of Christ or that of the Antichrist.

In his reaction to the attack leveled against him, Elipando used similar, though less imaginative, images. He denounced Beato's writings as spreading a fetid smell, the venom of which had polluted the hearts of those who had joined Beato's cause.[63] Beato himself was a new Arius, Elipando claimed in a letter to Alcuin, a reference to the father of Arianism, the Christian heresy that had held sway in Iberia until the end of the sixth century.[64]

The images of contagion employed by Beato are distinctly different from those of Isidore. Instead of being primarily a disease, contagion is here embodied, literally and figuratively, in the language of heretics and the pollution of the body of Christ. Beato's use of the analogy of the adulterated wine is reminiscent of commentaries on 1 Corinthians 5:6–8. But it is in the exploitation of *semen* to mean both seed and male semen that he departs most clearly from Isidore. Although the saint from Seville used *semen* in both ways in different works—one exegetical, one medical—Beato uses this image to a much greater extent. However, he never refers to "seeds of illness," using the word *semen* almost exclusively to refer to human, and not plant, reproduction.

An Interlude: Leprosy Turns Contagious, and the Reconquista Advances South

Between the ninth and the thirteenth century, the significance of both heresy and contagion itself changed significantly in Christian Iberia. François-Olivier Touati, in his exhaustive study of lepers and leprosariums in eleventh- to fourteenth-century France, has argued forcefully and convincingly against previous opinion that leprosy was not considered a contagious disease by either physicians or scholars until well after Gerard of Cremona's translation of Ibn Sīnā's *Canon* into Latin in 1187 in Toledo.[65] Indeed, in the authors examined thus far, while heretics were often referred to as lepers, and leprosy was equated with sin or disease, there was no explicit mention that leprosy was transmissible from one person to another.[66] In his *Qānūn,* the eleventh-century Persian physician and scholar Ibn Sīnā (d. 428/1037) explained how leprosy could be acquired through proximity to lepers and that it was in fact contagious (*fa-inna al-ᶜilla muᶜdiyya*).[67] Further, it could be inherited through the effect of the sperm (*al-nuṭfa*) in the womb under certain conditions: "If the blood clots (*al-ᶜulūq*) are the result of menstruation and if the heat of the air coincides with the food being vile—[including] fish, dried meat (*qadīd*), fatty meats, the flesh of the donkey and lentils—it is probable (*kāna bi-l-ḥarī*) that leprosy will occur."[68]

It was during the ninth to thirteenth centuries that the danger of heresy also shifted. Whereas for Isidore and Beato, the greatest danger faced by Christianity—heresy—was internal, for later Christian authors in the Iberian peninsula it was no longer possible, as it had been for Beato, to ignore the threat posed by Islam.[69] As Christian kingdoms emerged in northern Iberia in the eighth–ninth centuries and entered into an uneasy relationship with the Umayyad caliphate to their south, Muslims were initially depicted as pagans and the Prophet Muhammad as the Antichrist. After the First Crusade at the end of the eleventh century, however, this depiction began to change, and Muslims were increasingly seen to be Christian heretics, corrupted by the heresiarch Muhammad, who had in turn been led astray by a heretical monk.[70] Simultaneously, the balance of power on the peninsula began to change. The Umayyad caliphate collapsed at the beginning of the eleventh century, and despite the inclusion of al-Andalus within two Berber North African empires, after the defeat of the second of these, the Almohads, by a coalition of Christian kings in 1212, the Muslim presence in Iberia began to seem increasingly tentative. As Muslim political fortunes waned, an increasingly large number of Muslims came to live under Christian rule, especially in the kingdom of Valencia. It should not be surprising, then, that contagion and the tropes associated with it were employed in these later texts in a way that reflected the changing circumstances of Christian scholars and Latin scholarship.

The Alphonsine Corpus: The Arian Heresy of Islam

The Alphonsine corpus, written under the auspices of Alfonso X (d. 1284), is one of the earliest extant medieval bodies of vernacular literature. The number of works produced, their variety, and the influence of translated Arabic works on them have attracted considerable scholarly attention. The interest in Alfonso has been compounded by his ruling over a Christian Iberia where a definitive change in the political relations between Christians and Muslims had taken place. The balance of power had almost completely reversed itself since the time of Beato five centuries earlier. By the time Alfonso came to the throne, the only remaining Muslim state in Iberia was the Naṣrid kingdom of Granada, and it stood in tributary relation to Castile. Islam no longer posed a true military threat, and for the majority of his reign, Alfonso X was able to focus on consolidating the territories added to Castile by his father, Saint Ferdinand III (d. 1252). Although recent scholarship has begun to reevaluate Alfonso's political legacy in a much more favorable light than had earlier analyses, he remains best known for his cultural legacy.[71] A remarkable number of scientific, cultural, and literary texts were translated from Arabic and Hebrew into Castilian under his supervision, and an impressive array of legal and historical pieces were also brought out under his own name. His cultural enterprise served thus not only to transmit but also to create and to disseminate knowledge.

In the considerable writings attributed to Alfonso, contagion is seldom mentioned. Certain continuities with the writings of Isidore and Beato are apparent. Whereas Elipando had slandered Beato by comparing him with the heretical Arius, in Alfonso's *Estoria de España* it is Islam and Muslims in general who are associated with the Arians. A full consideration of the *Estoria de España* is beyond the scope of this study, but it is worth briefly considering the manner in which Islam is represented as a Christian heresy and Muhammad equated with Arius. After all, if heretics are the offspring of the Devil and contact with corrupted doctrine is broadly considered to be contagious, then characterizing Muslims as heretics has consequences for the interactions of Christians with Muslims. Alfonso's portrayal of Muhammad was typical of the Christian biographies of the period, combining elements taken from the early-thirteenth-century writings of Don Rodrigo Jimenez de la Rada and Lucas de Tuy.

Early in Alfonso's biography of Muhammad, the heresy of Arianism is mentioned three times.[72] The first is in the chapter preceding the one that contains Muhammad's genealogy. In the second, Arianism is placed alongside Judaism and Christianity in the *Estoria*'s depiction of the religions present in Arabia before Muhammad. In the third, Arabia is juxtaposed with a description of the evils of Arianism in Iberia at that time and how the Gothic king Leovegildo persecuted those who refused to convert to his heresy. A little further on, the historical narrative again tacks between an Arian Iberia and a Muslim Arabia, placing the eradication of Arianism in Iberia immediately before Muhammad's marriage to Cadiga (Khadija). Arianism's initial presence strongly suggests that Islam in the *Estoria* was considered a heresy and Muhammad first and foremost a heretic. The later disappearance of Arianism immediately before the rise of Muhammad to power suggests both a geographical and a narrative displacement of heresy.

David Hanlon, in his study of the *Estoria,* has concluded that Muhammad is identified with two heretical forms of Christianity, Simonism and Nicoltanism, with reference respectively to his aspirations to secular wealth and his sexual libertinism.[73] While not disputing the importance of these possibilities, I believe Arianism is at least as relevant if not more important. Like Islam, Arianism denies the divinity of Christ while continuing to hold him in high esteem. Marginalized within the Church by the end of the fourth century after the promulgation of the Nicene Creed, Arianism remained present in Iberia until a little before the arrival of Islam, which could therefore easily be seen as a heretical recurrence. If we understand the *Estoria* as employing Islam as a heresy, the two passages in which Muhammad is characterized as somewhat less wicked—the passage reporting his belief that it was Gabriel and not the Devil who came to him and the first-person account of his trip to heaven—also make more sense. These passages are read, then, not as sloppy editing on the compilers' part, one possible explanation, but as representations of a misguided and very human subject: one who believed that he received divine guidance but was actually afflicted with disease (epilepsy) and influenced by the Devil. This, and not simply condemnation, is the Islam that the *Estoria* offers its audience, a depiction that could have been targeted at both Christians and Mudejars.[74]

If, as Kenneth Wolf has suggested, early Christian historical responses to the presence of Islam in the Iberian peninsula de-emphasized religion and stressed the worldly success Muslim rulers brought Iberia, in the much later *Estoria,* religion provides the means to explain and delimit the meaning of the presence of Muslims within Iberia.[75] The two strategies reflect the shift in military primacy, for in part it was Christian predominance that allowed Islam to be recognized in history, albeit as a corrupted form of Christianity.

The Alphonsine Corpus: Contagious Leprosy or the Contagion of Leprosy?

In Alfonso's famous legal work *Las siete partidas,* compiled around 1265, in a discussion of the nature of treason, we find the following passage:[76]

> Treason is one of the greatest errors and grave injuries into which men can fall. The ancient scholars, who knew things well, held it to be so bad that they compared it with leprosy (*gafedad*): this because [it] like leprosy is an evil (*mal*), that affects the entire body, and after it has taken hold, it cannot be shaken loose, or weakened, so that the one who has it can recover. And so, what happens to a man, after he is leprous, [is that he] is separated and removed from all others. In the end, it is such a strong disease (*maletia*) that it doesn't just do harm to the one who has it, but also to those who are his direct descendants, and those who live with him. So in the same manner, treason affects the reputation (*fama*) of a man, harms it, corrupts it in such a fashion that it can never be put right, and leads to a great distance, an estrangement from those he knows. In truth, it disgraces and ruins the reputation of those who descend from this line—even though they have no fault in it—in such a fashion that all are disgraced because of this.[77]

While the Alphonsine text fails to mention that having sex with a menstruating woman can cause leprosy, it otherwise follows Ibn Sīnā in describing the disease as both contagious and inheritable.[78]

The metaphor of leprosy as treason has interesting implications. The text continues by defining treason as a tremendous sin, causing a man's heart to become so sick that he errs against God and the natural order. The punishment for treason is death, but as with leprosy, the effects of the sin carry over into the next generation, denying the traitor's male offspring any inheritance, the right to knighthood, or any other office or dignity.[79] There is no mention here of how the disease is transmitted, only that those who live with the one infected with it are prone to get it themselves. It can be assumed that it would be better to avoid those afflicted with the disease of treachery and not to speak with them.[80]

The subject of leprosy occurs again in the other Alphonsine history, *General estoria,* a history of the first six ages of man that contains many passages of scripture translated into Castilian.[81] In an annotated commentary on Leviticus 13:45—"And the leper in whom the plague is, his clothes shall be rent, and his head bare, and he shall put a covering upon his upper lip, and shall cry, Unclean, unclean"—the following reason is given for why the leper should cover his mouth and wear distinctive clothes: They cover their mouths with clothing "so that when they speak they do not cause harm to men, nor damage to those to whom they come with the fetidness of their bad breath. They should always say and show through these signs that they are sick."[82] Although not explicit, the passage strongly suggests that it is the breath of a leper that causes those who have contact with him to be harmed. The emphasis placed on the fetid quality of the air as the cause of sickness, a long-accepted explanation closely linked to the concept of miasma, is also found in the history's comments on the plagues of Egypt.[83] More extraordinary, however, is Alfonso's discussion of the anonymous accusation that Moses suffered from leprosy.

Alfonso's source for this accusation is the Jewish historian Josephus (d. ca. 100), who, in the third book of his *Antiquities,* summarily dismissed the suggestion that Moses had leprosy by asking why, if that had been the case, he should have made laws against it in Leviticus.[84] Alfonso, however, in his comments on Leviticus 13:45, spends more time on this charge, reflecting that the contagiousness of leprosy may well have caused the Egyptians to cast out the Jews, if they all had the disease. He begins by noting the magnitude of the affliction of leprosy: "From this the sick began to have signs indicating their sickness, to the point that they took up their wooden clappers (*tabliellas*), with which they now beg. Those [the lepers] they sent out of the whole town and the whole city, making them stay there separated, for there was no great difference between them and those nearly dead (*los muertos de lieue*). This was a grievous matter, a great shame for these men, a great dishonor and perfidy, for among both these and those there were many good men. . . . In addition it was a great loss."[85] The episode of Moses is then introduced:

> Now we will tell you here about some of the things Josephus tells, refuting Justin and Corneyo,[86] who wrote this story in Egyptian, and others [who wrote in] Arabic. We have here some events that we already told you in the story of the

> book of Exodus. There we did not tell them all, such as this one: they collected regarding the departure of Moses and the other Hebrews, wise men of the gentiles who dealt with similar events, in their histories in which they said that in the time of Moses it was perceived that many Hebrews were becoming lepers, Moses among them. Because leprosy is a sickness that is easily acquired (*malautia que se atrae mucho*), as we have said, we find in these histories that these wise men made, that the gentiles were on their guard (*que fueran en cueyta*) as they were afraid something bad would happen to them. They asked counsel from their idols, and they had the response that they should cast all of the sick out of their country and Moses with them.[87]

The story is of course denied by Alfonso. Alfonso cites Josephus's rejection of the slander and adds that it is hardly likely that God would have made Moses sick at all, much less afflicted him with leprosy.[88] Yet Alfonso's musing over the possibility that the Egyptians may have feared the contagiousness of leprosy is a striking addition to the debate. Josephus had seen in the accusation of leprosy an intimation of ritual impurity or dishonor, not a suggestion that Moses had been a health hazard.

In the Alphonsine corpus the significance of contagion had shifted yet again. It was now closely linked to leprosy and to the notion that disease could be transmitted from one person to another through the air. While the notion that corrupted air, miasma, was responsible for epidemic illness goes as far back as Galen, in the writings of Christian scholars, leprosy had only recently come to be seen as transmissible.[89] In a separate development, Alfonso associated Islam and Muslims with Arianism in his history of Iberia. We have seen in the works of earlier authors how heretics were commonly compared to lepers, an equivalence never made by Alfonso. Yet from the fifteenth century, looking back at the thirteenth, the pieces for rejecting Muslims (and Jews) as contagious were all present, if scattered and separate. All that remained was for them to be sewn together.

The Sermons of Saint Vincent Ferrer: Giving the Contagion of Jews and Muslims a Context

During the last decades of the fourteenth century and until his death in 1419, the Valencian Dominican Vicente Ferrer was the single most influential preacher in the Iberian Peninsula.[90] During the Great Schism, he was a vocal supporter of the Avignon papacy, advocating first Clement VII and then Pedro de Luna (d. 1423), who became Pope Benedict XIII at Avignon in 1394.[91] He traveled and preached in Italy and France, as well as in the closer Castile. In 1395, he was briefly investigated by the inquisitor Nicolau Eymerich (d. 1399) for heresy until Benedict XIII intervened in Ferrer's favor.[92] The extent of his reputation and influence can be measured by canonization proceedings introduced immediately following his death, resulting in his being declared a saint in 1455.[93] In recent scholarship, readings of Ferrer's sermons have generally focused on two areas: his millennialism and associated conviction that the Antichrist was born during his own lifetime, and his virulent attitude toward the Jews of Iberia.[94] The latter has been given special attention because it was Ferrer who persuaded Queen Catalina, mother of the infante Don Fernando, to decree the segregation of both Jews and Muslims.[95]

In the writings of Ferrer on contagion, as well as in other sermon collections from fifteenth-century Castile, the attitude toward Jews and Muslims plays an important role. In the following review of these texts, I attempt to describe the themes and images that enabled Ferrer's characterization of Jews and Muslims as contagious to make sense. Many of these have already been addressed in previous sections of this chapter: the equation of sin and disease, the association of leprosy with heresy, the contagiousness of leprosy and poor moral values, the juxtaposition of Muslims with heretics, and the importance of baptism as a sacramental purification. Ferrer drew on all these elements, adding to them and modifying them as he saw fit. It would be misguided, however, to attempt to force Ferrer's views on disease and healing, sin and salvation, into one reading. Part of the difficulty of ascertaining the exact relation of the various themes in his sermons lies in the nature of the material itself. While we are fortunate to have preserved for us a large number of Ferrer's sermons, most of them are based on the notes of people who listened to him.[96] That only a selection of his words has come down to us is also supported by reports that he spoke for several hours at a time, whereas the sermons we have are often only a handful of pages in length.[97] A more important reason for not trying to establish an ironclad series of equivalences between these themes is that Ferrer was not attempting to develop them systematically. These were not issues of doctrine or, as with his treatise on the papacy and his other writings, carefully crafted arguments. The sermons consist of individual occasions on which he spoke to different audiences in varied settings. It is only natural that he would have shifted emphases or used the same themes in different ways in order to make different points. It is precisely his variety of approach that suggests the merits of broadly classifying his themes in loose connection with one another instead of joining them into a linear development.

Although Ferrer was easily the most famous preacher of his generation, many other preachers were active at the same time. The number of Castilian sermons now edited and available for analysis has thankfully increased since Alan Deyermond sketched an overview of the state of the field in 1980. I have consulted two of the sermon collections published since then, both of them anonymous.[98] These sermons, as well as those of Ferrer himself, have come down to us almost exclusively in the vernacular, and insofar as they targeted a popular audience, they were certainly preached in the vernacular.[99] Offering more than an impression of the views of Ferrer and his fellow preachers, they hint at popular understandings of scripture, medicine, and religious minorities. We know, from Ferrer's ability to persuade Queen Catalina to issue her decree of segregation, that his words resonated with his audience and were acted upon. It is known that Ferrer directly influenced the segregation of Jews and Muslims in other individual cases as well.[100]

In order to contextualize Ferrer's employment of contagion, in the following sections I consider the concept in light of its relationship to other tropes that defined the significance of disease, and then I turn to how he used contagion to define the place of religious minorities within a Christian polity.

Christ as Doctor, Sin as Illness: Updating the Allegories

To fully understand the role played by contagion in Ferrer's sermons, one must first reflect on the relationship between Christ and disease. The characterization of Christ as *medicus,* the physician sent to cure humanity of its wounds and illnesses, reaches at least as far back as Augustine (d. 430), in whose writings it was developed at length.[101] Equating Christ with a doctor proved to be a rich metaphor, taken up by Augustine's opponents as well and adapted to their own purposes. Where Augustine saw in the comparison an indication of man's continual proclivity to sin, and thus the ongoing need for Christ's medicinal intervention, others saw Christ as having cured humanity once and for all.[102] Notable in Augustine's discussion is that Christ was not only a physician, *medicus,* but also medicine, *medicamentum,* and ultimately health itself.[103] As the Eucharist gained importance in the later Middle Ages, this line of thought aligned well with the perceived medicinal powers of the Host: the body of Christ as the ultimate medicine.[104] More immediately important for Augustine's discussion of sin was that "there was no reason for Christ to come, if it wasn't to save sinners; *take away the wound and the medicine has no purpose.*"[105]

Although the differentiation between God as surgeon and Christ as healer is not made by Ferrer or the Castilian preachers of his time, the trope of Christ as *medicus* is used often to discuss sin. Here, the emphasis is placed upon the importance of Christ's representatives, the preachers themselves.[106] Ferrer quotes Augustine on the nature of Christ as physician, come to cure our ills, and repeats this statement on his own authority.[107] These authors saw Christ's role as doctor prefigured in the Old Testament by Moses, among others.[108] The nature of the medicine brought by Christ is discussed by the preachers in two ways. The first consists of an explicit focus on the medicinal powers of the sacraments of baptism and the Eucharist; the second consists of explaining the spiritual significance of the medical terminology employed by Christ.[109]

Baptism was an especially important spiritual medicine in Ferrer's view. He repeatedly distinguishes between those who will go to heaven and those who will go to hell on the basis of whether they were baptized. Reflecting on John 4:53, in which Jesus healed a nobleman's son who was suffering from a fever, Ferrer states that the son signifies every Christian man and woman, born from the belly of the church and the font of baptism, into which the seed (*semen*) of God was given.[110] The fever, he explained, represents mortal sin, from which baptism saves the Christian.[111]

In the world to come, Jews, Muslims, impenitent Christians, and those who were not baptized will spend eternity in an infernal city.[112] Yet, baptism is not only the means by which former nonbelievers are brought into the body of Christ; the incorporation could also be accomplished in other ways, such as when Moses healed the lepers with blood and water in Leviticus 14:5–7.[113] This conflation of spiritual and physical illness is so common as to go uncommented upon, yet it brings lepers and religious minorities together in the same category of the sick who can be cured by the sacrament of baptism.[114]

When considering the exempla employed by Ferrer that deal explicitly with Jews and Muslims, it is worth remembering that these two groups, especially the Jews, were often forced to attend Ferrer's sermons, in the hope that they might be converted.[115] The following exemplum is a good illustration of this strategy. Ferrer relates a story in which a convert died before receiving baptism, only to be brought back from purgatory by Saint Martin. This account is then followed by the further episode:

> I'll tell you another, about a master of theology. Know that once there were two brothers. The one was worldly (*estave en lo món*) and had a slave with the

> name Muhammad. The other brother was religious and a master of theology. Know that the one brother sent the slave many times to the master of theology in another town with gifts. When Muhammad was there with the brother, the good master said to him: "Oh, Muhammad! Convert and become Christian!" The Muslim said: "I don't want to do it, I'll die Muslim." But one day or the other, know that God touched his heart. Thereafter, Muhammad fell gravely ill, and being in that state, he said to his master: "Christianity! Christianity! I want to go to your brother so that he baptizes me and I acquire the name Peter." "Go then, if you please." He mounted a horse and off he went. When he was riding, the horse threw him, Muhammad fell, broke his neck, and died. The soul went to the master of theology and appeared to him in the form of the slave Muhammad, so that the master, when he saw him, said to him: "Oh, welcome Muhammad." "No, don't say Muhammad," said the soul, "Rather, say: Peter, Peter." "How is that? Are you baptized?" The soul said: "No, but it was like this (*sic et sic*), and he told him everything that had happened, how it had been, and that he had the right to paradise with many angels. And this is why Jesus Christ said: "I will give unto him that is athirst the fountain of the water of life freely" (Revelation 21:6).[116]

The story should not be read as a deathbed conversion of dubious sincerity. That would, indeed, have delivered quite a different message to Ferrer's audience than he intended. Instead, God's touching of the Muslim's heart and infecting him with illness represents the means by which his soul was saved. Unlike other instances discussed earlier in this chapter, here God uses physical sickness to heal the spiritual body. Ferrer was deeply critical of those Christians who did not acknowledge the health of new converts—many of whom had entered Christianity en masse in 1391—and who did not treat them as full Christians. Insulting those Christians who had converted from Judaism, he argued, was equivalent to insulting the Virgin Mary and Mary Magdalene, both of whom had been Jews. Calling the newly converted "Oh, circumcised" was disrespectful to Christ himself, who also was circumcised.[117]

As with baptism, Christ heals Christians of their sins, especially original sin, through the Eucharist.[118] While the Host appears less frequently in the sermons than does baptism, Ferrer believed strongly in its curative properties.[119] Intriguingly, Ferrer does not seem to have believed in the doctrine of *fomes peccati*—which was not declared official by the Church for another century and a half—for he stated that those who believe baptism purifies one *only* of original sin were heretics.[120] Ferrer's reluctance to limit the effects of baptism may have been linked to the importance played by the sacrament in his conversion efforts. In 1391, when he decried the violent attacks against Jews in Valencia, he observed that the apostles had conquered the world, not with weapons, but with baptism.[121]

The sacraments of the Eucharist and baptism were only two, if the most effective, of the ways in which Christ exercised his role as doctor. In a sermon on Matthew 8:7 (*Ego veniam, et curabo eum*), Ferrer describes Jesus with detailed references to his methods as a physician: he looks at the patient in the face, ascertaining his sin; he feels his pulse, measuring his level of contrition; he studies the patient's urine in the act of confession; he advises abstention from sin in prescribing a diet; he gives him syrup (*eixarop*) mixed with warm water in the act of contrite prayer; he purges the patient of his evil humors by having him make restitution for his sins; and in his seventh act, he gives the patient the Host, the medicine.[122] One should not seek any coherence in Ferrer's equivalences. Confession can at one time be a reading of the urine, at another forcing the patient to vomit. As a preacher Ferrer sought to make the goal of spiritual health as vivid as possible, using what were, we can assume, methods commonly employed by a physician.[123]

Sickness as Both Punishment and Treatment

It is often stated, particularly in discussions of Europe after the Black Death, that illness was perceived as God's punishing man for his sins. One of Ferrer's anonymous contemporaries communicated a similar message when he retold a popular legend about how God sent a dragon against the sinning Romans. The dragon and its attendant snakes die in the Tiber, their bodies corrupting the air and causing a pestilence. It is only after Gregory leads a procession through the city, carrying an image of the Virgin Mary, that the air clears and the sickness ends.[124] Ferrer himself does not seem to have emphasized the role of disease as punishment; he was interested more in using disease to represent sin and its effects upon both individual and community.[125]

A contemporary of Ferrer's saw in plagues and illnesses not punishment but a divine temptation, a testing of man, and ultimately a device through which he can find spiritual health. In part such an understanding seems to have been based on a traditional distrust of the flesh, which exemplified the sinful nature of this world. By enduring sickness, one can achieve a greater reward in the world to come.[126] However, as depicted in Jesus's curing of the lepers, and as made clear in the spiritual medical counsel of Jesus, only those who show true contrition are worthy of his curing touch.[127]

Contagious Lepers, Dangerous Jews, and Muslims

Although Ferrer and others used leprosy as a figure for many sins, the disease was often most closely linked to sins spread through speech. One preacher glossed it as a disease of the mouth and noted that those who would not cease to speak ill of others resembled nothing as much as lepers, whose mouths also stank. The victims of leprosy were to be separated from the healthy, just as good people should keep their distance from those who speak ill of others. The case is similar to that of the sick pig that corrupts the healthy ones. For this reason, a speaker noted, Christ wanted us to have cleanliness in our mouths.[128] The focus on orality, on the potential for fetid words, like localized miasmas, to infect and corrupt, is striking. How easy, then, for the leper to represent the sinner who speaks falsely and whose internal corruption can potentially spread to others.[129] Jesus's healing of the lepers raises a problem, however: had the lepers themselves repented before he healed them? In a long passage from a sermon on Matthew 8:3 ("And Jesus put forth his hand, and touched him, saying, I will; be thou clean. And immediately his leprosy was cleansed"), a preacher suggests that lepers should not be healed if they are not repentant:

> Because of this, seeing how the words of our Lord Jesus Christ were holy, noble, full of virtue—as appears and is proven in this leper, whom, as the saints say, he healed physically and spiritually—it is a marvel that the Jews didn't understand that He was from heaven, not this world, and that He was the true God. . . .
>
> This leper, then, spiritually signifies the sinner, who through the pain and corruption of sin is corrupt and corrupts others. So you see the leper, who through the sickness is corrupted in himself and also corrupts others. Much the same does the sinner and because of this the lepers have to be distanced and thrown out of the company and the brotherhood of the good. We have this prefigured in the Old Law, *Leviticus,* chapter fourteen: "*Qui maculatus fuerit lepra erat separatus ad arbitrium saçerdotis, contaminatum ac sordidum se adclamabit. Omni tempore quo leprosus est et inmundus solus habitabit extra castra, ne sciliçet infiçidad alios*" ("everyone who is touched by leprosy will be separated from the others according to the judgment of the priest, and will call himself touched and wounded by this sickness for as long as he remains a leper, and will remain alone and separated, outside of the town so that he does not corrupt the others" [Lev. 13:44–46, Vulgate]). In the same manner the sick and mangy sheep corrupts the whole flock, and the sick putrid one corrupts the one who is healthy.

> This is according to what is written in the *Book of Kings,* in the fifth chapter: "*Lepra Naamán adherebit tibi*" ("the leprosy of Naamán has shifted itself to you"). God cures this leper many times, as one knows the sinner by the stains of his sins, from the tears of contrition and true remorse, as is written in *Leviticus,* fourteen: "*Lavabit leprosus vestimenta sua et mundus erit*" ("the leper will wash his clothes and he will be clean" [Lev. 13:6]). Because of this they say the first words with which I began with you: "*Extendens Jhesus manum suum,*" *et çetera.* The meaning is this: "Jesus reached out his hand and touched the leper, saying; "I want you to be healthy.' " In these words it is shown that it is very bad to heal the sinner of his sickness, and from the leprosy of sin. You should know that for the sinner to be cured of the sickness of sin, three things are needed, which are: a sign of capability, a work of piety and a word of truth.[130]

For much of this passage, the preacher seems to imply that being cured of leprosy is a good thing. That is, after all, what Jesus does in the cited passage of scripture. But in the closing section, he clarifies that healing a sinner is misguided if the sinner has not repented first. It is an awkward turn for the sermon to take, since we know nothing of the spiritual state of the leper in Matthew 8:3, beyond his belief in Jesus and his power.[131] The preacher seems to have been at pains to clarify that there is no quick way to salvation, despite Jesus's power to heal. It is instead incumbent upon the sinner first to repent and show proof of his repentance. Only then will Jesus heal him.[132] This reading is consistent with the spiritual explanations given of Jesus's work as a doctor, as shown above.

Ferrer's discussion of lepers follows much the same lines, with some notable exceptions. In a gloss on 1 Corinthians 5, he notes that if the disease is caught in its initial stages, doctors can still treat it. Once it spreads a little more, however, like the leaven mentioned by Paul, there is no remedy.[133] He also defines virtually all types of sin as spiritual leprosy, leading one to think that all of us, to some degree, could be considered to have leprous souls.[134] Yet, when considering the ways in which one can be cured of leprosy, after mentioning contrition and confession, he stresses the importance of separation, as in the case of Moses's sister Miriam. It is not enough to feel remorse. One must put the remorse into action. Particularly troublesome for him are those priests with mistresses, priests who, though contrite, stay with their women out of pity. He mocks their hypocritical attempts to follow the law: "Don't take this the way one presbyter in Castile did, where they left the common bed and arranged another bed, with nothing but a curtain between them. Ha! What separation! Roman leprosy (*Lebrós romanie*). So if you don't want to be a leper, separate yourself from bad company. [Consider] the [biblical] authority: '*Recedite, recedite* [*exite inde, pollutum nolite tangere, exite de medio ejus, mundamini, qui fertis vasa Domini*]' (*Isa., LII*° ca°). [Depart ye, depart ye, go ye out from thence, touch no unclean thing; go ye out of the midst of her; be ye clean, that bear the vessels of the Lord (Isa. 52:11).]"[135] Previous scholarship has noted how vehement Ferrer was on the subject of sexual relations, and Nirenberg has recently emphasized Ferrer's fear that sexual relations would occur between Christians and Jews or Muslims.[136] Ferrer's estimation of the danger of associating with women is seen especially clearly in his account of Saint Matthew's legendary trip to Ethiopia. After arriving in Ethiopia, performing miracles, healing lepers, and converting even the anachronistic Muslims to Christianity, Saint Matthew is faced with a dilemma when the recently converted king dies. The new king, a stranger and not yet a Christian, wishes to marry the former king's daughter. She had, however, already dedicated her life to Christ and so refuses the offer. Saint Matthew defends her choice and is subsequently killed for doing so. Ferrer remarks harshly: "You see why he was martyred: not for the Catholic faith, but for keeping the company of a lady."[137]

The sin with which Ferrer associates leprosy is rarely defined. The disease was a powerful image that illustrated both the spiritual corruption and the peril of associating with persons infected with sin, and one that offered many uses. At times Ferrer mixes his medical metaphors, as when he says that leprosy produces a tumor in the sinner's flesh, like the pride that inflates the soul.[138] It is difficult to hold the protean nature of his use of the trope against him, since the medical images are powerful and suggestive in their resonance and since the conception of the Church as the body of Christ reaches back to the time of Augustine. Nevertheless, his use of leprosy differed from that of his predecessors. Lepers were no longer only ritually impure, and as Ferrer explained, it was not only Christian sin that was contagious.

In his sermons in Castile in 1411–12, Ferrer presents his listeners with a vivid depiction of Islam within a genealogy of continual decline, expounding on the statue mentioned in Daniel 2:32–33 ("This image's head was of fine gold, his breast and his arms of silver, his belly and his thighs of brass, His legs of iron, his feet part of iron and part of clay").[139] Ferrer explained the passage's significance as follows: The golden age of early Christianity ended with the appearance of heresies, chief among them Arianism. Then the age of silver began. In order to treat the decadence and corruption that then set in, God sent the great doctors of the Church: Gregory, Augustine, Ambrose, and many others. This age lasted for more than five hundred years. Then, due to falsehoods, the Church "descended from the arms of silver to the stomach and thighs of copper." It was at that point that Muhammad appeared:

> In this time Muhammad came, he who infected (*enponçoño*) and corrupted all the earth of Barbary (*Verbería*). At that time they [the Christians?] didn't hear mass if they weren't forced to. They didn't pray and they denied God. The world was overcome by great evil and malice. Everyone consented to happily commit and perform vices and sins. They did not have justice, pity, or piety. They did not have faith and did not follow the commandments. Nor was there in them humility or any branch of good life.
>
> Because of this our Lord Jesus Christ wished to destroy the world. . . . Then the Virgin Mary achieved a brief extension, or a small petition regarding the end of the world, from her son Jesus Christ. That is, that he not destroy it until later, and that he wait for the preaching of the orders of Saint Francis and Saint Dominic. . . . It has now been more than fifty years since these two orders have failed to make inroads. Those who live in them don't abide by their institutions or rules. . . . Instead they are worse and more perverse than other Christians with regard to pride, luxury, avarice, gluttony, envy, fury, indifference, simony, vainglory, and all the other sins. . . . So the statue, which is the Church, descended from the thighs of copper to the shins of iron. This is the time in which we are now.[140]

Christ had almost destroyed the world when the infection of Islam first appeared, being prevented in this only by the intervention of the Virgin Mary. But it was not only the Muslims of the time of Muhammad who were corrupt. In terms similar to those used regarding lepers, Ferrer describes how only by cleaning himself or herself with prayers and tears that the Muslim, corrupt with sin, can become a Christian.[141] Yet there are many who do not wish to convert, just as there are many Muslims and Jews who sin in their pride and do not wish to do penance for their sins.[142] They may be proud now, and Ferrer acknowledges that the Muslims also have control over Jerusalem, but he assures us that after the Antichrist is defeated, they will go to hell and Jerusalem will return to the Christians.[143]

In his sermons Ferrer sometimes describes Muslims and Jews as corrupt and putrid and sometimes cajoles them to repent of their sins and join the body of Christ. With penance they can become free of contagion, but until then they are to be separated from Christians. The culmination of this logic is seen most clearly in Ferrer's comments on 1 Corinthians 5:

> It happened that Saint Paul, going through the world preaching, came to a city, Corinth, and converted it to the Christian faith. Among the things that he preached to them was that they put an end to their notorious sins, so that the city not be corrupted, and they not spread to other places. In a little time, due to a man who kept a whore in the city, from which the whole city was corrupted, it suffered great tribulations (*plagues*). They didn't know why. Among them was no one who had sinned in three years. They went to Saint Paul, who told them: "*Nescitis quia modicum fermentum totam massam corrumpit*" (*P*ª ad Cor., caº Vº). *Omnino auditur inter vos, dic totam causam.* Don't you know that a little leaven, if the dough is fermented (*posterada*), corrupts it all? Yes. So, throw the whore from that street, as it is because of her that so many tribulations have come upon you. Now you see that this sin angers God. *Ideo: "Expurgate vetus fermentum,"* etc. and you can say: "*In habitacione sancta coram ipso ministravi*" [Ecclesiasticus 24:14].
>
> The sixth virtue, which you have to tend, good people, is reasonable. Don't have Jews or Muslims among you, but [have them] in one part of the city, where they live according to your law. You Christians should not light a fire for them, as it has happened when a young Christian woman was raped by a Jew. If you display these virtues, you can say: "*In habitacione sancta coram ipso ministravi*" (In the holy dwelling place I ministered before him).[144]

In this passage, Jews and Muslims are grouped together with fornicators and sinners in general. The connection between the two cases is clear for Ferrer. The prostitute corrupts those around her with her sinning nature. Similarly, Jews and Muslims, by nature sinful, represent an imminent sexual menace to those Christians among whom they live. That which is sinful, corrupt, putrid, and infectious needs to be excised, cut off, or quarantined, so that it will not cause damage to those who are healthy.[145] Muslims and Jews are not dangerous solely due to the possibility of sexual aggression. Time and again Ferrer recounts how Jesus debates the Jews, who remain firm in the error of their ways because of the cardinal sin of pride.[146] Islam, for its part, is firmly set in a genealogy of heresy, following after Arianism. Like the Jews, Muslims are corrupt and corrupting by their very nature. The solution, for Ferrer, beyond the segregation he argued for and in many cases achieved, was the act of preaching itself. Despite his bitter attack on his own order, he sees in Saint Dominic a model for himself and others. Preaching on Matthew 5:13 (*Vos estis sal terre*), Ferrer identifies the salt with Dominic himself. As salt protects meat from corruption, so does the preaching of the saint protect the world from spiritual infection.[147] I do not think it goes too far to suggest that Ferrer saw himself following in Saint Dominic's footsteps, that he was himself purifying the Iberian Peninsula of the corruption of sin and quarantining the contagion of Judaism and Islam.

Conclusion: Revisiting the Metaphoric Richness of Contagion

> I find more delight in considering the saints when I regard them as the teeth of the Church. They bite off men from their heresies and carry them over to the body of the Church, when their hardness of heart has been softened as if by being bitten off and chewed. With very great delight I look upon them also as shorn sheep. . . . But it is hard to explain why I experience more pleasure in this reflection than if no such comparison were derived . . . , even though the matter and the knowledge are the same. . . . However, no one is uncertain now that everything is learned more willingly through figures.
>
> Saint Augustine, *De doctrina Christiana*

This chapter has traced the changing significances of contagion in Christian religious literature in the Iberian Peninsula. Beginning with the writings of Isidore in the seventh century, I showed how the concept of contagion was linked to both the plague and leprosy and how it was often used metaphorically to describe the heresy of Arianism. In the writings of the late-eighth-century monk Beato, contagion was increasingly employed to designate heresy, adoptionism in this case, and to represent a threat to the health of the Christian community. After the medical writings of the Muslim scholar Avicenna were translated in the twelfth century, leprosy began to be understood as contagious, and this shift was reflected in the thirteenth-century corpus of writings from the court of Alfonso X. Here, Muslims are depicted as heretics and explicitly compared with Arians, emphasizing the internal danger posed to Christianity by Islam. Finally, in the fifteenth-century sermons of Saint Vincent Ferrer, the explicit threat posed by the contagion of Muslims and Jews living under Christian rule is explored at length, as is the necessity of either excising or converting them. Whereas in the hadith commentaries discussed in chapter 1, Muslim scholars debated whether and how contagion existed, the Christian authors here examined struggled with how to best apply the metaphor of contagion in other contexts. They had no doubt that contagion existed, although they did not always agree on how and in what circumstances it occurred. What was important for them was not the place of contagion in a disease's etiology, but rather who was described as contagious and why.

If it were only a matter of Muslims or Jews being a minority under Christian control, both would have been considered contagious long before the fifteenth century. The designation of leprosy as contagious in the Latin translation of Avicenna's *Canon* at the end of the twelfth century played a role in how disease was used to describe both sin and heresy. Earlier it was mainly animals that were mentioned in religious writings as being contagious. It was particularly the supposed hereditary nature of leprosy and the belief that it was transmitted sexually that made it such a powerful metaphor with which to designate groups of heretics or Jews and Muslims. Heresy, of course, had been considered contagious several centuries before Beato sexualized it, declaring heretics to be the testicles of the Antichrist. But the force of an association corresponds to the explicitness with which it is proposed, and it was not until the sermons of the fifteenth century that Muslims and Jews living under Christian rule became truly contagious. I am not arguing that it was because of their perceived contagiousness that Jews and Muslims were segregated from Christians in fifteenth-century Castile and Aragon. Instead, by tracing the way in which the word and the concept were used in Christian Iberian texts of the Middle Ages, I have attempted to show that contagion played a role in the justification of this segregation. In part because contagion was not situated within a legal and theological context for Christian writers, it developed in a very different way than it did for Muslim scholars. In these texts it is even less defined and plays a more malleable role, adapting to the rhetorical and ideological needs of the authors who employ it. By examining the use to which contagion was put in the exegetical literature and within the texts here studied, I have shown the parameters within which it was used and the origin of the parameters themselves. Regardless of whether we agree with the social and cultural meanings assigned to disease—and here I think back to Sontag's impassioned if futile plea to strip disease of metaphoric significance—it is only by carefully following the rhetorical uses to which disease and disease transmission have been put that we can begin to comprehend the result of their encounter with society.

Contagion Contested

Greek Medical Thought, Prophetic Medicine, and the First Plague Treatises

As for what concerns children, al-Ṭabarī has said that if one suspends a fragment of elephant tusk around the throat of a child, it will be protected against the children's plague (*wabā' al-aṭfāl*).

al-Shaqūrī, eighth/fourteenth century

"Master, shall I mention the advice that al-Tabari gives on this topic, namely putting an elephant's tooth on children as a way of keeping the plague at bay?"

"Don't bother with that. Note down instead that 'prayer is the preferred weapon of the believer.' But God Almighty has said: *Say, O people, act in accordance with your station. I am acting, and you will know. . . .*

"There are specialists in law and hadith who claim that the plague is caused by a pinprick from the jinn and who deny the possibility of contagion as being contrary to observation, feel, experience, and research. Concerning such people I am reminded of an apt comment that Ibn al-Khatib made on several occasions: 'Ignoring the things that science tells us is an act of malice, a taunt against God Himself, and an insult to the hearts of all Muslims.'

"Just a minute more before we finish. It's not correct to attribute all the earthly causes of the plague to foul, humid air alone. Another factor involves symptoms of senility in a political regime, circumstances that are often characterized by unjust taxation and levies that oppress farmers and result in reduced activity and then total collapse. That in turn leads to food shortages, inflation and rebellion, followed by famines and plagues. Politicians bear a large responsibility for this chain of events. That's why human beings should, to the extent that they can, take all possible precautions."

Ibn Khaldūn in Bensalem Himmich's *The Polymath*

THE BLACK DEATH arrived on the Iberian peninsula near Almería in June of 1348 (Rabīᶜ I of 749), from where it spread throughout the Naṣrid kingdom of Granada, reaching Granada itself in the winter of 749–50/1348–49 and

Málaga in March of 750/1349.[1] While it is difficult to know how many people were killed by the epidemic—and its demographic impact may well have varied considerably regionally—what evidence we do have suggests that it was a devastating natural disaster, which lasted through the fall of 750/1349. Lirola Delgado, Garijo Galán, and Lirola Delgado have shown that more than half the number of scholars living in Almería during this period—twelve of twenty-one—died during the Black Death, though they rightly caution against deducing from this that the city in general suffered a mortality of 50 percent.[2] Similarly cautious, Calero Secall has suggested that at the height of the epidemic, more than three thousand people may have died in a single month in Málaga, close to one-fifth of the estimated population.[3] Regardless of the exact number who died, the plague was a catastrophic disaster for the Naṣrid kingdom and posed numerous challenges to its inhabitants. Among these were whether to attempt to flee the plague or not, how to care for those who had fallen sick with the disease, and whether the plague should be considered contagious. Numerous prominent Andalusī scholars rose to the occasion and wrote plague treatises in response to these questions, most notably among them Ibn al-Khaṭīb (d. 776/1374) and Ibn Khātima (d. 770/1369).[4] In doing so, they drew upon an understanding of the plague that was shaped by several discourses or fields of knowledge: Islamic medicine, Prophetic medicine, and Islamic law, the last of which included evaluating Prophetic traditions that related to the plague and contagion.

Although these plague treatises were important in their own time and, as we will see in chapter 5, were discussed and debated in the Islamic West for at least one hundred years after their authors died, their overall significance for later scholars pales in comparison with a work written in Egypt in the early ninth/fifteenth century by the famed scholar Ibn Ḥajar al-ʻAsqalānī (d. 852/1448), whose views on contagion we considered in chapter 1. Michael Dols, in his classic *The Black Death in the Middle East,* emphasized the importance of the work of Ibn Ḥajar, and rightly so, but also emphasized the exceptional nature of the Andalusi plague treatises, especially that of Ibn al-Khaṭīb. In this chapter I argue that the impression given by Dols's work and taken up by many scholars since, that Ibn Ḥajar championed Prophetic Tradition and Ibn al-Khaṭīb championed rationality—the works of the two appearing to enact a struggle between revelation and reason—is inaccurate and is rooted in projecting a laboratory understanding of plague onto the work of these premodern scholars. I will show that instead, although Muslim authors of plague treatises in the first hundred years after the Black Death held distinct views regarding whether the plague was contagious and interpreted empirical evidence in different ways, they are productively understood as engaging the same authoritative medical and scriptural sources. Their differences are the result of the richness of debate on the issue of contagion, rather than the product of a confrontation between conservative scripturalism and rational empiricism.

In chapter 1, we looked in detail at the Prophetic traditions pertaining to contagion in the early canonical collections of hadith and the commentaries that were written on these in the succeeding centuries. Both these collections and the commentaries were valuable sources for the authors of the plague treatises, but those authors also drew upon their knowledge of Islamic medicine. Before turning to the plague treatises themselves, then, we should consider how contagion had been discussed by the doctors of various religious backgrounds who lived in the Muslim world and wrote in Arabic.

Contagion in the Islamic Medical Tradition

The medical practices of Islamdom in the premodern period had their roots in the largely Galenic medicine practiced by Nestorian doctors living under Zoroastrian Sassanian rule in Iran (third–seventh centuries) and in Baghdad of the third/ninth century, to which some of these doctors moved to serve at the caliphal court.[5] This was an era in Baghdad when the ᶜAbbasid caliphs, well aware of the scientifically unsophisticated nature of their own Arab bedouin background, supported an immense translation project in order to acquire the scientific wisdom of the Hellenistic culture, which had flourished under both the Sassanian and the Byzantine empires.[6] We find, then, that during the third/ninth and fourth/tenth centuries, a preponderance of doctors who contributed to Islamic medicine were of either Nestorian or Ṣābi'ī origin.[7] This appropriation of Greek science by Christian and Muslim intellectuals, subsidized by the patronage of Muslim elites, occurred during the same era that produced the canonical collections of Prophetic Tradition. Since a not-insignificant number of these traditions related to medicine and sickness, it is not surprising that in the centuries following this period these two sources of medical authority at times stood in some tension to each other. This tension was addressed, though not necessarily resolved, in the eighth/fourteenth century with the full articulation of a Prophetic medicine.[8] The plague treatises discussed in this chapter are, to some extent, the result of this tension, for in them hadith and prayers can be found almost side by side with recipes for medicines and discussions of the effects of climate on the human body. Yet it would be a mistake to see the tradition of Greek medicine as foreign to Islam and Prophetic medicine as representative of the "authentic" practice of Islam; Muslims were active in the writing and practicing of both kinds of medicine.[9]

Physicians who worked and lived in the Muslim world—both Muslim and Christian—described a category of contagious diseases from at least the third/ninth century onward. Chief among these was leprosy, although others, such as scabies, smallpox, and the plague, are also mentioned. There was, however, no clear distinction between contagion and infection, and as with Isidore of Seville and those doctors in Christian Iberia who wrote plague treatises in the fourteenth century, it is not always clear what a given author meant when using the word *contagion* or referring to the concept of contagion.[10] In most cases contagion seems to refer to a disease's ability to be transmitted from one carrier to another, but how this takes place is often vague, and the concept is certainly compatible with disease etiologies based on the principle of miasma (the corruption of air) and even the agency of jinn.

Ibn Sahl b. Rabbān al-Ṭabarī (d. after 240/855), a Christian doctor and philosopher who lived in Baghdad and was a contemporary of Ibn Qutayba (whose views on contagion are discussed in chapter 1) makes several interesting observations regarding contagion in his *Garden of Wisdom concerning Medicine* (*Firdaws al-Ḥikma fī l-Ṭibb*).[11] While he does not explicitly claim that plagues are contagious—attributing their occurrence to the corruption of the air—he is clear regarding the contagious nature of leprosy: "Leprosy comes from a corrupt, black bitterness through which all the humors are corrupted and the corruption reaches the lung, the blood clots (*yajmud*), the hairs of the eyebrow fall out, the voice fails, the fingernails shrink (*tashannaj*), the tip of the nose falls off as well as the tips of the fingers. And perhaps this enters (*jarā*) into the sperm (*al-nuṭfa*), as because of this the child is not free of leprosy. It is one of the sicknesses that are contagious when one is close to them, like scabies (*al-ḥikka*), and smallpox (*al-judarī*). . . . Leprosy is usually found in cold countries with corrupt air, [stemming] from the eating of cheeses, milk products, the meat of cows, mountain goats (*tuyūs jabaliyya*), and fatty foods. It is a sickness that can almost not be cured."[12] This passage shows clearly the degree to which disease etiology before the advent of the laboratory was defined by numerous factors beyond transmission or contagion, including most notably the corruption of one's humoral balance through both climate and diet.

The extent to which contagion was far from a precisely defined concept but more of a signifier that could be applied to various phenomena is amply attested to in a treatise by Qusṭā ibn Lūqā (215/830–297/910 or 308/920), a Christian doctor who lived in Baghdad and later died in Armenia. Ibn Lūqā stands out among the doctors of Islamdom by having devoted an entire work to the phenomenon of contagion, his *Book on Contagion* (*Kitāb fī l-Iᶜdā'*).[13] At the beginning of his treatise, Ibn Lūqā offers his readers a precise definition of contagion or infection: "Infection is a spark (*qadḥ*) that jumps (*yanqadiḥu*) from a sick body to a healthy body, so there appears in the healthy body sickness (*min al-maraḍ*) similar to what appears in the sick body, and this is the definition of infection (*ḥadd al-iᶜdā'*)." After giving this precise definition, however, Ibn Lūqā notes that the subject of contagion is a controversial one and that opinions on the subject range from rejecting its existence to holding that sickness can be transmitted by a person who possesses great power of imagination (*wahm*).[14] Ibn Lūqā expresses astonishment over the views of the latter group and explains why it makes little sense to believe that the imagination can actually effect physical changes. Nonetheless, in the case of psychological states, contagion certainly does occur, he argues, citing the examples of sadness, yawning, and lust. Regarding lust, Ibn Lūqā notes that not only reading descriptions of sex can cause arousal, but also many people like to watch others have sex because it arouses them: "If there was not that which is disgusting in the narrations (*aḥādīth*) that are related of this type, then I would mention extraordinary and strange stories that I have heard from trustworthy people of our time."[15] Including the effects of pornography in a discussion of contagion reflects a somewhat broader understanding of the term than it was usually given in the premodern period.

When considering contagion in relation to sickness, Ibn Lūqā follows a Galenic understanding of "localized miasma" as the source of most contagious diseases: air corrupted by earthly (i.e., foul vapors from swamps or fires) or heavenly causes (the changing temperatures of the seasons, *not* astral origins) is inhaled through the lungs, nostrils, and pores of the skin, resulting in the corruption of the internal organs and the spirit. Once one has been infected by such vapors, one's body produces similar vapors that can infect those with whom one interacts.[16] The most exemplary of such diseases in Ibn Lūqā's opinion is leprosy, and he notes that it is because of the danger of interacting with those so afflicted that leper colonies have been created outside of cities such as Jerusalem and Damascus.[17] But Ibn Lūqā states that there are also other diseases that Galen has declared to be contagious, including hectic fever (*al-diqqa*) and scabies.[18] In seeming disagreement with Galen, Ibn Lūqā argues that ophthalmia (*al-ramad*) is not caused by a corruption of the air but occurs when the gaze of a healthy person meets that of a sick person. Here he seems to be drawing on a doctrine of rays as developed by his contemporary al-Kindī (d. ca. 256/870), the philosopher who argued that bodies transmit rays exhibiting the same characteristics as the bodies themselves.[19] It is striking that Ibn Lūqā fails to mention contagion in relation to epidemic diseases, much less the plague, because these were considered contagious by the majority of doctors following him. Yet he did comment on how diseases caused by the corruption of the air can have differing effects on those who are exposed to them, depending on the strength of a person's vital spirit (*al-rūḥ al-ḥayawāniyya*).[20] This is an important observation, for, as will be seen in the plague treatise of Ibn Ḥajar, one of the strongest criticisms that can be leveled against the miasma theory of disease is that if it were true, everyone exposed to corrupted air should die in an epidemic.

Two of Ibn Lūqā's near contemporaries, Muḥammad b. Zakariyyā al-Rāzī (d. 311/923) and Thābit b. Qurra (d. 288/901), went further than Ibn Lūqā by adding epidemic diseases to the list of contagious diseases given by Galen and by associating them closely with heritable diseases. In the first chapter of his *Book of Treasure in the Science of Medicine* (*Kitāb al-Dhakhīra fī ʿIlm al-Ṭibb*), Thābit b. Qurra states that the ancients declared seven diseases to be contagious: "leprosy, scabies, small pox, measles, ozaena (*bakhar*), ophthalmia and the epidemic diseases" and seven to be hereditary "leprosy, vitiligo, consumption (*diqq*), phthisis, melancholy, gout and epilepsy."[21] Al-Rāzī preserves this pairing in his influential *The Encompassing (treatise) on Medicine* (*Al-Ḥāwī fī l-Ṭibb*), citing Galen on the contagious nature of epidemic disease, mange, ophthalmia, ulcers of the lung, scabies, tuberculosis, epilepsy, and, surprisingly, baldness.[22] Drawing on al-Ṭabarī, he states that leprosy, tuberculosis, epilepsy, and hemorrhoids (*al-bawāsīr*) are inherited diseases, and, following al-Ḥarrānī and Ibn Lūqā, he includes leprosy among the contagious diseases.[23] As noted, al-Rāzī cites Galen's view that ophthalmia is contagious but seems to privilege Ibn Lūqā's view that it is transmitted by rays of vision themselves, stating that that to which a gaze is not turned is unaffected by this disease.[24]

It is clear from this brief survey of third/ninth- to fourth/tenth-century authors of the Islamic world that the transmission of diseases between humans was widely acknowledged by scholars of medicine and that they were comfortable referring to this process as contagion. It is also apparent that the process by which this transmission was thought to occur, when addressed at all, involved a localized miasma, or corruption of the air. With minor variations, including more detailed discussions of the effects of corrupted air on the body's humoral balance, this understanding of contagion continued in the Middle East (as in Europe) until the nineteenth century.[25] Considering the debates discussed in this chapter over whether, specifically, the plague (*ṭāʿūn*) should be considered contagious, it is important to note that none of these early sources ever single out the plague as contagious, although they do refer to it as the product of a corruption of the air.[26] While doctors of this period may not have seen a need to specify what they took for granted, this omission may have made it easier for later scholars, when faced with conflicting religious and medical sources, to claim that the plague is an exception among epidemic diseases and is not in fact contagious.

The Joining of Islamic Medicine with Prophetic Tradition

Prophetic medicine is often described as having its roots in the canonical collections of the Prophetic traditions and pre-Islamic local customs, but it did not come into its own until the eighth/fourteenth century, when three scholars living in Damascus, all students of the great Ḥanbalī scholar Ibn Taymiyya (d. 728/1328), presented their readers with a fully articulated and novel medical approach.[27] These scholars—Shams al-Dīn al-Dhahabī (d. 748/1348), Ibn Qayyim al-Jawziyya (d. 751/1350), and Ibn Mufliḥ al-Maqdisī (d. 763/1362)—while at times critical of Greco-Islamic medicine—also adopted its basic theoretical premises, including the existence of four humors (yellow bile, blood, phlegm, and black bile), which stand in relation to the four elements (fire, air, water, and earth) and, in times of health, rest in a harmonious relationship to each other. Life depends upon an individual's innate heat (*ḥarāra gharīzīya*), which is maintained by three types of spirits (*arwāḥ*)—natural, animal, and psychic—that nourish corresponding faculties (*quwāt*).[28] Each individual's temperament (*mizāj*) is determined by the relationship of the elements within him, and these vary according to a person's "age, sex, habits, profession, and the climate of his native area."[29] Disease results when the harmonious relation of an individual's humors is disturbed, but because each person's temperament is different, physicians had to consider that the harmonious relationship of the humors is different in each patient.

Irmeli Perho's detailed discussion of Prophetic medicine effectively refutes many of the previous characterizations of the genre. If one relies on common descriptions of Prophetic medicine in the secondary literature, one expects the treatment of both the plague and contagion in Prophetic medicine to be entirely based on Prophetic traditions and folk remedies.[30] Indeed, the oft-cited denouncement by Ibn Khaldūn (d. 808/1406) of Prophetic Tradition as a source of medical knowledge seems to have been uncritically accepted by scholars as a comprehensive and sufficient critique of the genre.[31] It is precisely because Prophetic medicine as found in the work of the three Damascene authors of the fourteenth century is not simply a compilation of hadith that Ibn Khaldūn's remarks fail to apply fully to it.

Perho argues convincingly that Prophetic medicine, especially as found in the work of Ibn Qayyim al-Jawziyya, is an attempt of traditionists who disagreed with Ashᶜarī theology and its denial of causality to explain the medical relevance of the Prophet's traditions to a broad audience.[32] Because these authors followed their teacher Ibn Taymiyya in his refutation of Ashᶜarism and its stance on causality, they had little trouble accepting that diseases can be transmitted, although they were confronted by the Prophet's apparent denial of contagion.[33] Of central importance to this discussion, instead, is the doctrine of relying upon God (*tawakkul*), which attracted especial attention in Sufi circles and had to be placed in correct relation to medicine and the phenomenon of contagion. Perho suggests that in fact the genre of Prophetic medicine, which had its beginnings in the third/ninth century, was a response of the scholars who felt that an excessive interpretation of *tawakkul* had failed to take the Prophet's own attitude toward medicine into account.[34] These early works, little more than lists of what the Prophet had said on matters relating to medicine, were taken up in the seventh/thirteenth century by scholars with medical knowledge, such as ᶜAbd al-Laṭīf al-Baghdādī (d. 629/1231) and al-Kaḥḥāl ibn Ṭarkhān (d. 720/1320), who provided the earlier collections with a Greco-Islamic frame.[35] The full theological implications of this reconciliation of two rather different traditions were then explored in the eighth/fourteenth century, when Prophetic medicine was fully articulated in the work of al-Dhahabī, Ibn Qayyim, and Ibn Mufliḥ.[36]

These three authors wrote in the years immediately preceding the Black Death and presented in their work a cogent case for the transmission of disease between humans in the case of the plague. Yet, unlike the Andalusī authors Ibn al-Khaṭīb and Ibn Khātima, they have tellingly not been described as exceptional voices of rationalism in a world dominated by orthodoxy. This discrepancy can likely be attributed to their working within a framework that largely accepted Prophetic Tradition, instead of rejecting its validity when confronted with contradictory empirical evidence. In the following pages I will examine the treatment of contagion in the treatises of Ibn Qayyim al-Jawziya and al-Dhahabī, both of whom enjoyed continued popularity, which continues today.

Ibn Qayyim's work on Prophetic medicine forms a section of his longer work *Zād al-Maᶜād fī Hady Khayr al-ᶜIbād* (*The Provisions of the World to Come on the Guidance of the Best of Men*).[37] The author deals with contagion in chapters 5 ("Treatment of Plague [*ṭāᶜūn*] and Precautions against It") and 27 ("On the Progression of Illness and Contagious Disease").[38] Ibn Qayyim begins his chapter on the plague with a series of Prophetic traditions, including one that describes the plague as a martyrdom for every Muslim who dies from it, but he then continues by discussing how doctors have described the plague and its symptoms. He acknowledges the veracity of the observations made by the doctors but goes on to argue that because they have not taken the Prophet's comments on the matter into full account, they have missed the heart of the matter. The plague is, as the Prophet stated, a martyrdom for Muslims, yet Ibn Qayyim does not say it is the result of the actions of jinn. His explanation of the disease's etiology is worth quoting at length:

> The physicians have nothing whereby to repel these illnesses and their causes, any more than they have anything to explain them.
>
> The prophets give information about hidden matters. On the other hand the physicians have no reason to deny that these symptoms which they understand about the plague should be caused through the mediation of spirits (*arwāḥ*). For the influence of spirits upon the body's constitution, its illnesses, and its eventual destruction, is only denied by people who are quite ignorant of spirits and their influences and the reaction they produce in bodies and constitutions. God, praised be He, can give to these spirits power over the bodies of the sons of Adam, during the occurrence of an epidemic (*al-wabā'*) and through corruption of the air. In the same way, He gives them power to act in the predominance of unhealthy substances, which produce an evil condition for souls, especially in the disturbance of blood, black bile, or semen.
>
> Now the satanic spirits have a power working upon the person who is affected by these conditions in a way which they cannot regarding others. Their power continues as long as they are not repelled by some defence stronger than their causes, such as *dhikr* (remembrance of God) and prayer, supplication and entreaty, almsgiving and recitation of the Qur'ān. . . .
>
> In short, corruption of the air is one part of the overall effective causes of plague, and corruption of the essence of the air is the prerequisite to the occurrence of pestilence. Its pollution comes about because its essence changes into an unhealthy state; one of the negative qualities predominates over it, such as putrefaction, decay or poison. It is true at any season of the year, although it occurs mostly in the latter part of the summer and most frequently in the autumn. The reason is that the sharp, bilious superfluities and others collect during the summer season, and they are not dissolved at the end of summer. In autumn,

> the miasma occurs because the air is cold, and the vapours and superfluities which were wont to dissolve freely during the summer now become thick and murky. Thus they are constricted, become heated, and putrefy, bringing about the putrid diseases. This is especially so when the body which they encounter is susceptible to them by being flaccid, sedentary and replete; such bodies can hardly hope to escape unharmed.[39]

While Ibn Qayyim argues for the ultimate authority of Prophetic Tradition, he places it within the humoral framework of Galenic medicine. It is precisely because the etiology of the plague is unclear (and contemporary remedies against it ineffective) that Ibn Qayyim is able to propose a composite causality for the epidemic that is rooted in an acceptance of secondary causation: God grants spirits the ability to influence one's humoral composition, and it is only through invoking God's protection that one can save oneself from the plague. Strikingly, Ibn Qayyim does not seem to be arguing for the agency of external spirits (i.e., jinn) that pierce their victims, but rather for an imbalance of spirits within each human.[40] This stance is quite different from that later taken by Ibn Ḥajar in the ninth/fifteenth century.

Simultaneously, Ibn Qayyim emphasizes that the corruption of the air is a necessary precondition for the occurrence of the plague, thus clearly rejecting the standard Ashᶜarī understanding of occasionalism. Such a reading is borne out by his brief comments on contagion, made within the framework of the famous Prophetic tradition of not entering or leaving a plague-afflicted area.[41] Regarding the latter, Ibn Qayyim insists that one should not leave such an area, because one should trust in God, but also because the doctors have argued that in a time of plague the body is weakened by unnecessary movement and becomes more susceptible to the disease. With regard to entering a plague-afflicted area, the order of Ibn Qayyim's authorities is reversed, and he begins with a series of medical considerations: remaining outside such a place helps one avoid harmful causes, seek out good health, avoid harmful airs, and most strikingly, avoid coming into contact with the sick, who might transmit their sickness.[42] Only after listing these factors does the author state, relying on Prophetic tradition, that a belief in either augury or contagion can harm the soul. This chapter ends with the listing of several traditions on the caliph ᶜUmar's turning back from the plague at Sargh.

In chapter 27 of his work, Ibn Qayyim takes up the subject of contagion again, beginning with the Prophetic traditions on leprosy.[43] He presents the Greco-Islamic view that leprosy is both contagious and inherited as consistent with those

Prophetic traditions that caution against proximity to lepers. Contagion can be understood as a combination of predisposition, the weakening of the body through the power of fear on one's imagination (a concept reminiscent of Ibn Lūqā's discussion of mental contagion), and the influence of the breath of those already sick. Ibn Qayyim is adamant that those traditions from the Prophet that would seem to contradict the transmission of leprosy—including the Prophet's denial of contagion—are, in fact, not contradictory. To support this assertion, he casts doubt on the soundness of the traditions that deny contagion, cites Ibn Qutayba as an authority, and in the end settles on differentiating between contagion in the case of leprosy and in the case on the plague. Whereas the first case definitely involves the transmission of disease, the second case is more complicated. His discussion here is similar to those found in the hadith commentaries discussed in chapter 1, with Ibn Qayyim presenting the views of many different groups. Ibn Qayyim expresses, as an exegetical principle, a preference for the view that the Prophet addressed different statements on a given subject to different audiences, depending on their dispositions and capabilities: "If the person is strong in his faith and his trust in God, then the strength of his trust would repel the power of contagion, just as the strength of the constitution repels the power of the illness and makes it of no avail. Another person has no such strength, so he counseled him to be careful to take precautions. The Prophet himself practised both options: so that the Community might draw an example from both. . . . They are both valid paths—one for the firm believer, the other for the one whose faith is weak."[44] Following this passage, Ibn Qayyim presents several opinions—all similar to those discussed in chapter 1—and ends the chapter emphasizing the weakness of those traditions that would undermine a belief in contagion. His final comment refers the reader to a longer discussion of the same subject in another work of his, the *Kitāb al-Miftāḥ*. In this book, the *Key to the House of Happiness* (*Miftāḥ Dār al-Saᶜāda*), Ibn Qayyim clearly states that contagion was created by God as a cause (among several) of illness and that denying its existence entails a denial of God's law.[45]

This discussion strongly suggests that Ibn Qayyim supported both the existence of contagion and its place as a cause within a larger web of secondary causes that were created by God with causal power and attributes.[46] When Muslims who are strong in their faith ignore the fact that diseases are contagious, it constitutes not a denial of the existence of contagion but a belief that trusting in God and praying to him itself functions as a cause to protect them from disease. The role played by psychology in disease prevention is paramount for Ibn Qayyim: fear of contagion weakens one's constitution and should be replaced with fear of God.[47]

This harmonization of Prophetic with Greco-Islamic medicine is also found in Shams al-Dīn al-Dhahabī's *Al-Ṭibb al-Nabawī*.[48] Like Ibn Qayyim's book on Prophetic medicine, this work reveals considerable knowledge of the Greco-Islamic tradition, and authorities such as Ibn Sīnā are referred to favorably on issues such as plague typology.[49] Al-Dhahabī deals with contagion and the plague in two separate sections, the first entitled "Visits of the Sick to the Healthy" and the second "The Plague." In the first he relates a Prophetic tradition that the sick should not visit the healthy but specifies that this tradition refers to a person who has sick cattle, not a person who is sick himself.[50] He follows the example of the authors of the hadith commentaries examined in chapter 1 and explains that the Prophet said this in order to prevent anyone from believing in contagion. This statement is followed by the Prophet's repudiation of contagion. While al-Dhahabī seems to expand his own rejection of contagion to disease transmission in general, he first denies but then later affirms Ibn Qutayba's explanation that leprosy is transmitted by the smell of the leper. Regarding the etiology of the plague, al-Dhahabī, like Ibn Qayyim, lists the Prophetic traditions that assert that death by the plague is martyrdom for believers, that it is a remnant of a punishment sent down upon the Jews, and that prohibit approaching or fleeing it. However, al-Dhahabī surpasses Ibn Qayyim in his emphasis on the importance of the corruption of the air in causing the plague. The role of jinn is nowhere mentioned. Instead, the danger of proximity to the plague is repeatedly stated, with the explanation that plague is the result of "spontaneous putrefaction," which brings about the corruption of the body's humors.[51]

Based on the preceding reading of both Ibn Qayyim and al-Dhahabī, I argue that any simplistic distinction between Greek and Prophetic medicine—at least in the case of contagion and the plague—is false and misleading. Instead, Prophetic medicine as represented in these two works is best understood as a critical evaluation of Greek medical traditions alongside relevant Prophetic traditions and, in effect, a new medical tradition. While Prophetic Tradition is nominally preferred over its Galenic counterpart, many of the latter's presuppositions are accepted and at times privileged. This is clearly seen in the case of contagion, both al-Dhahabī and Ibn Qayyim accepting the phenomenon of disease transmission.[52] This evaluation is striking when one compares these writings with the treatise of Ibn Ḥajar al-ʿAsqalānī (see the section "Ibn Ḥajar al-ʿAsqalānī's Intervention"). Unlike Ibn Qayyim and al-Dhahabī, Ibn Ḥajar explicitly rejects the authority of the medical profession on the issue of the plague.[53] As has been shown here, this was certainly not the case for the authors of books on Prophetic medicine. The prevailing binary in much of the scholarship on Islamic medicine—elite and rational Greek medicine versus irrational, religiously narrow-minded, and popular Prophetic medicine—is insufficient to explain the variety of approaches in these texts. Instead, in the works of, for example, al-Ṭabarī, Ibn Qayyim al-Jawziyya and Ibn Ḥajar, we find at least three broadly different approaches to how to reconcile two medical traditions.[54] This variety of possible approaches to both contagion and plague can be followed into plague treatises written in al-Andalus following the Black Death of the eighth/fourteenth century.

Andalusi Plague Treatises of the Eighth/Fourteenth Century

In the historiography on the plague, Andalusī plague treatises written in the eighth/fourteenth century—specifically those of Ibn al-Khaṭīb and Ibn Khātima—have been consistently praised as scientific, rational, and (therefore) exceptions to the generally oppressive religious orthodoxy of the late medieval period.[55] Time after time, Ibn al-Khaṭīb, in particular, has been declared a shining example of what some authors have called a fourteenth-century rationality. Implicit—and at times explicit—in these narratives of exceptionality is that the majority of plague treatises are characterized by a slavish devotion to religious orthodoxy—that is, Ashᶜarī occasionalism. As evidence for this assertion, the example of contagion is often advanced with Ibn al-Khaṭīb's passionate support of the concept in the face of the majority of scholars' rejection of it. The overarching effect of this narrative has been to support the widely held thesis that the postformative period of Islamic civilization was characterized by intellectual rigidity, an aversion to rational inquiry, and an unchanging legal tradition.[56] That such an argument has serious weaknesses is already apparent from the preceding discussion of Prophetic medicine. Without wishing to detract from the intellectual achievements of Ibn al-Khaṭīb and his contemporaries, I argue that these plague treatises have been misread to support a larger historical narrative; as a corrective, I propose to present them in light of previous discussions of plague and contagion in both medical and religious/legal sources.[57]

Ibn al-Khaṭīb was the most prominent historian in al-Andalus of his time, and his biographical history of prominent inhabitants of, and visitors to, Granada, *Al-Iḥāṭa fī Akhbār Gharnāṭa,* is one of the most important sources for the history of al-Andalus during the Naṣrid period.[58] To his contemporaries, Ibn al-Khaṭīb was best known as Granada's most powerful political figure; he served as wazir first under Yusūf I (d. 755/1354) and then twice under Muḥammad V (d. 793/1391), both before and after the latter's exile in Morocco from 1359 to 1362.[59] Known for his learning as well as his political acumen, Ibn al-Khaṭīb ultimately fell victim to court intrigue and, after accusations of heresy were leveled against him, was summarily murdered in Fez in 776/1374.[60] The Granadan wazir was a prolific author, his works ranging far beyond history to include poetry, mysticism, geography, and medicine. In the wake of the Black Death of 750/1349, Ibn al-Khaṭīb wrote a treatise entitled *That Which Satisfies the Questioner regarding the Appalling Illness* (*Muqniᶜat al-Sā'il ᶜan al-Maraḍ al-Hā'il*), which dealt chiefly with the medical aspects of the plague. Included in its strong defense of the need to flee the plague, however, is an unabashed attack on legal scholars who deny the principle of contagion. For Ibn al-Khaṭīb, any Prophetic traditions and prior legal arguments that deny contagion must yield before the empirical evidence that supports the contagious nature of the plague. To think otherwise would be to expose the Muslim community to needless danger, which goes against the underlying principles of the *sharīᶜa*. Toward the end of Ibn al-Khaṭīb's plague treatise, we read:

> One principle that cannot be ignored is that if the senses and observation (*al-mushāhada*) oppose a revealed indication (*al-dalīl al-samᶜī*), the latter needs to be interpreted, and the correct course in this case is to interpret it according to what a group of those who affirm contagion say (*bi-mā dhahaba ilayhi ṭā'ifatun mimman athbata al-qawl bi-l-ᶜadwā*). In the Law (*al-sharᶜ*) there are many texts that support this (*mu'nisāt ᶜadīda*), such as his saying, may God pray for him and grant him peace: "The sick should not be watered with the healthy," and the saying of the Companion: "I flee from the will of God to His will." This is not the place for prolixity on this subject (*fī dhālik al-gharaḍ*).
>
> The discussion, based on the Law (*sharᶜan*), regarding the existence or non-existence of contagion, is not among the duties of medicine (*hādhā al-fann*), but instead it arises only parenthetically and by way of examples (*innamā jarā majrā al-jumal al-muᶜtariḍa wa-l-muthul*), and this is analyzed in its place.
>
> To sum up (*wa-bi-l-jumla*), to play deaf to such an inference is malicious (*zaᶜārah*), perverting blasphemy against God, and holding the lives of Muslims to be cheap. A group of pious people in the Maghrib have renounced [their previous view] to the people, bearing witness against themselves that they no longer give fatwas to this effect [i.e., not believing in contagion], in order to avoid being in the position of declaring it permissible for people to engage in suicidal behaviour (*mustaqillīn mushhidīn ᶜalā anfusihim bi-l-rujūᶜ ᶜan al-fatāwā*

> *bi-dhālik taḥarrujan min taswīgh al-ilqā' bi-l-yad ilā-l-tahluka*) [Q2:195]. God protect us from nonsense (*al-khaṭal*) and grant us success in both speech and action (*waffaqana fī-l-qawl wa-l-ᶜamal*).[61]

Despite Ibn al-Khaṭīb's claim that his plague treatise is not the place to expand on legal rationales for permitting Muslims to flee from the plague, he presents his reader with a dual-faceted legal argument in favor of the efficacy of contagion. The first aspect can be found in his selective citation of Prophetic Tradition: he chooses to mention two traditions that, when combined, strongly suggest the validity of contagion and the acceptance of this fact by the Prophet's Companions. The second aspect of his compressed argument can be found in his blanket refutation of legal arguments and Prophetic traditions that are detrimental to the Muslim community. In taking this step, he chooses to present his reader with a rationale implicitly based on the welfare of the Muslim community (*maṣlaḥa*). In doing so, he draws on a legal principle that, though controversial, had gained prominence by the fifth/eleventh century.[62] It is worth remembering that it was in Ibn al-Khaṭīb's lifetime that the doctrine of *maṣlaḥa* was given its most comprehensive reformulation since al-Ghazālī (d. 505/1111) as *maqāṣid al-sharīᶜa* by al-Shāṭibī (d. 790/1388).[63] Generally defined as the preservation of religion, life, mind, wealth, and progeny, the *maqāṣid* of the law provides jurists with a method to privilege general objectives over specific injunctions. In this respect, they overlap in scope with the principle of communal good (*maṣlaḥa*). At issue here is the degree of importance given to *maṣlaḥa* as a legal principle. While al-Ghazālī acknowledged *maṣlaḥa,* he treated it as a type of *qiyās* (reasoning by analogy), refusing to see in it an independent source of legal reasoning.[64] Al-Shāṭibī's innovation lay in being able to separate *maṣlaḥa* from the classical theory of law, which had four sources (Qur'an, Sunna, Ijmāᶜ, and Qiyās), and relate it directly to Qur'an and Sunna.[65] Yet while al-Shāṭibī's discussion of *maṣlaḥa* had ramifications for later generations, Ibn al-Khaṭīb, who never mentions *maṣlaḥa* explicitly, makes no reference to his contemporary.

Of central importance to Ibn al-Khaṭīb is the question of the appropriate ethical behavior in a time of plague. In this, he took up the same task as his teacher Ibn Lubb (d. 782/1381), whose views are discussed in detail in chapter 5. That Ibn al-Khaṭīb and Ibn Lubb came to diametrically opposite conclusions was largely the result of their differing attitudes toward the value of empirical evidence. Accepting the occasionalism promoted by Ashᶜarī theology, Ibn Lubb saw no reason to believe in contagion, and indeed he believed that supporting such a belief would lead to abandoning the sick and dying.[66] More confident about the connections between the events he had observed, Ibn al-Khaṭīb saw no benefit to staying in a plague-struck area. He went so far as to equate a decision to do so with stretching one's hands toward self-destruction (an implicit reference to Q2:195).[67] He bitterly attacked those legal scholars who advocated placing oneself in danger, noting that some of them had in fact recanted their former views. For Ibn al-Khaṭīb, the only proper response to the plague is to advise all Muslims to avoid people who have been infected and to flee from an area in which the plague is found.

Although he was probably not a practicing physician, Ibn al-Khaṭīb had received medical training, and besides his treatise on the plague, he wrote other works on medicine, displaying his knowledge of the Greco-Islamic tradition.[68] He shared this medical background with his friend and contemporary Ibn Khātima, who wrote a justly celebrated treatise on the plague entitled *The Attainment of the Goal of the Seeker for Information concerning the Epidemic* (*Taḥṣīl Gharaḍ al-Qāṣid fī Tafṣīl al-Maraḍ al-Wāfid*).[69] Previous scholarship has at times represented Ibn Khātima's treatise on the plague as markedly different from Ibn al-Khaṭīb's on the subject of contagion, claiming that the former accepted and the latter rejected religious orthodoxy. It has even been suggested that Ibn al-Khaṭīb may have written his treatise in response to that of Ibn Khātima.[70] While Ibn Khātima engaged with the Prophetic traditions at much greater length than Ibn al-Khaṭīb did, and evaluated them differently, there is little doubt that he believed in the transmissibility of the plague. He may have denied the existence of "contagion" per se, but he did so in a manner similar to that of the previously examined authors on Prophetic medicine: he denied the existence of contagion as it was understood during the Jāhiliyya, but he affirmed disease transmission. This can be seen in the following passage:

> What is clear and cannot be concealed is that this disease's evil spreads and its damage transmits itself (*yataᶜaddā ḍarruhu*). Custom has borne witness to this and experience has confirmed it (*aḥkamat-hu al-tajriba*). A healthy person does not touch a sick person and draw out the interaction with him in this affair without its damage most always (*ᶜādatan ghāliban*) penetrating to him and afflicting him with a disease like the sick person's. The disease is caused by God, the most high (*ajrāhā Allāh taᶜālā*) and this act first and foremost attests to the truth of His splendor, [He], the creator of everything. He denied the generation (*tawlīd*) [of the disease] claimed by some of the people of error, and rejected the contagion in which the Arabs of the Jāhiliyya believed. . . .

As the damage occurs according to the meeting of their breaths, so it occurs from the vapors rising from their bodies, though these are less than the others in effect (*wa-in kānat dūna tilka fī-l-ta'thīr*). In this manner [damage] also [occurs] from their clothes and their linens (*furūshihim*), in which they tossed and turned due to their sickness, when these are used as undergarments (*idhā istuᶜmila dhālik ᶜan shiᶜārin*), lying close to the body when they were exposed for a length of time to their breathing. To all of this knowledge (*ᶜilm*) and experience bears witness.

I have witnessed most of the people of the old-clothes market (*ahl sūq al-khalaq*) in Almeria die, those who used to traffic (*yabtāᶜūna*) there in the clothes of the dead and their furnishings. Until now, none of them remained well, and only a few of those who followed after them [have remained healthy]. The state of merchants (*min arbāb aswāq*) other than them is like that of the rest of the people.

I have been informed of the state of countries whose people were careful not to let anyone enter upon them from the areas struck by the plague. In this manner, they remained healthy (*istaṣḥabū al-salāma*) for a time until they were overcome. The majority of the people of the fortresses that are close to Almeria, when this incident occurred, date the time of its occurrence among them from the arrival of someone from the countries of the epidemic and his death in their midst. They remember this and preserve stories of their experiences during it, which have been widely related (*tawātarat bi-intishārihā*), so there is no point in denying them.

And the most wondrous of what contemplation and reflection made clear through repeated experience (*ᶜalā ṭūl al-tajriba*) is that he who associates with one who is sick through the occurrence of this incident is afflicted by the same disease and the same symptoms appear in him. So if the first sick person spits blood, the second spits blood, or if the first suffers from diphtheria (*dhibḥa*), the second comes to suffer from the same, or buboes appear on the first in the groin or armpits (*maghābin*) of his body [and] exactly the same appear on the second in that same place. Or a sore appears on the first's body [and] the second becomes sick from a similar sore, and in the same fashion with those with whom the second associates. Even so in the case of a family, one disease spreads among them, its symptoms being similar. If the sickness was deadly [*mahlikan*] [for one], they follow him in death or if his case regains health, so in their cases as well.[71]

As in the writing of Ibn al-Khaṭīb, and in greater detail, Ibn Khātima's treatise emphasizes empirical observation as proof for the transmission of disease. Emphasizing God as the origin of all acts, his description of the spread of the plague strongly implies an acceptance of secondary causation and contagion. Unlike Ibn al-Khaṭīb, however, who summarily dismissed Prophetic traditions that did not fit with his understanding of the plague's etiology, Ibn Khātima devoted chapters 7 through 10 of his treatise to a detailed examination of relevant Prophetic traditions.[72]

In these chapters Ibn Khātima takes up the discussion of contagion as it was found in the hadith commentaries. Central to his discussion, as in the commentaries examined in chapter 1, is how to harmonize apparently contradictory Prophetic traditions. Unlike the authors of the works on Prophetic medicine examined before, he explicitly accepts the tenet that God is the only creator and that the causes he has created do not have natures of their own.[73] For Ibn Khātima, there exists no contradiction between the traditions on contagion, and he takes the view that the most convincing interpretation of the "No contagion" tradition is that it is simply a denial of pre-Islamic bedouin beliefs.[74] Despite these comments, Ibn Khātima makes a case for secondary causation, arguing that the caliph ᶜUmar had turned back at Sargh because "he sought the causes that are the antecedents (*sawābiq*) of the decree (*al-qadar*) and the secrets of the decree (*al-qaḍā'*), just as we have been ordered to take refuge from the enemy in fortifications, and to avoid places of fear and danger (*al-makhāwif wa-l-mahālik*) and everything by which the decree (*al-qadar*) is preceded."[75]

Like al-Yūsī (d. 1102/1691) much later, Ibn Khātima comes to an acceptance of the transmission of disease within the framework of Ashᶜarism. While professing a belief in occasionalism, he simultaneously attacks the validity of the arguments of those who did not experience the very epidemic he himself had lived through.[76] Such a person "assumes (*yaẓunn*), but assuming is the least credible form of reasoning, and for those who know (*arbāb al-ᶜuqūl*), there is no contradiction between what is rational (*al-maᶜqūl*) and what is revealed and transmitted (*al-manqūl*)."[77] Concluding his commentary on the tradition against watering healthy with sick animals, Ibn Khātima cites a tradition carrying similar import: "Hobble the camel and trust in God." He continues: "This is the secret of serving God (*sirr al-ᶜubūdiyya*)."[78]

Ibn Khātima was able to walk a fine line, stating his adherence to Ashᶜarism and acknowledging the transmission of the plague from one person to another. He avoided claiming that God created sickness in each and every case, instead alluding to a web of causes that God had created and which exercised influences of their own that, in the case of the plague, one can perceive empirically. He was careful not to get too involved in explaining exactly how secondary causation takes place, and he denied that secondary causes had independent natures while at the same time emphasizing the extent to which one could depend on their regular behavior. Although he was certainly not as abrupt as Ibn al-Khaṭīb, like him, he based his acceptance of disease transmission on empirical evidence. It is true that, unlike his contemporary, but like the authors who wrote on Prophetic medicine, Ibn Khātima was concerned to show in detail how Prophetic tradition and medicine were compatible. I argue that it is not therefore what Ibn al-Khaṭīb said regarding contagion or the value of empirical evidence that has made him such an object of acclamation in both Arab and European scholarship, but the vehemence of his rhetorical attack on Prophetic Tradition. It is precisely because the figure of Ibn al-Khaṭīb has served a larger historiographical argument that equates a rejection of religious authority with scientific advance that he has been held up as a paradigm of rational thought. In order to make this argument, however, Ibn al-Khaṭīb's own brief but vital engagement with Prophetic tradition has been ignored, as has his larger intellectual and social context.[79]

A few words should be addressed to the third of the Andalusī plague treatises. In the eighth/fourteenth century, Ibn al-Khaṭīb and Ibn Khātima were joined in al-Andalus as writers of plague treatises by al-Shaqūrī (d. 749/1348), the only one of the three who may himself have perished in the Black Death, and that at the young age of twenty-one.[80] We possess only an abridgment of his longer treatise, in which he comments on the etiology of the plague. Al-Shaqūrī spends some time defending the discipline of medicine, using arguments similar to those found in works of Prophetic medicine, and like the authors of these works, he implies the existence of secondary causation.[81] The cause of the plague, for al-Shaqūrī, is the corruption of the air. The subject of contagion is not addressed in this treatise.[82]

Ibn Ḥajar al-ᶜAsqalanī's Intervention: The Blessings of the Plague and the Unreliability of Empirical Evidence

In both the Mashriqī works on Prophetic medicine and the Andalusī plague treatises of the eighth/fourteenth century, the existence of disease transmission in the case of the plague was accepted, and the potential conflict between empirical observation and Prophetic tradition was resolved. Nonetheless, as Michael Dols has shown, plague treatises written in the Muslim East following the Black Death by scholars such as Ibn al-Wardī (d. 749/1349) and al-Manbijī (d. 785/1383) denied that the plague could be transmitted, drawing on arguments similar to those discussed in chapter 1.[83] However, not all treatises written in the East were inimical to the transmissibility of the plague, for as Dols observed in passing, Ibn Abī Ḥajalah (d. 776/1375), who himself died of the plague in Cairo, believed that proximity to persons afflicted with plague was to be avoided, just as one would avoid lepers, because the air around them had been corrupted.[84]

This balance of supporters and deniers of the transmissible nature of plague changed in the following century in the Muslim West, with the majority of plague treatises denying contagion in the case of the plague until the nineteenth century.[85] While the exact extent to which the plague treatise *An Offering of Kindness on the Virtue of the Plague* (*Badhl al-Māᶜūn fī Faḍl al-Ṭāᶜūn*) of Ibn Ḥajar al-ᶜAsqalānī was responsible for this shift is difficult to assess, it can be assumed that it played a significant role.[86] The author was a prominent and highly respected scholar whose command of hadith won him great acclaim. The influence of his views on later authors can be seen in the numerous favorable references to the *Badhl al-Māᶜūn* and his commentary on Bukhārī, *Al-Fatḥ al-Bārī,* in the plague treatises written in the Maghrib from the seventeenth to the nineteenth centuries.[87]

The later influence of Ibn Ḥajar's plague treatise was arguably due to its structure and comprehensiveness. Few of his opinions are novel: (1) dying of the plague is martyrdom for believers, (2) the plague is caused by jinn, and (3) there is no contagion of any kind. All of these statements had been made many times before. What distinguishes Ibn Ḥajar's arguments from those of previous authors is the sophistication of his discussion of Prophetic traditions and his adamant rejection of the claims of doctors to control the interpretation of empirical evidence.

Like Ibn al-Khaṭīb and Ibn Khātima, whose empirical observations on the plague have often been linked to their personal experience of it, Ibn Ḥajar lived through repeated incidences of the plague. Three of his daughters died in outbreaks of the plague, two in 819/1416 and the third, while pregnant, in 833/1429. Aḥmad ᶜAṣṣām, the editor of the *Badhl al-Mā'ūn,* suggests that Ibn Ḥajar composed his work on the plague between these two dates.[88]

At the beginning of *Badhl al-Mā'ūn,* Ibn Ḥajar describes the content of the book's five chapters: (1) a general introduction to the subject of the plague, (2) a discussion and definition of the plague, (3) how dying of the plague constitutes martyrdom for Muslims, (4) comments about any land in which the plague occurs, and (5) what is to be done following the outbreak of the plague. The book also includes an appendix that summarizes the plagues that have broken out in Islam. At the very end of his book, Ibn Ḥajar provides his readers with a full quotation of the treatise of Ibn al-Wardī (d. 749/1349) on the plague, a work of which he highly approves, doubtless in part because the author agrees with most of his own positions.[89] References to contagion and the etiology of the plague, found throughout the treatise, can be summarized as follows: the plague is different from other epidemic diseases in that it is not caused by the corruption of the air or by astronomical events but by the piercing of jinn.[90] Since this piercing occurs internally, Ibn Ḥajar notes that the opinion of the doctors that the plague is caused by a poisonous substance or boiling of the blood hardly contradicts the agency of jinn, for these symptoms could simply be the effects of the internal piercing.[91] While knowledge of the role of jinn could only have been received from God, Ibn Ḥajar argues, it is borne out by the fact that if the plague were really caused by the corruption of the air, it would affect the entire body and not just certain parts.[92] He presents the following empirical evidence to support his argument: "If it [the plague] were from the air, then it would comprehensively include people and animals (*la-ᶜamma al-nās wa al-ḥayawānāt*). We find that the plague strikes many people and animals, while next to them are those of their kind, whose temperament (*mizāj*) is similar who are not struck. It has been witnessed that it takes all the people of a house in a country, and does not enter a house of their neighbors at all, or that it enters a house and doesn't strike but some of them. It has also been witnessed to perhaps be less when the air is corrupt than when it is well balanced. And while the corruption of the air requires a change of the humors (*akhlāṭ*) and a multitude of sicknesses and illnesses, this kills without sickness or with only a mild sickness."[93] In short, Ibn Ḥajar argues that there is no conclusive or even convincing evidence to support the Galenic thesis that miasma causes the plague. On the contrary, he claims that the plague could not have a natural origin like other diseases, for if it had, it would have a cure and the doctors would not have been thwarted in their efforts.[94] To support his position, he cites the sound tradition on how God did not send down a disease without also sending down a remedy. If doctors are unable to find a cure for it, that suggests that the plague is produced by nonnatural causes. Ibn Ḥajar offers what he describes as a credible anecdote related to him by the sharīf Shihāb al-Dīn ibn ᶜAdnān (d. 833/1429),[95] the sultan's private secretary, to fully explain how jinn would carry out such a piercing: "At one time the plague broke out and I went to visit a sick person. I heard someone saying to another: 'Pierce Him.' And the other said: No. And the first repeated [the order]. The second said: Leave him alone because he benefits people. The first said: It is necessary. The second said: In the eye of his horse. He said: And during all of this I turned and couldn't see anyone. I visited the sick person and returned and I saw a horse that had escaped from its riders and they were following it to bring it back. And its eye had disappeared without a trace of a visible blow. He said: Thus, I confirmed the truth of what was related regarding the plague being from the pricking of jinn."[96]

While this anecdote may appear incredible, in Ibn Ḥajar's text it supports his assertion that the cause of the plague lies outside the realm of knowledge of doctors and medicine. Ibn Ḥajar finds support for such a conclusion in the Prophet's statement that death by the plague was a martyrdom for his community.[97] A great deal of the *Badhl al-Māʼūn* is devoted to explaining the precise implications of this last statement, especially the exact requirements to be fulfilled to guarantee the status of martyr.[98] In this context, it is not surprising that Ibn Ḥajar would reject the existence of contagion completely,[99] although it is striking that he would criticize earlier legal authorities of the stature of al-Shāfiᶜī (d. 204/820)—reputed founder of the eponymous law school—for having given credence to doctors' statements that leprosy is often transmitted between spouses: the founder of the Shāfiᶜī school had erred in giving more credence to those who rely on experience (*ahl al-tajriba*) than to the Prophet's denial of contagion.[100] The majority of Ibn Ḥajar's arguments against contagion are based on close readings of Prophetic tradition and are similar to the discussion found in his *Fatḥ al-Bārī* (discussed in chapter 1).[101] It is in his comments on the authority of the medical profession that he breaks new ground. After complaining that the doctors of his age have been delinquent in avoiding bloodletting as a treatment of plague victims, he cites the view of the famous scholar Tāj al-Dīn al-Subkī (d. 771/1370) that if two knowledgeable, just, Muslim doctors declare that interacting with a plague victim is a cause of harm, it is permissible to avoid those afflicted with the plague.[102] Ibn Ḥajar has little patience for such a statement: "The testimony of one who bears witness to this is not acceptable because the senses (*al-ḥiss*) give the lie to it. These plagues have repeatedly occurred in the houses of Egypt and Syria, and it has rarely happened that a dwelling was emptied due to them. There are those struck by the plague who were surrounded by their family and close ones—whose interactions with the sick are closer by far than those of strangers—and the majority of these stayed healthy from it. So that anyone who bears witness that a reason for harm is interaction [with the sick], he is obstinate in his error (*mukābir*)."[103] Continuing his refutation of al-Subkī, Ibn Ḥajar attacks the former's attempt to explain the existence of contagion through the Ashᶜarī notion of God's habitual action (*al-ᶜāda*). For Ibn Ḥajar, it is true that God causes plague to occur in each and every case, but reason, observation, and reliance on Prophetic tradition have shown him that this happens not in conjunction with interacting with the sick, but because of jinn.[104]

Ibn Ḥajar's argument against contagion is hardly irrational or an example of blind adherence to orthodoxy. Taking both empirical evidence and Prophetic tradition into account, and subjecting both to intense scrutiny, he decides that by far the most reasonable explanation for the plague is that it is caused by jinn. Today, at first glance, this claim seems ridiculous, and because a belief in spirits seems to be anathema to science and medicine, it is easy to reject Ibn Ḥajar's treatise as superstition. In an age before the microscope revealed bacteria, however, identifying jinn as the causative agent in plague was as rational as believing in the effects of miasma. Finally, it is important to remember that Ibn Ḥajar did not reject medicine as a discipline and that in accordance with contemporary medical wisdom, he approved of bleeding plague victims liberally in order to prevent a superabundance of poisoned blood.[105]

Conclusion

In the second half of the fourteenth century, the plague (*Yersinia pestis*) swept repeatedly through the Mediterranean region, devastating both the Christian and the Muslims worlds. Significant attention has been devoted to the numerous plague treatises that were written in the aftermath of the Black Death. Previous characterizations of the plague treatises have largely been confined to seeing them as an application of Prophetic traditions to the plague, almost always written by religious scholars with no medical training.[106] Considering the breadth of views on the issue of contagion expressed by authors such as Ibn al-Khaṭīb, Ibn Khātima, and Ibn Ḥajar and the wide variety of sources upon which they drew, such a description is insufficient. Instead, the authors of the plague treatises, like those of works on Prophetic medicine, attempted to reconcile a variety of authoritative sources—Prophetic Tradition, Islamic medicine, and empirical evidence—in order to explain the puzzling phenomenon of the spread of the plague. That they differed in their analysis, some affirming the plague's contagious nature, others arguing for its ability to be transmitted while refraining from the term *contagion,* and yet others seeing it as the work of jinn, speaks not to a deep epistemological division between these scholars, so much as it emphasizes the ambiguous nature of the evidence they sought to interpret. Ibn al-Khaṭīb, Ibn Khātimah, Ibn Ḥajar, and the other authors discussed in this chapter were all shaped by the same general curriculum and scholarly environment that characterized the world of Muslim intellectuals of their era. This world was broad enough to contain the variety of views they expressed and to facilitate the continuation of their ongoing conversation on the subject of contagion into subsequent generations.

In our world today, the fields of law, medicine, and religious studies are all highly specialized and disciplinarily distinct. When dealing with the authority of experts in a matter that touches on all three of these fields, we are not surprised that there are tensions between the opinions of authorities; and, precisely due to the highly specialized nature of these disciplines, we are generally suspicious of claims that any one person has mastered more than one of these disciplines. While the Muslim scholars discussed in these chapters certainly recognized disciplinary differences between the fields of hadith studies, medicine, and law, they also felt capable of synthesizing them, and in a matter of practical ethics such as the response to epidemic disease, they responded to the moral imperative of protecting the Muslim community from a natural disaster and of shaping the communal response appropriately. The theological and ethical dimensions of the debate surrounding contagion are discussed in greater depth in chapter 5; in chapter 4 we will turn to the place of contagion in Christian thought in Iberia in the years following the Black Death.

Situating Scholastic Contagion between Miasma and the Evil Eye

Sympathy is an instance of the *Same* so strong and so insistent that it will not rest content to be merely one of the forms of likeness; it has the dangerous power of *assimilating,* of rendering things identical to one another, of mingling them, of causing their individuality to disappear—and thus of rendering them foreign to what they were before. Sympathy transforms.

Michel Foucault

Yet these people in the past did know what plague was and how it struck: they just knew these things differently from how we know them, because the laboratory way of thinking did not exist.

Andrew Cunningham

THE AUTHORS of the plague treatises written in Christian Iberia and much of Christian Europe following the Black Death had little doubt that the disease that had ravaged their communities was contagious. It is, however, much more difficult to determine what it meant to them that the plague could be transmitted from one person to another. The difficulty of the issue is marked by the fact that even the form in which the question of the nature of contagion is posed is determined by late-nineteenth-century notions of disease that distort late medieval and early modern notions of the nature of illness and health.[1] Epidemic disease today is primarily conceived of as an external agent that enters into the body, an agent whose identity can be authoritatively established only in the laboratory. For such a description to persuade both practitioner and patient of its accuracy and usefulness, it has to be understood that diseases are caused by microbes, invisible to the naked eye, identifiable only through a microscope. This understanding of disease is barely 150 years old, and when it is projected—consciously or subconsciously—onto earlier periods, it not only facilitates an anachronistic reading of earlier sources, but it can also suggest a teleological understanding of the importance and significance of medieval and early modern texts.[2] Past descriptions of diseases and their etiologies may then become of interest to a historian only insofar as they can be shown to mark a slow but gradual progress toward our contemporary medical understanding. This type of reading has determined much of the writing on the subject of contagion in the plague treatises written in the centuries after the Black Death; despite occasional weak caveats, authors have seized upon the word *contagio* or its variants as evidence for, well, contagion.[3] Words, however, have histories of being used in a variety of ways, and the meanings behind them can shift and be transformed almost entirely while the word itself stays deceptively the same.

In this chapter, I explore a neglected aspect of the concept of contagion, both as it was employed by the authors of the plague treatises in the fourteenth century and as it continued to be discussed in Iberia throughout the fifteenth century. In the writings of the authors examined here, the concept of contagion referred not only to the transmission of disease between people through contact or proximity, but also to the transmission of disease between animals or even the corrosion of inanimate objects. Most strikingly, contagion was used to describe the transmission of disease or malignancy by gaze or the meeting of the eyes, a phenomenon usually known as the evil eye. While the individual elements of the argument presented here have been previously discussed, the implications of the fact that the word and the concept of contagion were used to refer to processes qualitatively distinct from those now associated with the word have not been fully explored.

Recent studies on the subject of contagion have gone to considerable lengths to help us understand the nature of the multiple conceptions of contagion that existed in competition with one another in Europe from the fourteenth to the sixteenth centuries.[4] It is now clear that there never was any simple division between a popular belief in contagion and a scholastic preference for astrological influence and miasma theory. In fact, medical practitioners saw no contradiction between contagion and miasma.[5] But what did "contagion" mean to those who used the word? All of the medical practitioners writing during these centuries adhered to some form of the Galenic understanding of health as rooted in a balance of the four humors (blood, phlegm, black bile, and yellow bile). Disease was not an independent entity but an imbalance of these humors, and because each person's humoral balance was different, illnesses and diseases were thought to manifest themselves differently in each person. Pestilential sickness, in which many people were simultaneously afflicted, was widely linked to the corruption of the air, the only common factor that practitioners could identify as being shared by the sick. And yet, during the fourteenth and fifteenth centuries, it was generally not thought that the air itself brought the disease into the body, but rather that an influence represented by the air caused the body's humoral balance to become corrupted. As opposed to the laboratory model of the late nineteenth century, disease very much affected the body from the inside out, not the outside in.[6] Although in the sixteenth century, doctors such as Fracastoro assigned to "seeds of disease" a primary role in the transmission of disease, the causation of disease remained much debated well into the nineteenth century, and understandings of it were shaped, as has been shown, by social, religious, and political factors as much as by medical or scientific ones.[7]

Visual Contagion in the Plague Treatises

Beginning with Karl Sudhoff's exhaustive efforts to edit and publish plague treatises written in Europe during the 150 years following the Black Death, a great deal has been written on the reaction of European physicians to the pandemic that first struck Europe in 1346–53.[8] Both Anna Campbell and Dominick Palazzotto have devoted monographs to analyzing the treatises written in response to the initial outbreak of the Black Death, and numerous valuable articles have been devoted to these initial treatises as well.[9] Perhaps because it was assumed that later plague treatises merely repeated earlier approaches and material, much less has been written about the later waves of the pandemic that continued to strike Europe through the fourteenth–eighteenth centuries.[10]

The concept of contagion is well represented within the roughly twenty extant treatises written immediately after the Black Death.[11] In general it is situated within a complex web of causality in which it plays only one part. While Cunningham's terminology is taken from nineteenth-century medicine, the framework he describes can be equally well applied to the fourteenth century:

> There were *predisposing* causes, such as the particular constitution of the patient, the weather, the season of the year and the state of the soil. There were *external* (procatarctic or preceding) causes, such as the six "non-naturals": the state of the air around a patient, and the nature, quality and quantity of his food and drink, his sleep and watch, his inanition and repletion, his movement and rest, and the passions of his mind. There were *antecedent* causes, such as some obstruction within the body. And there were *immediate* causes, such as a particular state of the blood. In plague, as in every other illness, these causes were operative. Some, such as the "non-naturals," the physician could regulate to ward off or repel the disease; others he could not. Some causes were obviously

> not necessarily unique to a particular disease. Moreover, pre-lab plague did not have a *specific causal agent.*[12]

Here Cunningham emphasizes, rightly, that contagion was never the only factor considered in the transmission of the illness, even when the disease was considered to result, in part, from the effects of a poison upon the body, as was the case with two Iberian authors, Alfonso of Cordoba (fl. 1348) and Jacme d'Agramont (d. 1348).[13] Nonetheless, while administrative action against the plague, leading to the organizing of quarantines from 1378 onward, does reflect a heightened emphasis on contagion, the ways in which contagion was conceived and represented did not change significantly from the fourteenth to the fifteenth century.[14] My sympathies in this matter are with those scholars who argue against the existence of a clear break between the scholarly reactions to the first experience of the Black Death and to later outbreaks in the fourteenth and fifteenth centuries.[15] Yet instead of engaging with the historiographical debates on the issues surrounding the changing nature of scholastic medicine and the place of experimental practice in medieval medicine, I wish to focus here on the presence of a belief in visual contagion among several of the doctors who belonged to the first generation of scholars who responded to the Black Death.[16]

Many of the authors of plague treatises emphasize the importance of the patient's mental state during the time of pestilence. They explain that thoughts of death, sickness, fear, or anger may affect the constitution, making it more susceptible to disease.[17] It is even possible for a person to acquire the plague simply by thinking too much about it, according to an eloquent description by the Valencian doctor Jacme d'Agramont, who wrote in 1348:

> But among the other influences that must be avoided in such times are especially those of fear and imagination. For from imagination alone, can come any malady. So one will find that some people get into a consumptive state solely by imagination. This influence is of such great force that it will change the form and figure of the infant in the mother's womb. And to prove the great efficacy and the great power of imagination over our body and our lives, one can quote in proof first the Holy Scripture, where we read in Genesis, chapter 30, that the sheep and goats that Jacob kept, by imagination and by looking at the boughs which were of divers colors put before them by Jacob when they conceived, gave birth to lambs and kids of divers colors and speckled black and white. Another proof of this proposition can be made by the following experiment: When somebody stands on a level board on the flat floor, he can go from one end to the

> other with nothing to hold on to, so as not to fall off, but when this same board is placed in a high and perilous position, no one would dare to try to pass over the said board. Evidently the difference is due wholly to the imagination. In the first case there is no fear, and in the other there is. Thus, it is evidently very dangerous and perilous in times of pestilence to imagine death and to have fears.[18]

Jacme's invoking of Genesis 30:37–42, where Jacob placed white-streaked rods in front of those cattle that he wished to bear speckled offspring, suggests a strong link between the power of imagination and that of sight.[19] And indeed, while Jacme may not have made this link explicit, there were other fourteenth-century medical authorities who believed the plague could be transmitted with a glance: Gui de Chauliac (d. 1368), author of *Inventarium seu Collectorium in parte Cyrurgicali Medicine,* and the anonymous practitioner of Montpellier (fl. 1349).[20] Gui de Chauliac refers briefly to the transmission of disease by sight as an example of the extreme contagiousness of the plague, and the anonymous practitioner of Montpellier pursued the topic in greater detail. In addition, whereas Gui de Chauliac is vague regarding the means by which the plague can be transmitted visually, the author from Montpellier presents a precise depiction of how the gaze of the infected is the cause of transmission:

> But the greater strength of this epidemic and, as it were, instantaneous death is when the aërial spirit going out of the eyes of the sick strikes the eyes of the well person standing near and looking at the sick, especially when they are in agony; for then the poisonous nature of that member passes from one to the other, killing the other. Whence whoever has seen the *Book on Mirrors* of Euclid about burning and concave and reflex mirrors will not wonder, but will grant that this epidemic can occur, and pass from sick to well, and the latter be killed naturally and in the nature of the case, and not miraculously; since a thing is miraculous when there is no reason or natural cause for its occurrence. But the aërial and subtle nature going forth and reflected from two mirrors, by means of the heat and brightness of the sun, immediately takes fire and, as it were, acts suddenly, contracting the diaphanous air by virtue of the brightness simply generated from solar rays and mirrors; from which brightness buildings and houses and fortified places and trees, situated in that vicinity, are burned and destroyed; example of which may be had in the book of Euclid. Thus also by corruption of the air attack is made on human bodies, and more quickly on them than on any other anywhere because [*prope*] of the first soft matter of which they are composed. . . . Then the sick die soon afterward; and sometimes the brain expels this

> windy and poisonous material through the concave optic nerve to the eyes, and then the sick person is in agony, holding his eyes as if they could not be moved from place to place, and there the first ventosity receives a marvelous property, in that, thus standing and permanent, that toxic spirit is continually being made, and seeks a dwelling-place in some nature into which in can enter and lie quiet. And if any well person looks upon that visible spirit, he receives the attack of the pestilential disease, and the person is poisoned more quickly than by inhaling the air of the sick man, because that diaphanous poison penetrates more quickly than the heavy air.[21]

In this passage, the author is drawing on a theory of visual emission, in which the eye projects spirits or rays onto the objects it perceives, imparting to them its own quality and nature. While this theory enjoyed widespread acceptance in the medieval Christian and Muslim worlds, by the fourteenth century it had been superseded in some circles by the cogent articulation by Ibn al-Haytham (d. ca. 430/1039) of a theory of visual intromission, according to which seeing is the result of rays entering and not exiting the eye.[22] The work of Ibn al-Haytham (known in the West as Alhazen) was largely accepted by scholars in Europe writing on optics, although the possibility that the eye also, though not principally, emitted rays was posited by Roger Bacon and John Pecham in the second half of the thirteenth century.[23] However, whether these writers on the plague in the fourteenth century proposed a theory of visual emission or intromission, they agreed that disease could be spread by sight. In this they were joined in the fifteenth and sixteenth centuries by Iberian Christian scholars writing on the plague, leprosy, and the evil eye.

Contagious Houses and the Leprosy of Trees

Contagion in the fourteenth century is often depicted as entailing the effect of corrupted or poisoned air on those who inhale it. As has been shown in the previous section, while contagion does refer to the detrimental effects of localized miasmas, it can also refer to the visual transmission of disease from the sick to the healthy. Although such a belief may seem difficult to accept today, within the general understanding of disease etiology at the time, it was certainly an arguable possibility. And, as will be discussed, a theory of visual contagion was not only compatible with but also supported efforts by scholars in the Iberian peninsula in the fifteenth and sixteenth century to justify—from within the framework of scholastic medicine—a belief in the evil eye.

Enrique de Villena (d. 1434), a Castilian and Aragonese noble, had an interesting life and left a perhaps even more interesting legacy.[24] At age twenty he had his marriage annulled so that he could ascend to the position of grand master of the military order of Calatrava.[25] His election to the order was controversial, the pope revoked the annulment of his marriage ten years later, and in 1416 at age thirty-two, Villena retreated from public life to devote himself to scholarship and literature. Today, he may be chiefly remembered because his library was seized after his death by order of Juan II of Castile, and as a result more than fifty of the volumes were burned for containing material related to the occult.[26] He is also renowned as the author of the first translation of Virgil's *Aeneid* into Castilian and for playing an important role in fifteenth-century humanist circles in Castile and Aragon.[27] Of interest here are two of the shorter treatises he wrote, his *Tratado de la lepra,* written in response to a request from well-known physician, Alonso de Chirino (d. between 1429–31), and his treatise on the evil eye, *Tratado de fascinación o de aojamiento.*[28] Alonso de Chirino was himself the author of two works on medicine and advised Enrique de Villena on the latter's *Arte de cisoria.*[29] In both of these treatises, Villena expounds understandings of contagion that differ significantly from theories of miasma and corruption of the air.

Villena begins his treatise on leprosy by stating that he has been asked by Alonso de Chirino to comment on Leviticus 14, where leprosy is described as afflicting not only people but also houses and clothes. To his query on how it is that leprosy is found in inanimate objects as well as humans, Alonso suggested three possible answers, drawing explicitly on the authority of the *Talmud* for the first and the third answers: (1) that God had chosen to place leprosy in walls and clothes in order to instill a belief in the supernatural, (2) that it is possible that things happened in the past that no longer occur, and (3) that if after speaking poorly of others one does not repent, one can become infected with leprosy and that by contact with bodies, clothes, and even buildings one can acquire the disease. Alonso doubts that this last explanation has much validity, but he affirms that in any case leprosy "is a contagious sickness and abominable, but not to the degree that one would think, considering its nature" ("es enfermedat contagiosa e abominable, pero non en tanto grado segúnt natura").[30]

In his answer, Villena begins by providing a wide variety of learned citations to show that leprosy has indeed been shown to be present in humans, plants, and inanimate objects.[31] While the modern reader might understand these references to be figurative—how can the oxidization of iron be considered truly leprous?—Villena and the authorities he cites show no inclination to view them as metaphoric.

For these authors, leprosy is not an external agent, which has penetrated the body and which can later be isolated and identified, so much as it is a corruption of the air, bringing about a change in the humoral composition of the victim's body that results in lesions. Considering that similar processes occur within trees and metals, why should the cause of those changes not also be called leprosy? Similarly, like authors of many of the plague treatises of the fourteenth century, and appropriately for a commentary on Leviticus, Villena does not differentiate clearly between moral and physical disease. Citing Psalm 106:29–30 and Leviticus 14, he describes how the plague and leprosy, respectively, can result from man's moral failings and how in the latter case, not only the houses of Canaan but also the very earth itself became infected with leprosy.[32] Villena extends the parallel between moral and physical causes of disease by comparing the effects of the sin of gluttony to the effect of putrid air on the radical humidity of the wall.[33] As eating excessive amounts of meat creates an internal putrefaction, so corrupted air drives out the wall's dryness, disturbing its balance with the wall's humidity and bringing about leprosy. Important for the concept of contagion in Villena's treatise is that it is not just corrupt air that can transmit the disease but infected clothes as well, and that they can convey leprosy not only to walls but to people too. Citing Leviticus 13:47–59, Villena argues that the only cure for clothing infected in this manner is to burn it, and if an infected wall still shows blotches after a week, it should be dismantled and thrown outside the city.[34]

For Villena, it seems that the line between physical and moral disease, between metaphoric language and sympathetic relationships, is a fine one, if present at all: "Leprosy in the soul is moral sin. And when it is in the will or intention, it is in the wall of our house, which becomes healthy through the dryness of good thoughts and is corrupted through idle behavior."[35] If such a moral leprosy goes untreated, and the victim fails to confess his sins and his sinful thoughts to a priest, the disease will spread to his clothes and jewelry, which represent his personal habits and customs. Citing 1 Corinthians 15:33, Villena completes the arc from literal to metaphoric disease by asserting that interacting with those who exhibit evil habits can lead to a corruption of one's own good ones.[36] His response to Alonso concludes with a statement that the leprosy of the house is no longer to be feared and that now one needs to fear only spiritual leprosy, from which one can guard oneself through confession. Not to place one's faith in the Church and to fear physical more than spiritual leprosy would be to "judaize" (*judeizar*). Before invoking God's protection from spiritual leprosy in the final lines of the treatise, Villena remarks cryptically that the learned will understand from his response what is to be done and will know what can be explained through implicit references.[37]

Whether Villena's final division of leprosy into a physical Jewish affliction and a spiritual Christian one is read as sincere or as indicative of a desire to demonstrate his own orthodoxy (understandable for a man who was known for his study of the occult and the Talmud), or as both, in his treatise the concept of contagion describes the physical and spiritual transmission of disease between people, clothes, and houses. The importance placed by the authors of plague treatises on restricting one's imagination and thinking to positive matters in order to prevent being struck by the plague is reflected here in Villena's care to emphasize the importance of trusting in God and in the confession of one's sins. In another of his treatises, this one on the nature of the evil eye, Villena expanded the concept of disease transmission yet again.

Poisonous Eyes, Visual Contagion, and Evil Old Women

In *Menor Daño de la Medicina,* one of his two published works on medicine, Alonso de Chirino, Enrique de Villena's correspondent and contemporary, described the transmission of epidemic diseases in terms that parallel those of his fourteenth-century predecessors who believed in visual contagion: "Every person should protect himself from those sicknesses that are known to be able to strike those who are well when they are close to the infected, or when they sleep with them or when they are with them in one of those narrow houses. Among these sicknesses are leprosy, cancer, and phthisis, from which bad smells are emitted, and pestilential fevers, variola, measles, the great redness of the eyes which can afflict one if one looks at them [i.e., the eyes] (*que se puede pegar catando en ellos*) and the ugly sores with bad smells and in general all of the sicknesses that smell bad."[38] Whereas Alonso confined his understanding of visual contagion to diseases that affect the eye itself—implicitly professing, as did the physician of Montpellier, a theory of visual emission—Villena discussed the nature and mechanics of the evil eye in a more general fashion in his *Tratado de facinación o de aojamiento.* Although he does not address the question of the transmission of sickness from one person to another by sight, he does comment on those who become sick because another person looks at them. This, then, is not a case of contagion in the narrow sense, but it is rooted in a logic similar to that of the authors examined previously, and it adopts an understanding that sickness is the result of poison.[39] Above all, Villena's discussion of the evil eye shares with authors writing on contagion the understanding that the transmission of a negative influence from outside the body changes the internal composition of the body. It also represents a precedent for the later attempt of sixteenth-century medical scholastics to legitimate the belief in the evil eye.[40]

Villena wrote his *Tratado de aojamiento* at the request of Juan Fernández de Valera, the same courtier who asked Villena to write his *Tratado de consolación* for him after he lost much of his family in an outbreak of the plague in 1422.[41] Villena begins the treatise noting that many scholars have previously dealt with the topic, describing people, especially women, who are so poisonous that they can kill you with a glance.[42] Similar examples of the power of sight to kill have been attributed to the basilisk, Villena notes, citing a long list of authorities.[43] His description of the mechanism by which the eye is able to cause such damage is reminiscent of the passage cited previously from the practitioner of Montpellier: "Such is the constitution's venomous nature that it works more through sight than by any other way, through the subtlety of the visual spirit diffusing its impression far through the air. It has various degrees, depending on the power of the possessor of the eye (*catador*) and the disposition of the one affected (*catado*). This is the reason why it causes more damage among children, who are disposed to receive the impression (of the glances) due to their being looked at by damaging glances, and due to the openness of their pores and the heat and delicate nature of their abundant blood."[44] The classical example of this type of venomous sight is the case of the poisonous maiden sent to kill Alexander the Great.[45] This episode and the example of the basilisk had been referenced by the anonymous practitioner of Montpellier and continued to be cited as a credible datum into the sixteenth century.[46]

Villena was clearly aware of a need to insist that there is nothing unusual or irrational in believing that gazes could poison, and, citing the *Astronomía* of Felipe Elefant, he took pains to emphasize that the evil eye occurs according to mechanisms supported by natural science.[47] In his discussion of the evil eye, divided into three parts—preservation, diagnosis, and cure—Villena displays his wide reading, citing Greek, Jewish, and Muslim authorities, with several references to methods used by Kabbalists.[48] After giving many types of treatment, including the use of an emerald to ward off the evil eye, in a rhetorical move similar to that of the conclusion of his treatise on leprosy, he asserts that in accordance with Church practice, one should live virtuously in mind and body. In part, drawing on the authority of Saint Jerome, this demands avoiding the company of those who speak ill, in order to be able to conserve one's own good habits.[49] Villena's discussion thus moves from a detailed consideration of the phenomenon of the evil eye to a rather traditional admonition to shun the company of those whose beliefs are dangerous and whose morals are reprehensible.

The subject of the evil eye and the manner of the transmission of its influence was the subject of some discussion during Villena's lifetime. His treatise achieved substantial popularity during the fifteenth century, and as Salmón and Cabré have shown, it served as an important precedent for other treatises written on the evil eye in the sixteenth century. It has been suggested that Alfonso Fernández de Madrigal (El Tostado) (d. 1455), was in part refuting Villena's treatise in the section of his *Las çinco figuratas paradoxas,* completed in 1437, in which he addressed the question of the evil eye extensively in the fourth paradox.[50] Most striking in El Tostado's treatment of the subject is that he chooses to explain the evil eye through the example of contagious disease and the transmission of the plague by corrupt air. He, like Villena, is convinced that the evil eye exists and is able to spread disease. It is Villena's theory of visual emission with which he disagrees, and to which he offers numerous objections.

When Alfonso Fernández de Madrigal was asked by Queen María, first wife of Juan II of Castile, to write a book on the metaphoric references to Christ and the Virgin Mary in the Bible, he had served as professor of moral philosophy at the University of Salamanca and had devoted himself to the study of theology.[51] While much of his work was exegetical, he was able to use the genre of exegesis to address a variety of subjects associated with natural science.[52] His discussion of the evil eye and contagion is an excellent example of this trend, for it is found in his book in his discussion of the fourth paradox, largely based on his previous biblical exegesis, in which he discusses the prefiguring of Christ in the serpent of brass used by Moses in Numbers 21:9 to cure those who, after they had murmured against God and Moses, were bitten by fiery snakes sent down upon them by God.[53] El Tostado's long digression on the evil eye was thus placed within his discussion of how it was that the sight of the brass serpent cured those who saw it.

Like other humanists of the fifteenth and sixteenth centuries in Iberia, El Tostado believed that the gaze of the basilisk could kill, the stare of a wolf could prevent one from speaking, and the glance of a menstruating women could cause beads of blood to appear on a mirror.[54] The question that was unsettled was how this occurred. Unlike Enrique de Villena, El Tostado rejected the notion of visual emission and marshaled numerous arguments against it. He differentiated between seeing as an act in which rays are emitted by the eyes and the evil eye as an act in which hot and humid spirits are emitted by diseased and corrupted organs and, transmitted through the air, strike and infect delicate tissues.[55] The first case, the idea that the eye sent out rays, he rejected emphatically; the second he proposed as an explanation for the phenomena under discussion. El Tostado's argument against the evil eye's being caused by visual stimuli can be summarized as follows:[56] for the evil eye to cause anything, it would have to actively emit spiritual bodies. Visual emission is a Platonic concept that Aristotle criticized on the grounds that vision is passive, not active. If our power to see were based on actively emitting spirits, we would never be able to see as far as we can, nor would we be able to see clearly or straight when there was a wind, or under water, for that matter, since the emitted bodies would be distorted by the currents. Similarly, since spirits are subtle (*sotiles*), humid bodies, if there were visual emissions, they would condense as drops in cold weather, as blood does on a mirror stared at by a menstruating woman. Since this does not occur, and neither do these supposed spirits condense when we look at the heavens— under which is found a layer of cold air that would cause them to condense, making it impossible for us to see the sky—visual emission cannot be accepted. Finally, the author notes that if spiritual bodies were emitted from the eyes, then after the eyes had been closed and then opened, it would take some time for them to reach their object and return with an image. Instead, once our eyes are opened, we see immediately.

But if the evil eye is not to be understood as an exceptional result of a natural process of visual emission, how is it (and the basilisk, the wolf, and menstruating women) to be explained? The answer is that the objects in question are infected, diseased, and that whereas sight is the result of images entering the eye, these in fact do emit spirits, albeit of a tactile and not a visual nature.[57] This distinction is important not only because it clarifies the nature of vision but also because it explains the natural origin of the phenomenon of the evil eye, believers in which faced criticism from the Catholic Church. As El Tostado patiently explains, the evil eye is not a phenomenon caused by an inherent power possessed by some people, but rather one brought about by the natural propensity of diseased eyes to emit putrid smells or corrupt spirits in the fashion of other diseased parts of the body. Instead of a supernatural phenomenon, and regardless of the name given to it, this is actually quite a natural phenomenon, rooted, although El Tostado does not say so explicitly here, in a Galenic understanding of contagion.[58] The culmination of El Tostado's explanation of the evil eye is found in the 275th section of the fourth paradox, which deserves to be translated in its entirety, for it uses the concept of pestilential disease to help fully explain the workings of the evil eye:

On how the evil eye (*aojar*) is caused by touch and why epidemics are infectious diseases (*enfermedad apegadiza*), and on some of its properties.

There is another basis for this, namely that the doctors call some diseases "contagious," which is to say "sticky" (*apegadizas*), and this because they travel (*se apegan*) from one man to another like eczema, plague, leprosy, and similar diseases. This may also be the case with the eye, that if someone has a sickness in the eye, his eye strikes others with the like. Because if a man has eczema and approaches another, even though his head doesn't touch the head of the other, it will cause eczema on it. It is the same if a man is leprous and speaks, eats, or drinks with a healthy person: if this happens for any length of time, it will bring about leprosy in the healthy person, even though he didn't physically touch the healthy person. So, if in these cases leprosy is caused by interaction with lepers, and eczema by interaction with those who have it, even though they do not touch physically, why is it that he who has diseased or infected eyes could not harm those who were close to him? This they call the evil eye (*aojar*). Thus, it follows that one can give another the evil eye. This appears more clearly in the case of an epidemic (*pestilençia*), which occurs through the corruption of the air. When a man is fetid with pestilence, if he speaks with others, he brings harm to them and many of them die. In this fashion, most often in somewhat large epidemics, in a house where one has died, many more die after him. So as in an epidemic, one who is corrupted corrupts others, so in the corruption of poor disposition of the eye, when one has been corrupted, it will harm the others. It appears even more so that the corruption of the epidemics is of this kind: that the air may be corrupted through the influence of the heavenly bodies or through some mixture of the elements from which a corrupting smell is emitted. We receive this air through the mouth, and it enters and corrupts the entrails, passing to the heart and killing people. And after a man has been corrupted, all the air that he inhales and exhales is corrupted by the corruption that he carries within him. When this man emits air from himself, all the air that is around him will be corrupted, and those men who receive of this air will be corrupted if they do not possess an excellent constitution (*si no fueren mucho bien complexionados*). So it is that when one possesses corruption of the eyes or other parts of the body from which it has to exit from the eyes, there exit from the eyes some very slender, hot, and humid bodies, which due to their subtlety (*sotileza*) cannot be seen. And the things to which these bodies attain and affix themselves, if they are disposed to corruption, they corrupt. And this they call the evil eye. In this fashion it is certain that the evil eye exists, and we should not deny such a thing.[59]

In this passage, building on the argument advanced in the preceding pages, El Tostado succeeds in naturalizing the phenomenon of the evil eye, thus rendering belief in it permissible for Catholics concerned about its orthodoxy.[60] Crucial to El Tostado's argument is his shifting of the effective cause of the evil eye from the supernatural realm to that of disease. Here the concept of contagion explains the transmission of corrupt humors, and animals such as basilisks can be reframed as being inherently pestilential but not endowed with magical sight.[61] The susceptibility of some to the evil eye—usually children—and not others can be explained in the same way that some can be exposed to pestilential disease but, due to their robust constitutions, remain healthy.[62] This long digression of El Tostado on the subject of the evil eye, along with the treatise of Villena, provided inspiration for writers in Spain into the seventeenth century to devote treatises to the phenomenon.[63]

Conclusion

As the discussion in this chapter has shown, during the fourteenth and fifteenth centuries in the Iberian Peninsula and southern France, but in other parts of Europe as well, the concept of contagion had a much broader field of signification than the mere transfer of disease from one person to another. During this period—and up to the second half of the nineteenth century—epidemic disease was not conceived as an invasive entity but largely as an unbalancing of the body's humors. For the authors examined here, contagion was far from the transmission of a germ from one person to another through touch. To emphasize certain similarities between the statements of the authors of the plague treatises of these centuries and modern laboratory conceptions, while ignoring the substantial conceptual differences between the two, would be to indulge in a myopic misreading of history. As this chapter's focus on theories of visual contagion has emphasized, the meaning and significance of "contagion" in the texts examined suggest that it covered what from a modern perspective would appear to be a disparate variety of phenomena. The material presented here functions, then, as a caution to those who would search for the roots of modern notions of contagious disease in the plague treatises and literature written in the wake of the Black Death and in the following centuries. Before the microscope and the "discovery" of the plague in the laboratory, it was, after all, as reasonable to consider that the plague was transmitted by sight as it was to see the transmission as the work of invisible creatures. Yet, despite my warning not to read these texts teleologically as prefiguring nineteenth-century germ theory, I should not be understood as implying that the authors discussed above did not believe they were engaged in the pursuit of an accurate understanding of the phenomena at hand. Quite the contrary was the case. While the conceptual tools available to the scholars of the fifteenth and the nineteenth centuries who grappled with the task of explaining contagion differed significantly, the two groups of intellectuals can productively be seen as being inspired by a similar desire for an accurate and clear grasp of how disease could be transmitted.

In this context it is necessary to add that one should not think theories of visual contagion flourished in Iberia during this period and not in Italy or northern Europe because the Renaissance or the development of modern science was somehow slower to arrive there. Recent scholarship has placed Enrique de Villena firmly at the beginning of the Castilian Renaissance, and the work of Jorge Cañizares-Esguerra, among others, has contributed to a substantial reevaluation of the place of Iberia in both the Renaissance and the Scientific Revolution.[64] The consideration of the evil eye and the transmission of disease together under the rubric of "contagion" is not evidence for the scientific ineptitude of those fourteenth and fifteenth century scholars examined here but the result of their honest attempt to explain the world to themselves and their contemporaries. That this attempt did not necessarily prefigure modern conceptions of contagion and disease should not be taken to mean that it was in any way lacking by contemporary standards. These scientists knew what contagion was with as much confidence and conviction as do today's scholars, but they based their discussions of it on a different set of data and conceived it according to a different logic.

Contagion between Islamic Law and Theology

In short, the *mutakallimūn* struggled for a solution to the central issue the Koran had imposed on the Muslims: to bring into agreement worldly causality (and thus responsibility for one's actions) and the one Creator's incessantly manifesting omnipotence.

Tilman Nagel, *The History of Islamic Theology*

THIS CHAPTER takes up the issue of how Muslim jurists in al-Andalus and North Africa responded to the Black Death and how theological considerations influenced the way these jurists addressed the issue of contagion. The material considered here is distinct from, though related to, that discussed in chapters 1 and 3, where contagion is explored first as an exegetical problem posed by apparently conflicting Prophetic traditions and then as a complicated medical phenomenon related to the plague. The juridical opinions presented here approach contagion and the possible transmissibility of the plague from a different angle and principally consider two questions. The first relates to proper action: Can one flee the plague? The second has to do with correct belief: Does belief in the contagious nature of the plague violate an accurate understanding of the unity of God? Far from being a mere compilation of exhortations and prescriptions, Islamic law represents a moral and ethical discourse that endeavors to balance justice and mercy while explaining the intention of God's revealed law and maintaining the public good. When framing their responses to queries regarding the plague and contagion, jurists considered not only the physical and spiritual well-being of the questioner but also the broader social consequences of their answer. In addition, within the framework of law, while relevant Qur'anic verses and Prophetic traditions were certainly considered authoritative, the opinions of prominent jurists of one's legal school (*madhhab*) were seen as equally if not more important.

Islamic law is far from monolithic: by the third/ninth century, numerous loosely defined schools existed; by the fifth/eleventh, four of these—named after their putative founders, Abū Hanīfa (d. 150/767), Mālik b. Anas (d. 179/795), al-Shāfiʿī (d. 204/820), and Ibn Ḥanbal (d. 241/855)—had become dominant in the Sunni world. While the later defunct school of the Syrian scholar al-Awzāʿī (d. 157/774), introduced to al-Andalus in the late eighth century by the jurist Ṣaᶜṣaᶜa b. Sallām (d. 180/796, 192/807, or 202/817), enjoyed some early prominence there, by the middle of the third/ninth century the Mālikis had established themselves as the prevalent school of law.[1] Thus, when the Black Death struck al-Andalus in the eighth/fourteenth century, Muslim jurists both there and in North Africa, where the Mālikī school had similarly prevailed, formulated their responses to the epidemic by reference to earlier Mālikī views on contagion and the plague.[2]

Mālikī jurists of the eighth–ninth/fourteenth–fifteenth centuries did not draw only on the foundational works of their school—Mālik's *Muwaṭṭā'* and the *Mudawanna* of Saḥnūn (d. 240/854–55)—and the associated commentaries and epitomes of Mālikī jurisprudence that formed the body of Mālikī law; they were also influenced in their rulings by the Ashᶜārī school of theology, which had spread to North Africa by the fourth/tenth century and to al-Andalus by the fifth/eleventh century.[3] Central to the Ashᶜarī school, as briefly addressed in the introduction, is the argument that God's unity implies the utterly contingent nature of his creation. With some notable exceptions, this assertion entails denying secondary causation and explaining observable regular occurrences in the natural world as the result of God's regular and reliable tendency to cause things to happen in a certain fashion, his habit (*ᶜāda*). Of course, investigating the nature of God's habit hardly prevents accurate interpretations of empirical evidence as far as ascertaining the precise "occasions" chosen by God to create an event are concerned. Those occasions were, however, from a theological point of view, less important than correctly understanding how causality works in relation to them. To take an example favored by Ashᶜarī theologians, bringing wool into contact with flame does indeed have the result that the wool burns, but this is not, as commoners and philosophers jointly and mistakenly believed, due to the flame itself; it happens because God made contact with flame an occasion for many (though hardly all) things to burn. Admittedly, thinking about causation is notoriously confusing, and this confusion is reflected in language itself, as can be seen in the Arabic word used by jurists to signify "occasion"—*sabab*—which also carries the meaning of "cause."[4] What is meant by the word *sabab,* then, is highly contextual and reflects the degree to which causation itself is the focus of the discussion. In some contexts, for example, the same scholar who strenuously denied the existence of secondary causation in his works on theology or law, could, for the sake of convenience, speak easily of causes in the context of the effects of certain medicines.[5] The ability of language to suggest a dangerously misguided understanding of causality is reflected dramatically in the argument of al-Raṣṣāᶜ (d. 894/1489), discussed in the section "Continued Perplexity," that the word *contagion* should not be used in any case, since no matter how nuanced an understanding of it scholars might be able convey, the general public would always associate it with secondary causation.

In order to convey the diversity and richness of the discussion of contagion in the Maghrib during this period, I trace the debate in Mālikī legal writings from the work of Ibn Rushd al-Jadd (d. 520/1126) in the sixth/twelfth century down to the writings of al-Yūsī (d. 1102/1691) in the twelfth/seventeenth. Along with demonstrating a lasting preoccupation with the subject of contagion, this debate also casts light on the influence of Ashᶜarī theology on the way Mālikī jurists increasingly chose to frame their legal opinions, on the authoritative sources within the Mālikī school, and on the influence of other legal schools on Mālikī thought during this period.

Mālikī Discussions of Contagion and Causation before the Black Death

Ibn Rushd al-Jadd, grandfather of Averroes, was without a doubt one of the most important jurists in the history of al-Andalus. While he tolerated Ashᶜarism, he did not cultivate theology himself.[6] Much of the importance of Ibn Rushd in the centuries following his death was due to his magisterial reformulation of Mālikī law, *Al-Bayān wa-l-Taḥṣīl.*[7] In this work, Ibn Rushd took it upon himself to review and update one of the most popular sources of Mālikī law in his time, the *ᶜUtbiyya* of Muḥammad al-ᶜUtbī al-Qurṭubī (d. 255/869).[8] The *ᶜUtbiyya* consists largely of Mālikī legal opinions that are not found in the *Mudawwana,* and it was initially structured according to the relations of individual disciples of Mālik.[9] It was subsequently restructured by Ibn Abī Zayd al-Qayrawānī (d. 386/996) along lines similar to the *Mudawwana,* reflecting the consolidation of the Mālikī legal school.[10] In his *Al-Bayān wa-l-Taḥṣīl,* Ibn Rushd restructured the book once again in order to comment upon it. Since the *ᶜUtbiyya* itself disappeared subsequent to the widespread reception of the *Bayān,* it is only in the writings of Ibn Rushd that this material is preserved. The *ᶜUtbiyya* was not accepted as a legitimate source of law by all, and some prominent Mālikīs, including contemporaries of Ibn Rushd such as al-Qāḍī ᶜIyāḍ (d. 544/1149), held it in low esteem.[11] The split between supporters and critics of the *ᶜUtbiyya* can be understood in part as a difference between those who believed in early Mālikī applied law (*furūᶜ*) and those who emphasized the centrality of Prophetic Tradition in the legal process (*ahl al-ḥadīth*). The former group relied to a large extent on the opinion (*ra'y*) of prominent Mālikī jurists, first and foremost Mālik himself. It took time for the proponents of Prophetic Tradition to win out in the Islamic West, and their initial attempts to introduce a hadith-based legal methodology into al-Andalus resulted in their persecution in the second half of the third/ninth century.[12] It was precisely at this moment, when the supporters of earlier Mālikī legal opinions were forced to respond to the challenge of the proponents of Prophetic Tradition—the generation of al-ᶜUtbī—that Fernández Félix sees the consolidation of the Mālikī school taking place.[13]

It was in part because of its wide popularity that Ibn Rushd chose to devote his time to writing a commentary on the *ᶜUtbiyya.* However, in methodological terms, the *ᶜUtbiyya* was sadly dated and indeed could be seen as representing the losing side in a struggle within the Mālikī school. In the end, the proponents of Prophetic Tradition carried the day, forcing Mālikī jurists to increasingly justify the positions of their school with traditions ascribed to the Prophet. A turning point, in which Mālikī jurists made increasing use of the methodology of the supporters of Prophetic Tradition—*uṣūl al-fiqh*—can be tentatively dated to the end of the fourth/tenth century.[14]

In his *Bayān,* Ibn Rushd took a classic of Mālikī law that predated the methodology in vogue in his day and brought it up to speed. If he had not done so, it is possible that the *ᶜUtbiyya* would have disappeared entirely. In the generation of his grandson Averroes, the Almohads conquered al-Andalus and initiated a policy of strongly encouraging the study of Prophetic tradition. A great deal of earlier Mālikī *furūᶜ* was burned during the rule of Abū Yūsuf Yaᶜqūb al-Manṣūr (480/1184–595/1199).[15] Encased in the reputable legal theory (*uṣūl al-fiqh*) of Ibn Rushd, the *ᶜUtbiyya* survived the shift in methodological approaches, although it changed substantially in the process. In the *Bayān,* Ibn Rushd's practice is to quote a passage from the *ᶜUtbiyya* in which the opinions of Mālik and his disciples on a specific subject are given. He then discusses these opinions in light of relevant Prophetic traditions and analogical reasoning (*qiyās*), at times rejecting them but often reaching conclusions in support of the older views.[16] His commentary found favor with later generations down to and well beyond the time of Ibn Lubb in the eighth/fourteenth century, and the prominence it enjoyed encourages a closer examination of Ibn Rushd's discussion of the subject of contagion. Since the *Bayān* includes the text of the earlier *ᶜUtbiyya,* such a reading also offers insight into third/ninth-century Mālikī views on the issue.

Contagion in the Writings of Ibn Rushd

Following the *ᶜUtbiyya*'s contents, Ibn Rushd discussed contagion numerous times in the *Bayān:* in the contexts of epidemic disease, evil omens, and above all, leprosy. Leprosy was of special relevance to jurists, for the problem of how to deal with lepers was an ongoing one, unlike the matter of epidemic disease, which occurred only intermittently. Nevertheless, it is Ibn Rushd's discussion of entering or leaving a plague-struck area that is first addressed here. It is this passage that greatly impressed a jurist from Malaga, a certain ᶜUmar, in the ninth/fifteenth century when he wrote a poem, discussed below, on the plague; and it was also this passage that is tacitly rejected by scholars such as Ibn Lubb (d. 782/1381), who categorically denied the transmission of the plague. The tension between the views of ᶜUmar and Ibn Lubb reflects a similar tension between the opinion of Mālik and that of the proponents of Prophetic tradition. While Ibn Rushd is not able to bring the views into complete accord, he does employ arguments from the hadith commentaries to make Mālik's view more palatable. Notably, causality as discussed by Ashᶜarī theologians makes no appearance in this discussion.

In the *ᶜUtbiyya,* Mālik was asked about the case of a man who was loath to enter a country where disease was rampant and many were dying.[17] After answering that he did not see any harm in either departing or staying in such an area, Mālik compared his stance to what the Prophet had said regarding the plague. To confirm that he understood correctly, his listener asked him if he saw the two situations as being similar, and Mālik responded in the affirmative. This stance could not but seem contradictory to the *ahl al-ḥadīth,* for as we have seen in chapter 1, ᶜAbd al-Raḥmān b. ᶜAwf had related from the Prophet that one should neither leave nor approach the plague. How did Ibn Rushd reconcile the apparent contradiction?

He began by giving a summary of what had occurred when ᶜUmar reached Sargh and heard of the plague in Syria. His account differs from the canonical account of the incident. He relates that while some say ᶜUmar returned because of what ᶜAbd al-Raḥmān b. ᶜAwf had said, others said that ᶜUmar and his generals had already decided to return when ᶜAbd al-Raḥmān related the tradition. Ibn Rushd does not pursue the implications of this second version, for which he gives no source, but it stands in contradiction to what by his time had become the standard version of the episode.[18] In the traditional account offered by the hadith commentaries, ᶜUmar's companions, the Muhājirūn of Mecca and the Anṣār of Medina, were split regarding whether to continue or to return, and it was the quotation of the Prophetic tradition that settled the issue. By suggesting that ᶜUmar could have returned based on the authority of his own point of view, Ibn Rushd may have been offering an earlier example in which informed opinion (*ra'y*) was sufficient to decide a legal issue. Such a reading is conjectural, however, and Ibn Rushd did not expound on the matter.

Ibn Rushd then takes up the tradition related by ᶜAbd al-Raḥmān b. ᶜAwf on neither advancing toward nor fleeing from the plague. Drawing on what were by now traditional interpretations of the Prophetic traditions for not watering sick and healthy animals together and for fleeing from lepers, Ibn Rushd interprets the tradition not as a prohibition but rather as humane guidance and advice intended to spare people the temptation of thinking that the plague actually causes anything.[19] It was because Mālik trusted so deeply in God that he did not see anything wrong in approaching the plague:

> There is no protector (*mujīr*) for anyone from what is decreed (*qadar*). Because of this Mālik said: "I don't see any harm if he advances or stays." That is, since it is not an interdiction that amounts to prohibition, it is not a sin (*ḥaraj*) if, contrary to the interdiction (*al-nahy*), he advances toward the area. Instead, there is a reward for him, God willing, if he advances toward it certain (*mūqinan*) that what already afflicts him was not because of his advancing . . . (*mā aṣāba-hu lam yakun li-yukhṭi'a-hu*). He is rewarded if he advances toward it in this fashion and is rewarded if he doesn't advance toward it, following the interdiction of the Prophet, peace be upon him. This is the preference of Mālik in this matter.
>
> Likewise the saying of the Prophet, peace be upon him: "If it occurs in a country in which you are, do not leave in flight from it" [this saying] does not carry an interdiction of prohibition. Instead it is an order to stay. This is better, due to its involving submitting to what has been decreed. Staying is better in two ways: The first is that it corresponds to the hadith, and the second is that it involves submission to what has been decreed. Leaving is permitted; there is no sin in it, God willing, save that it is reprehensible (*makrūh*) due to its contradicting the hadith.[20]

The words of Mālik are brought into harmony with the beliefs of the *ahl al-ḥadīth* by showing that their intention is one and the same: both agree that God is the only actor and that only he can cause disease. In neither case, then, is there contagion. It is true, Ibn Rushd notes, that one should try to avoid doing something expressly forbidden in a Prophetic statement, but if one's intention is correct and one relies on God, then there is nothing wrong with leaving or entering a plague-struck area.

In any case, the intention of the tradition related by ᶜAbd al-Raḥmān b. ᶜAwf was directed to those whose belief was not strong enough to rely on God in a situation as extreme as the confrontation of the plague. Ibn Rushd's reasoning is identical to that of those hadith commentators who argued that sick animals and lepers present occasions for crises of faith, not dangers of contagion.[21] Seen in this light, the ingenuity of the jurist ᶜUmar of Málaga, who in the ninth/fifteenth century cited Ibn Rushd to justify flight from pestilential air, becomes clear. While he did not change the words of Ibn Rushd, he placed them within a context that gave them a substantially different meaning.[22]

Ibn Rushd rounds out his section on the plague by giving details on the debates between ᶜAmr b. al-ᶜĀṣ, Muᶜādh b. Jabal and Shuraḥbīl b. Ḥasana. In a nice touch, he explains that ᶜAmr b. al-ᶜĀṣ's desire to flee the plague was out of a concern for the faith of Muslims who might fall into temptation because of the plague, and because he believed the plague was dangerous in and of itself. This not only shows that all of the Prophet's Companions were equal in their reliance on God—if distinct in how they expressed this reliance—but it also shows how Mālik's later views coincided with their intentions. Ibn Rushd concludes his treatment by restating that there is no sin or offense in approaching or leaving the area of an epidemic, even though the early scholars took different positions on the issue. The most preferable option is to follow the Prophetic injunction and to neither approach nor depart from the plague, but it is striking how for Ibn Rushd—without employing techniques such as abrogation or questioning the reliability of traditions—the hadith simply indicates a preference for a believer to behave in a certain way and is not an authoritative directive.

Noncontagious Lepers

In his *Bayān* as well as in his fatwas and in his commentary on the *Mudawanna,* Ibn Rushd firmly rejected both the contagious nature of leprosy and the effective power of evil omens.[23] With few exceptions, Ibn Rushd follows traditional wisdom by interpreting the injunction to avoid lepers as arising from fear for the faith of the believer, who might be tempted to think that something other than God causes disease. At one point he does cite the opinion of Mālik's companion Muḥammad b. Dīnār (d. 182/798) on the question of whether leprosy can be inherited: the answer is that one should seek the opinion of doctors, and if they agree that in general it is inherited, then the son of a leper should not be allowed to engage in trade.[24] Despite citing this opinion, Ibn Rushd does not seem to have agreed, for in a fatwa he gave to the people of Sabta, he argued that because the Prophet had denied contagion, a leper may conceal his sickness from people and both sell to and buy from them.[25] He took a different stance on whether it is allowed for a leper to have sex with one of his slaves. Early Mālikī scholars disagreed on the issue, with Ibn al-Qāsim arguing that it was not permitted and Saḥnūn arguing that it was. Ibn Rushd sided with Ibn al-Qāsim, noting that in light of the known traditions advising against approaching lepers, sex with lepers should certainly be avoided. The deciding factor for Ibn Rushd seems to have been the degree of interaction to which the healthy person would be exposed. With dark humor or astute insight into the misogyny of his predecessor, he noted that Saḥnūn's opinion could be explained by the latter's belief that it was a greater harm for the leper to go without sex than for a woman to have sex with a leper.[26]

Ibn Rushd was able to update Mālik's views on contagion and present them within the framework of an increasingly hadith-oriented legal tradition. Two centuries later, when the Black Death struck al-Andalus, the most prominent legal scholar of the time differed from the view of Ibn Rushd and supported his own view with arguments from Ashᶜarī theology. Yet before we turn to the fatwas of Ibn Lubb, it is worth considering the influence of Ashᶜarī theology on the contagion debate in the Maghrib before the Black Death.

An Early Eighth/Fourteenth-Century Ashᶜarī Discussion of Contagion

In the late seventh/thirteenth or early eighth/fourteenth century, the Tunisian scholar Abū ᶜAlī ᶜUmar al-Sakūnī al-Ishbīlī (d. 717/1317) touched on the subject of causation in two of his works.[27] As his *nisba* reveals, his family was originally from al-Andalus, and in the decades following the dissolution of the Almohad Empire in the first half of the seventh/thirteenth century, his ancestors emigrated to Tunis. Abū ᶜAlī al-Sakūnī belonged to a family of scholars: his great-uncle Yaḥyā b. Aḥmad b. Khalīl al-Sakūnī (d. 627/1229) wrote a commentary on al-Ghazālī's *Mustaṣfā,* and his grandfather Abū al-Khaṭṭāb Muḥammad b. Aḥmad b. Khalīl al-Sakūnī (d. 652/1254), possibly the most prominent member of the family, distinguished himself in *kalām* and *uṣūl* while living in Seville.[28] Abū ᶜAlī al-Sakūnī grew up in Ḥafṣid Tunis in the midst of an Andalusī immigrant community. A staunch proponent of Ashᶜarī theology, he was concerned about the popular tendency to believe in secondary causation. In his *Solecisms of the Commoners in Matters concerning Theology* (*Laḥn al-ʻawāmm fīmā yataᶜallaq bi-ᶜilm al-kalām*), he focused on widespread sayings that carried heretical connotations.[29] Like many Ashʿarī theologians before him, al-Sakūnī was vehement in his condemnation of astrologers and their belief in the connections of habitual phenomena (*rawābiṭ al-ʿādāt*).[30] Of greater pertinence, however was his repudiation of the saying "God creates a cause for everything" (*Allāh yajʿal li-kull shay' sababan*).[31] For al-Sakūnī, the expression implies a belief in secondary causes that have actual influence. This, in turn, presupposes an infinite chain of intermediary causes and ultimately the eternity of the world (a central tenet of philosophers, shared by Averroes, for example). Such a belief could be equated with outright unbelief. At the end of the work, al-Sakūnī gives the concerned reader a list of books to avoid opening if one wishes to avoid trouble: al-Ghazālī's work demands care; Zamakhsharī's *tafsīr* often extends beyond pure Muʿtazilism to strident unbelief (*kufr*) and is thus to be avoided; and one should shun the works of Ibn Ḥazm, Ibn Rushd (Averroes), and al-Kindī.[32]

Al-Sakūnī also took up the subject of contagion in his *Collection of Choice Debates* (*ʿUyūn al-Munāẓarāt*). In his introduction to the book, he lists seven sources of unbelief that lead to sinning in one's social interactions. The fourth of these is placing the judgment of the mind (*ḥukm al-ʿaql*) above that of Revelation (*ḥukm al-sharʿ*), and the fifth consists in seeking an intermediate cause (*al-ʿilla*) in the judgment of God (*ḥukm al-ʿazīz*), an attempt that creates needless confusion (*taḥyīr*).[33] For al-Sakūnī, the Zoroastrians were the first who were led into polytheism by inquiring into the causes of God's dispensation, and they had many successors, including those who believed that things had natures proper to themselves (i.e., natural philosophers).[34] The philosophers had similarly gone astray, for among many other reprehensible things, they believed that some acts had effects, whereas God was the only true actor.[35]

It is in his fifty-third debate that al-Sakūnī comes to contagion.[36] He opens the section with the tradition "No Contagion" and continues with the account of the Prophet's refutation of the bedouin who questioned him regarding the transmission of disease between mangy camels. Al-Sakūnī interprets the Prophet's words "Who infected the first?" as a refutation of secondary causation, for the existence of the disease in the first place is unthinkable if not explained by the action of God. The answer to those who believe in the nature of objects lies in noting that the concept of "nature" implies an infinite series of intermediate causes, a view that contradicts the status of God as sole actor. He notes that the same logic can be used to argue against the existence of evil omens.

Immediately following this section, al-Sakūnī pauses to reflect more generally on the value and richness of Prophetic Tradition. Without referring to individual traditions, he wonders how, in the light of Prophetic tradition, one can believe in the eternity of the world, a series of intermediate causes, or a single independent cause. He believes that Prophetic Tradition clearly shows the flaws in the concepts of natural disposition (*al-ṭabīᶜa*) and efficient cause (*al-ᶜilla*). In closing he address the question of why, if this is so, the law should forbid approaching an area struck by plague. Drawing perhaps on the arguments contained in the hadith commentaries, al-Sakūnī argues that the purpose of this injunction (an implicit reference to *sadd al-dharīᶜa,* a legal principle defined in the next section) is to prevent believers from confusing the action of God with the phenomenon of contagion (*al-iᶜdā'*), thereby falling into polytheism. By staying away from an area of illness, one would not fail to assign all acts to God, the only Creator.

Two Fatwas of Ibn Lubb: A Muslim Jurist Struggles with Contagion, Causation, and Plague in the Eighth/Fourteenth Century

In the eighth/fourteenth century, the Granadan jurist Abū Saᶜīd Faraj b. Qāsim b. Aḥmad b. Lubb, one of Ibn al-Khaṭīb's teachers, wrote two legal opinions (fatwas) in which he argued that one should not flee from the plague.[37] The fatwas were later copied by the North African legal scholar al-Wansharīsī (d. 914/1506) into his massive collection of legal opinions, the *Miᶜyār,* the only source in which they are preserved.[38] These fatwas are of interest because they show not only how the debate on contagion carried out in the hadith commentaries extended into legal literature, but also how one of the central debates of Islamic speculative theology (*kalām*), that regarding causality, was used by Ibn Lubb and others to argue against the existence of contagion. The conclusion reached by Ibn Lubb was no different from that reached by many of the hadith commentators: contagion does not exist; God causes the occurrence of disease directly in each and every case. Yet, by choosing to justify the nonexistence of contagion with theological arguments, Ibn Lubb refined the debate on the issue and offered a consistent though not highly innovative rationale for why one should not flee the plague. He also justified this argument by emphasizing the social and moral importance for Muslims to help each other. His appeal to social responsibility, which can be understood as an implicit reference to the *maqāṣid al-sharᶜīa,* or purposes of the law, offers an instructive example of how legal scholars were able to deal with divergent traditions by appealing to their understanding of the overarching spirit of the law.[39]

In addition, we find in the writings of Ibn Lubb and other jurists in al-Andalus in the eighth/fourteenth–ninth/fifteenth centuries an emphasis on the importance of the legal principle of *sadd al-dharī^c^a,* or the forbidding of something that is in itself permissible because it may lead to negative consequences.[40] This principle, already implicit in the arguments of the hadith commentators discussed in chapter 1, is of critical importance in the theological discussion of contagion, for it justifies keeping one's distance from plague victims even though, in the eyes of jurists influenced by Ash^c^arī theology, they are not in themselves dangerous. For these scholars, the risk is that proximity to the plague-sick and the ensuing unrelated occurrence of plague may lead believers to believe in contagion and doubt that God is the only source of causation.

Ibn Lubb's two fatwas are found in al-Wansharīsī's *Mi^c^yār* without any reference to who requested them or when and where they were written.[41] We know that Ibn Lubb lived through the Black Death and witnessed the recurring effects of the plague. In view of the plague's epidemic nature in the fourteenth century, it is likely that the questions raised and discussed in these fatwas were of relevance to all Muslims at the time.[42]

The essential question addressed by both opinions is how a Muslim should behave when the land in which he lives is afflicted by the plague. In order to respond to this question, Ibn Lubb had to summarize previous opinions, address Prophetic traditions that appeared to advocate disparate courses of action, and justify his ultimate conclusion. In the first of the two fatwas, he considers the issue of contagion carefully, drawing on the debates found in the hadith commentaries, and, using strategies taken from Ash^c^arī theology, argues against the existence of contagion. In this fatwa Ibn Lubb makes repeated reference to the *^c^Utbiyya* and Ibn Rushd al-Jadd's commentary thereon, the *Bayān.* In his second, much shorter fatwa, he addresses the question of a Muslim's duty to help fellow Muslims in times of epidemic disease; here he cites no earlier works, dealing solely with individual Prophetic traditions. The two fatwas repay close reading. While advancing both theological and moral arguments against contagion, Ibn Lubb concedes—however briefly and with numerous caveats—that proximity to disease may be used by God as an intermediary cause through which he brings about a further case of the disease. This concession, however, applies only to leprosy and mange, not to the plague.

Unfortunately, the first fatwa does not include the actual query (*istiftā'*); al-Wansharīsī notes only that Ibn Lubb was asked about epidemics and the flight of people from each other during them. Ibn Lubb begins his answer by giving a selection of Prophetic traditions: the no-contagion-or-evil-omen tradition, juxtaposed with the Prophet's recommendation not to intermingle healthy with sick animals and the Prophet's injunction to flee lepers as if they were lions. Ibn Lubb observes that scholars have differed regarding these traditions and that there are three schools of thought on the matter. None of the schools support the existence of contagion, and Ibn Lubb's ultimately cautious support of the third school is best understood as a matter of emphasis and expression.

With a nod to Ashᶜarī theology, followers of the first school emphasize that association (*iqtirān*) should not be mistaken for causal connection:

> Consider the fact that the strong gale of wind in summer on the [otherwise] still sea in the evening is often of this type (*min hādhā al-bāb*). It is not right that you say that the evening caused [it] to move (*ḥarraka*) or to happen, nor that the early morning caused [it] to be still. These are only events associated with times and are the continuation of the norm and the prevailing condition [*ghalabat al-wujūd*]. This [association] does not necessarily contradict [the idea that these things occur without earthly causation], nor does it detract [from the validity of this view], since the association of one thing with another does not mean that it is its cause, nor that it has influence on it or connection with [its] existence. The belief in contagion, according to this view, becomes one (*shay'*) of the sicknesses of which nothing can be said (*rajman bi-l-ghayb wa-hawā bi-lā dalīl*) [an allusion to Q18:22], especially when the hadith has informed differently (*bi-khilāf*) from this concerning these [sicknesses].[43]

Those who believed in contagion would sin, spreading heresy and ignoring the nature of reality as described in Revelation. Their behavior would lead them to contradict the Prophetic tradition that says: "The believer loves for his brother what he loves for himself. And you don't believe until you love each other."[44] Supporters of this school think the Prophet here referred to the believer's duty to take care of the sick, to stay by their side and tend to them. Believers in contagion flee from the sick, with the result that the afflicted die of thirst and hunger and go unburied, without having been ritually washed after death. Thus, this group sins and fails to give their fellow believers what they are owed. How does this school deal with the traditions that advocate avoiding sick animals and people? Like many of the authors of hadith commentaries, its adherents explain that in the case of the sick animals, the tradition was revealed in order to prevent believers of weak faith from mistakenly associating proximity to illness with its transmission.

The second school presented by Ibn Lubb avoids theological arguments, relying almost entirely on Prophetic tradition, although it too concedes that the smell of lepers may be dangerous. This school holds that Islam abolished the belief that disease may be transmitted through proximity to the sick and that this was a beneficial act, for thereafter people no longer had reason to avoid each other in times of sickness. Two Prophetic traditions are advanced to support this view: "A Muslim is brother to a Muslim; he does not forsake or oppress him,"[45] and "The Muslims in their love and mercy for each other (*fī tawāddihim wa tarāhumihim*) are like the body: when part of it complains, it afflicts the rest of it with sleeplessness and fever (*al-sahar wa-l-ḥummā*)."[46] Further traditions are cited to argue against the necessity to avoid lepers: the Prophet ate with them and ᶜĀ'isha argued against the validity of the tradition that advises fleeing them, citing the "No contagion" tradition for support. At the end of Ibn Lubb's description of this school, however, he shows its adherents acknowledging that lepers can be harmful, although the harm is related to the lepers' smell and not contagion. Their position on this issue hardly seems consistent unless one reads their disparate positions in the context of the traditions applying to two different groups of believers: one for those of sufficient faith to remain near lepers as the Prophet did, and the second for those of lesser faith, who may not be able to undergo such a trial without being harmed.[47] In essence, the second school rejects the notion of contagion entirely, while allowing the smell of lepers to be harmful. As with the first school, moral arguments are here advanced through the citation of Prophetic hadith that encourage believers to stay with the sick and care for them.

Ibn Lubb's description of the third school begins with its members' interpretation of the "No contagion" tradition: nothing is transmitted from anything to anything by any actor but God. This is a sentiment that any good Ashᶜarī occasionalist might proudly echo, and this line of argument is bolstered with the citation of the Prophet's refutation of the Jāhilī belief that contagion represents a denial of any role of intermediary causes. This rejection of contagion is made additionally clear by the tradition already cited by the first school: the Prophet's response to the bedouin, Who infected the first? The argument here is that although sickness may sometimes seem to be transmitted by interacting with sick animals or people, in reality God causes sickness to come about in connection with proximity to sickness or without any such circumstantial association at all.

The confusion is not cleared up in the third school's argument that sick animals should be kept from healthy animals because God might use them "as a cause" (*ka-l-sabab*) for the spread of the illness. Indeed, since we have been given to understand that God might cause sickness with or without the association of sick animals, this position makes sense only if one assumes that seeing sick animals as a cause is a Satanic temptation that should be avoided.

It is at this point in the fatwa that Ibn Lubb declares his preference for the third school, stating that it is the only one that enables one to meet one's religious obligations by taking care of the sick. Seeing that the first two schools, and not the third, emphasized the importance of looking after one's fellow Muslims, taken at face value this statement makes little sense if not simply understood as a preference for the third school's attention to theological aspects of the debate.

In his writing, Ibn Lubb treats with respect some of the views of Ibn Rushd al-Jadd, citing them even if they rest uneasily next to his own discussion. He notes that the author of the *Bayān* had written that whether one leaves or approaches the plague, there is no sin or fault in the matter. Despite the incongruence with the rest of his discussion, he stops short of explicitly refuting Ibn Rushd's opinion in *Al-Bayān wa-l-Taḥṣīl.* He is less generous with the view expressed by Ibn Rushd in his *Muqaddimāt,* where the latter warned against associating with one who had left a plague-afflicted area.[48] No one holds this opinion, observes Ibn Lubb. No doubt having in mind the plight of the sick, he goes on to make a telling statement: "There is [here] a refuge in God from a clash between [on the one hand] the rights that establish through the book of God a secure state of affairs among Muslims (*allatī tathbut li-l-muslimīn baᶜḍu-hum ᶜalā baᶜḍ thubūt al-ḥāl*), and [on the other] the tradition of the Prophet of God, may God bless Him and grant him salvation. The Muslims found consensus in this [matter] along these lines."[49] The goal of his exploration of the issue of contagion, as Ibn Lubb describes it here, is not simply to bring apparently contradictory Prophetic traditions into harmony. That is only half of the equation. Equally if not more important is to guarantee the social and moral stability of the Muslim body politic, a stability that would crumble if one deserted one's fellow believers in a time of need.[50]

It is only at this point that Ibn Lubb mentions the Prophetic tradition that someone struck down by the plague is considered to be a martyr (*al-maṭᶜūn shahīd*) if he did not flee from it and trusted in God. It is curious that this tradition, which could have been used to clear up much of the confusion in the preceding sections, is not introduced until now. Ibn Lubb does not give it as much credence as the highly respected Egyptian scholar Ibn Ḥajar al-ᶜAsqalānī, who used it as the basis for his long treatise on the value of the plague.[51] Instead, Ibn Lubb uses the tradition to emphasize the importance of relying on God and placing one's trust in him.

In comparison to Ibn Lubb's first fatwa on the subject of contagion and epidemic disease, his second is succinct and clear. The material he uses to answer the question posed to him is much the same as in the first fatwa, with greater detail in some cases. In part, the greater coherence found here can be linked to the query itself—summarized by al-Wansharīsī—which clearly states which points need to be addressed: "He was also asked about those among whom an epidemic broke out and they fled from each other. What is owed to them with respect to their brothers when they see the spread (*sarayān*) of the epidemic among the majority? Are there various possibilities or not (*hal fī dhālik fusḥa am lā*)? They had observed in some places the perdition of all." The formulation of the question betrays a strong anxiety regarding epidemic disease, and it would be hard not to imagine that the questioner would have liked to be told that yes, in fact, there are certain cases in which one can legitimately flee from the plague. If so, then the answer of Ibn Lubb would have been far from reassuring.

In the first sentence of his response, Ibn Lubb emphasizes that helping the sick is a duty incumbent on the believer, a duty that was specified by Revelation and cannot be avoided. The injunction not to approach a plague-struck country is merely that—a prohibition from entering a specified area. It does not imply that the plague itself is contagious, a matter regarding which only God has secure knowledge. Nor does it advise failing to care for the sick if one is in an area ravaged by the plague. To do so would entail a violation of the rights of the sick person. Ibn Lubb then compares someone who advocates fleeing from a plague-struck country to ᶜAmr b. al-ᶜĀṣ, who was in Syria when Jābiya, a small village near Damascus, was afflicted with the plague.[52] On hearing of the plague, ᶜAmr b. al-ᶜĀs, the future conqueror of Egypt, is said to have stood and called for people to flee from it, comparing it to a conflagration (*huwa bi-manzilat al-nār*). No sooner had he spoken, however, than his view was challenged by Muᶜādh b. Jabal, who related the following tradition from the Prophet: "It is a mercy for this community," adding, "Remember Muᶜādh among those you mentioned regarding this mercy (*udhkur Muᶜādhan fīman dhakartahu fī hadhihi al-raḥma*)." Ibn Lubb takes Muᶜādh's death soon thereafter in the plague of ᶜAmwās as a sign that his prayer was answered and that God had indeed created the plague to be a mercy for his community.[53] There is no direct statement here that dying of the plague results in martyrdom, but it is not far from the surface. ᶜAmr's call for flight is thus refuted; Muᶜādh wins the argument and achieves success in the world to come.[54]

Causality in the Writings of the Contemporaries of Ibn Lubb: Ibn Khaldūn and al-Shātibī

Ibn Lubb was not the first to consider the issue of causality in connection with the plague. A handful of other contemporary North African and Andalusī scholars at least mentioned the topic briefly, and their writings testify that Ibn Lubb's own stance fell well within the range of the views of his time. With the exception of some intriguing details, all of the authors discussed in this section rejected the concept of secondary causation. Their rejection, like Ibn Lubb's, was closely linked to theological issues in which the presence of intermediary causes was considered primarily in the context of correct belief. This stance is especially clear in the case of Ibn Khaldūn, whose famed theoretical introduction to history, his *Muqaddima,* reflects an acceptance of the principle of causality on almost every page. That he rejects in the same work the attempt to ascertain causal processes because of the potential damage such a search could cause a believer can be understood only by limiting the discussion of causality to relationships between physical phenomena. Even then, it seems that the danger Ibn Khaldūn saw in a belief in causality is more closely tied to doctrine than to attempts to understand nature. Between the lines of the writings of all these authors, and sometimes expressed explicitly, is the understanding that many people—especially philosophers and the ignorant masses—do believe in secondary causation and that this belief needs to be corrected and controlled in order to preserve the integrity of faith.

Al-Shāṭibī (d. 790/1388), the famed legal theorist and student of Ibn Lubb, addressed both causality and contagion in his inquiry into the intentions of the law (*maqāṣid al-sharīᶜa*), the *Muwāfaqāt* and his treatise on heresy, *Al-Iᶜtiṣām.* A contemporary of Granada's vizier Ibn al-Khaṭīb as well as Ibn Khaldūn, al-Shāṭibī taught law, hadith, and a variety of other subjects in the Great Mosque of Granada. His chief contribution to Ashᶜarism's rejection of contagion and causality is his argument that one should not inquire into causation because doing so is not in accord with God's intention.[55] Al-Shāṭibī begins this section of his discussion by explaining that it is legally incumbent upon him to perform the five pillars of Islam *and* to inquire into the reasons of the Law (*al-tasabbub*). He quickly specifies that causes are not effective on their own and that results occur in conjunction with them but not because of them. That al-Shāṭibī is addressing not just causality but also the human capacity for action is made clear by alluding to the doctrine of *kasb* ("God is the Creator of the reason and the worshipper acquires it from him").[56] He proceeds to offer an array of Qur'anic citations attesting that God is the sole actor and man is dependent on the power of God.[57] These are followed by the Prophet's words "Who infected the first?" and ᶜUmar's retort to ᶜAmr b. al-ᶜĀṣ, "We flee from the will of God to the will of God."[58] Al-Shāṭibī explains that causes do not cause results and that, as is seen when the course of habitual occurrence is interrupted (possibly a reference to miracles), it is God who may or may not effect the results in conjunction with causes.

It is in his *Al-Iᶜtiṣām* that al-Shāṭibī made his most original and interesting contribution to Muslim scholars' discussion of contagion. In a discussion of heresy, he chooses to do something that would have been mundane for a contemporary Christian scholar but was highly unusual for a Muslim jurist: he compares heretical beliefs to a contagious disease. While the passage under consideration is an almost verbatim quotation from *Kitāb al-Bidaᶜ*, of Muḥammad b. Waḍḍāḥ al-Qurṭubī (d. 287/900), al-Shāṭibī chooses to frame heresy differently from his Cordoban predecessor.[59] The passage in Ibn Waḍḍāḥ's text dealt with the spiritual danger of spending time with innovators and heretics. Al-Shāṭibī introduces the topic as follows:

> The elucidation of this is that in the sickness of a dog there is something that resembles contagion, and the root of rabies (*aṣl al-kalab*) is present in the dog. Then, when this dog bites another, it becomes like him, and the disease usually cannot be separated from him until death. It is the same with the innovator (*al-mubtadiᶜ*) when he presents his opinion and his doubt (*ishkālahu*) to another, so that the other seldom escapes ruin, but either falls with him [the innovator] into his school of thought and becomes one of his party, or doubt takes root in his heart, doubt that he desires to separate from himself but cannot.
>
> This is different from other sins (*sā'ir al-maᶜāṣī*), for the one afflicted by them (*ṣāḥibu-hā*) is not harmed or does not enter into them save after a long period of companionship and intimacy with an afflicted one, and with repeated practice of his sin (*al-iᶜtiyād li-ḥuḍūr ma'ṣiyati-hi*). There is among the traditions (*al-āthār*) something that indicates this meaning, for the pure ancestors prohibited access to the innovators' society (*mujālasata-hum*) and their conversations, and forbade imitating their speech. They spoke harshly on this matter (*wa-aghlaẓū fī dhālik*). Many traditions have been presented on this in the second chapter.
>
> Regarding this [matter] there is [also] what was related from Ibn Masᶜūd: He said: Who wishes to honor his religion, let him withdraw from interaction with

> Satan and the society of heretics (*aṣḥāb al-ahwā'*), for their society is more contagious than mange (*alṣaq min al-jarab*).[60]

The fact that Ibn Waḍḍāḥ had put the matter similarly indicates that the sentiment expressed by al-Shāṭibī had been present among some scholars for centuries, though it had not been put quite so forcefully.[61] The metaphoric implications of describing heresy as disease in Christianity are explored in chapter 2. As a trope, it was in less favor among Muslim scholars, but al-Shāṭibī used it in much the same way as Saint Vincent Ferrer:

> This draws attention to the reason why the innovator remains far from repentance: the sins present in the doings of humans (*al-ᶜibād*) in speech, act, or opinion are like the sicknesses that descend in their bodies or souls. The medicines of physical sicknesses are known and the medicines of sicknesses in deed (*al-ᶜamaliyya*) are repentance and pure acts. And as with physical sicknesses, some of which cannot be treated, and some of which are very hard to treat, thus it is the case with rabies (*al-kalab*), which is of the sicknesses [that manifest themselves in] deeds. For there are some of them in which repentance is normally not possible, and some in which it is not possible [at all].
>
> With all sins, except heresy, repentance is possible, from the highest of them, and these are mortal sins (*al-kabā'ir*), to the lowest of them, which are venial sins (*al-lamam*). We have been given two messages regarding heresy, both of which speak to there being no repenting of it. The first: What preceded regarding the censure of innovation, that there is no repentance for the heretic, with no exceptions. And the other: That which we are explaining, which is the likening of heresy to those sicknesses with which it most favors comparison, such as rabies. If there is no repentance—especially for him whom heresy (*al-hawā*) accompanies as rabies does the one sick with it—there is in general no favorable outcome from heresy.[62]

Although he capitalizes on the metaphoric potential of contagious disease, al-Shāṭibī was, as we have seen, a strict occasionalist when it came to the subject of contagion itself. That he was able to deny contagion for theological reasons while using the term *contagion* to refer to some diseases (rabies, but not the plague) is perhaps best explained by saying that the latter was the result of a temptation to avail himself of the rhetorical power of the trope of infectious disease in his discussion of heresy.[63]

Of the same generation as al-Shāṭibī and Ibn al-Khaṭīb, Ibn Khaldūn is famous among students of Islamic theology for stating that by his time theology was no longer a necessary science, having fulfilled its original purpose of refuting heretics and innovators.[64] Writing in the century following Ibn Khaldūn, al-Sanūsī was far less sanguine about the dangers of heretics and innovators, and the writings of the other scholars examined in this section show that he was not alone in this. Yet, if Ibn Khaldūn considered theology to no longer be a necessary discipline, with respect to causality he was influenced by Ashᶜarism. His position on the matter is unique. While arguing for the existence of an extensive web of intermediate causes through which God acts, Ibn Khaldūn states that understanding how these causes interrelate is beyond the ability of man. Like some of the Ashᶜarī thinkers examined here, he connects this inability to the belief that the seat of man's perception is in the soul. Obvious and straightforward causal links can be apprehended, but more complicated ones belong to the realm of the intellect, beyond the ability of the soul to reach. Therefore one should avoid speculating about them:

> Furthermore, the way in which causes exercise their influence upon the majority of things caused is unknown. They are only known through customary (experience) and through conclusions which attest to (the existence of an) apparent (causal) relationship. What that influence really is and how it takes place is not known. Therefore, we have been commanded completely to abandon and suppress any speculation about them and to direct ourselves to the Causer of all causes, so that the soul will be firmly coloured with the oneness of God.
>
> A man who stops at the causes is frustrated. He is rightly (said to be) an unbeliever. If he ventures to swim in the ocean of speculation and of research, (seeking) each one of the causes that cause them and the influence they exercise, I can guarantee him that he will return unsuccessful. Therefore, we were forbidden by Muhammad to study causes. We were commanded to recognize the absolute oneness of God.[65]

Considering that the author of this passage was a scholar who developed a detailed theory of the causes of the rise and fall of empires, it is tempting to read this passage only as an injunction not to inquire into theological issues associated with causality. Instead of a general prohibition, then, Ibn Khaldūn may be read as proscribing attempts to define theologically sensitive issues and not, for example, the sort of sociological inquiry in which he himself engaged. Such a reading is admittedly tentative, and as far as later theologians such as al-Sanūsī were concerned, by admitting the existence of secondary causes—even if claiming to be agnostic regarding their effectiveness—Ibn Khaldūn had already come close to placing himself outside the community of believers.

The *Muqaddimāt* of al-Sanūsī

In his two fatwas on the plague, Ibn Lubb laid down a series of arguments against contagion that can be roughly summarized as follows: (1) God is the only true agent, and he causes each and every event at every moment, (2) believing in the causal connection of events that follow upon others is a fallacy stemming from overly optimistic trust in sensory perception, (3) it would be a violation of one's fellow Muslims' rights to abandon them in a time of need and not to care for them, and (4) God created the plague as a mercy for Muslims, and patiently enduring it leads to a reward in the afterlife. Nonetheless, several inconsistencies remained in Ibn Lubb's argument: unlike plague, but like mange, leprosy is described as being able to cause harm through its smell, and twice Ibn Lubb indicates that the issue of contagion is one understood by God alone (*min ᶜilm al-ghayb*). While the famed theologian Muḥammad b. Yūsuf b. ᶜUmar al-Sanūsī (d. 895/1490), a contemporary of al-Mawwāq and al-Raṣṣāᶜ, whose correspondence on contagion is discussed in the section "Continued Perplexity," did not address contagion specifically in his writing, he dealt at length with the problem of causality. In his work we can see that the above-mentioned tension between legal and medical experience continued, even as the arguments against secondary causation were rehearsed at length.

Al-Sanūsī does seem to have believed in the causal power of certain medicines (or at least an apparent habitual effect). Despite his coherent refutation of both contagion and causality, there were cases in which both were acknowledged to exist. This division continues in al-Sanūsī's explicitly theological writings, in which he explains in detail why those who believe in causality and the independent natures of objects should be considered reprehensible innovators, if not outright unbelievers. While this ability to propose two different and apparently contradictory views can be seen as hypocritical, I argue that al-Sanūsī was responding to the dictates of different situations, which he considered to belong to separate domains that did not need to be harmonized. Admittedly, this may be an unsatisfactory attitude for the modern reader looking for a consistent position regarding causality.

Al-Sanūsī expounds his understanding of Ashᶜarī theology in his *Muqaddimāt,* in what has generally been seen as a standard, though not particularly innovative, demonstration of the issues at hand.[66] He begins the treatise with a series of definitions of the different types of decrees or judgments (*aḥkām*) that he will employ in his discussion. As an example of a habitual decree he mentions oxymel, which is claimed to calm yellow bile. This is, however, one of two types of habitual judgments, for they can be divided into intuitive (*ḍurūrī*) and inductive (*naẓarī*) judgments. Al-Sanūsī explains as follows:

> An example of habitual intuitive judgments (*al-ḥukm al-ᶜādī al-ḍurūrī*): fire burns, the robe covers, and so on. An example of habitual inductive judgments (*al-ḥukm al-ᶜādī al-naẓarī*) is what preceded regarding the example of oxymel and unleavened bread. Most of the decisions of the doctors (*aḥkām ahl al-ṭibb*) are habitual and inductive. The benefit of knowing [what is] intuitive and [what is] inductive in legal judgment (*al-ḥukm al-sharᶜī*) lies in knowing which principles, if denied, would result in unbelief (*mā yūjib inkāruhu al-kufr wa-mā lā yūjibuhu*). He who denies what he knows intuitively regarding religion is an unbeliever, different from him who denies the hidden, what is known only by the few. The latter is not judged to be an unbeliever in the opinion of many authorities (*ᶜinda kathīr min al-muḥaqqiqīn*).[67]

Al-Sanūsī differentiates between two different types of knowledge and two different types of people. While he has not yet addressed causality, which will help to clarify exactly what he means by the "denial" of intuitive and inductive judgments, we can see a distinction here that will play an important role in his determination of what type of causality one can believe in and still be a Muslim, albeit an innovating, reprehensible Muslim.

According to al-Sanūsī, habitual decrees in general can be defined as the relationship between things whose existence or absence is conjoined, though one has no influence upon the other.[68] This will no doubt seem counterintuitive to some readers, for how can two things be conjoined without some degree of mutual influence? The examples offered by al-Sanūsī reveal exactly what he is worried about. He notes that the masses have become confused regarding this matter of habitual decrees, to the extent that they have come to believe that the things are *necessarily* conjoined, instead of merely resting in a state of association in which neither influences the other. This is certainly the case with those who believe in contagion and have asked Ibn Lubb—in vain—for legal comfort. But theirs is not the case that al-Sanūsī is worried about here. Instead, it is the status of miracles that he sees endangered by believers in secondary causation: "Because of this ignorance, the resurrection and the raising of the dead from the grave is denied as is the eternity in the fire. . . . all of this is for them in contradiction to the continual observed habitual occurrence [of events] and [their] associated connection."[69] Here, al-Sanūsī cites Abū ᶜImrān al-Fāsī (d. 430/1038) as an authority for his argument; this is a fitting choice, for this scholar played an important role in introducing Ashᶜarī *kalām* into North Africa.[70] Yet the example of miracles—the defense of which admittedly played an important role in theology—seems disingenuous. While a strict belief in causality would indeed rule out the miracles cited by al-Sanūsī, miracles are easily explained as a violation of secondary causality—exceptions that hardly rule out the existence of secondary causality in the first place. Instead, it seems more probable that al-Sanūsī is concerned with establishing God's authorship of each and every occurrence. This would be in accordance with his classical portrayal farther along in the *Muqaddimāt* of the Ashᶜarī doctrine of *kasb,* in which God creates acts that man then acquires.[71]

Before reaching the doctrine of *kasb,* however, al-Sanūsī returns to the example of oxymel and its purported ability to calm yellow bile, emphasizing the degree to which one can depend in this matter on the opinion of doctors: "This judgment is not proved save by means of repetition and experience, to the point where it is known that it is not accidental (*ittifāqī*). If you say that we rely on this judgment regarding oxymel by blindly following the opinion of the doctors (*taqlīdan li-l-aṭṭibā'*) and that we have not repeated it or experienced it, I would say: We have relied in this judgment on our estimation of the doctor's experience. This is not a case of our experience of habitual judgment, but it consists of relying on the ascertaining of habitual judgment in the case when it is through the experience of one in whom one can place faith (*wa-in ḥumila min baᶜḍ al-mawthūq bi-tajribatihi*)."[72] Here, the concept of "habitual judgment" comes tantalizingly close to that of natural law, in which God works regularly through secondary causes whose properties can be ascertained through repeated observation. Although this example does not necessarily lead one to conclude that al-Sanūsī's conception of causality was contradictory, it does suggest that he was far more willing to concede the possibility of admitting causality into the contemplation of purely medical topics than those related to theology.[73]

Al-Sanūsī was also the author of several works in which he defended the medical properties of medicines and their ability to heal but never raised the subject of theology or causality.[74] He may, however, have felt it necessary to justify his interest in medicine. On the Prophetic tradition "The stomach is the house of sickness, diet is the head of the cure, and the origin of every sickness is poor digestion (*al-barada*)," he wrote a book entitled *Khayr al-Bariyya min Ghāmiḍ asrār al-Ṣināᶜa al-Ṭibbiyya,* where he recounted a dream that he had. He saw both the Prophet and Abū Bakr and was told by Abū Bakr that the Prophet approved of his (al-Sanūsī's) book.[75] In this work the existence of natural law goes unchallenged. The stomach is shown to be the location where unpleasant humors (*akhlāṭ*) can form, which then affect the rest of the body.[76] The author describes how individual foods have their own natures that possess properties, which have corresponding effects.[77] Of greatest interest, however, is al-Sanūsī's explanation of the etiology of skin diseases such as leprosy, mange, scabies, mild leprosy (*al-bahaq*), and jaundice: these occur when the body's innate nature (*al-ṭibāᶜ*) repels undigested food to the surface of the body, protecting itself from this food's putrid condition. The Ashᶜarī theologians had long been suspicious of the notion of nature, and "natural philosophers" (*al-ṭabīᶜiyyūn*) were considered heretics of the first order precisely because they believed in secondary causality.[78] That al-Sanūsī, an Ashᶜarī scholar of note, could so blithely invoke the concept of "nature" in a medical treatise suggests that when comparing his medical and theological writings, we are dealing with separate discourses that rarely overlapped and that the different bases of the discourses were even more seldom consciously discussed.

In the *Muqaddimāt,* when al-Sanūsī presents his full theoretical treatment of the errors of those who believe in causality, he does it in his account of the different types of polytheism (*shirk*). The fifth of the six types he examines is believing in habitual causes (*al-asbāb al-ᶜādiyya*), an error of both philosophers and natural philosophers (those who believe that things have an intrinsic nature).[79] Though long, his metaphoric exploration of how one can be misled into a belief in causality is worth quoting:

> The cause of the polytheism of habitual causes (*al-asbāb al-ᶜādiyya*) is blindness of sight and the way in which the senses are deceived (*ightirār bi-mā ẓahara li-l-ḥiss*) when they apprehend the conjunction (*iqtirān*) of an event with another event and their concurrence (*dawrānuhu*) in terms of presence or absence, according to what the Lord, Most Blessed and Most High, wished. An example is found in the concurrence of the cooking of food when it is close to fire, and another in the covering of nakedness with the wearing of clothes. There are more examples of this type than can be given. One who looks into this, if he is blind of sight, thinks that the habitual cause is what effects the presence of that which it coincides with (*mā iqtarana maᶜahu*) and that it is not of the act of the Lord, Most Blessed and Most High. This is like the deception of a blind, stupid

beggar (*faqīh*) to whom it habitually occurs (*jarrat ᶜādatuhu*) that whenever he comes to one of the doors of the house of the King, there is placed in his hand when he stands next to the door something to eat or to drink or something to wear, etc., of those things he needs. Due to his stupidity and the blindness of his sight—for he did not witness who placed this in his hand—he does not doubt that it is that door that gave him his desires by means of its nature (*bi-ṭabᶜihi*) or through its power. So his heart is filled with love for it, and even more so, his tongue is eloquent in appreciation of it and he recites poems in the door's praise. [Thus] he forgets to mention the King and his excellence (*faḍluhu*) and His unique ability to grant gifts. On the contrary, there is not much space in his (the beggar's) heart for Him. Contained in (*fī-l-maᶜna*) the polytheism of habitual causes is the polytheism of the Qadariyya due to their belief in the influence of the power that God created for animals in association with [their] acts (*fīmā yuqārinu-hā min al-afᶜāl*). The elucidation of their foolishness (*bayān hawasi-hum*) has preceded.[80]

As al-Qurṭūbī had argued more than two centuries previously, the radical error of those who believe in causality lies in their trust in sensory perception.[81] Al-Sanūsī is able to expand on this criticism by using the metaphor of the beggar and the king to emphasize the true danger of a belief in intermediary causes, namely that one would forget to praise God or even, hyperbolically, forget God. Nevertheless, it should be pointed out that, strictly speaking, al-Sanūsī's example *supports* secondary causation: after all, it is not the King himself who places the gifts in the beggar's hands; it is a servant. The beggar may have a skewed understanding of *which* secondary cause is at work here, and he may confuse the secondary with the primary cause, but unless it is the King himself who comes to the door to give the beggar food, al-Sanūsī seems to have slipped into the same mistake as those he is criticizing. Emphasizing this point may be bordering on the pedantic, for the thrust of al-Sanūsī's simile is clear enough, but his difficulty in finding an appropriate simile is perhaps the best illustration of how easily one can slip into the heresy of believing in causality.

The denial of causality is first and foremost motivated by an anxiety regarding the maintenance of correct belief. Similarly, the chief reason advanced by Ibn Lubb for his denial of contagion in the case of the plague was his fear that Muslims might forsake their fellow Muslims and not take care of them in a time of need. Here as well, an Ashᶜarī theologian was motivated by a desire to preserve, or perhaps recover, an ideal of proper action and faith within the Muslim polity.

So did a believer in secondary causation still have a place within Islam? There are four positions one can take on the influence of habitual causes, al-Sanūsī writes, giving them in order of reprehensibility. If one holds that intermediate causes exert influence through their own nature, then one has crossed the line and become an unbeliever.[82] Those who see intermediate causes as the vehicle for the power of God, however, are merely impious and blameworthy innovators and can still be considered as Muslims.[83] Denying that these causes have any influence but nevertheless seeing them as necessarily linked to events that occur in association with them is still dangerous, for it can lead to the rejection of miracles, as explained above. The belief of all correct believers (*ahl al-sunna*) is that habitual causes have no effect or power, either of their own or of power placed in them. They are instead indications and marks of God's creation, without any connection, for God can break his habit (*al-ᶜāda*) at any time.

There is, naturally, a strong argument that could be made that it is precisely the habit of God that constitutes natural law. But as we have seen, al-Sanūsī identified the danger of a belief in causality to lie in its threat to the moral fabric of society. As in his discussion of miracles, the identification of a system of secondary causes, whose workings God may interrupt any time he wished, may have seemed to al-Sanūsī to threaten God's central role as the only true cause. It was therefore better to deny the workings of intermediary causes altogether. The exception was of course medicine, where, in a defined realm—the effectiveness of individual medicines—secondary causation was implicitly admitted to have a place.

An Exceptional Voice: ᶜUmar of Málaga

In the seventeenth century, the Moroccan scholar al-Maqqarī (d. 1041/1632) wrote two encyclopedic works on the history of al-Andalus, paying especial attention to the generation of the eighth/fourteenth-century Granadan vizier Ibn al-Khaṭīb, to whose life he dedicated half of the longer of his two books. In the second of al-Maqqarī's works, *Azhār al-Riyāḍ,* a reader interested in contagion finds an intriguing prose poem (*maqāma*), in which the sultan of Granada is advised to leave Granada for Málaga due to the former's pestilential air.[84] The outbreak of the plague that occasioned this advice took place in 844/1441, and the legal scholar who addressed himself to the Naṣrid ruler is the only author of the ninth/fifteenth century in the Islamic West in whose extant writings we find an argument for fleeing the plague.

Al-Maqqarī is aware that the opinions expressed in the poem are not in accordance with the standard views on the subject of epidemic disease, for in his introduction he notes that not all of its content corresponds with "the schools of the scholars." In addition, the poem's author is clearly aware that his views are in need of defense. He omits any reference to the tradition "No contagion," which he doubtlessly would have been aware of, considering his knowledge of other Prophetic traditions on the subject of the plague, and cites Ibn Rushd as an authority to interpret his way around the injunction not to enter or leave a plague-struck area. There is a more important issue, however. Perhaps the poem's author was aware of the writings of Ibn ᶜĀṣim, who was still alive at the time. In any case, how was he able to justify advising flight from the plague in light of previous scholarship that stressed the importance of reliance on God? In part, ᶜUmar was able to draw selectively on Prophetic Tradition, asking rhetorically: "What does the one who submits do with body and soul when he is told, Flee from the lion?"[85] In addition, ᶜUmar was able to compare flight from the plague to fleeing other dangers, such as that of houses collapsing in an earthquake. This was appropriate, but hardly enough in light of the traditions surrounding the episode of the caliph ᶜUmar at Sargh. As we have seen, Ibn Lubb interpreted the second caliph's retreat from the plague as in accordance with the words of the Prophet as related by ᶜAbd al-Raḥmān b. ᶜAwf: do not enter or leave a plague-struck area. For Ibn Lubb, this order had nothing to do with contagion and was instead in accordance with the duty of a Muslim to take care of his fellow believers in a time of disease. So how was the author of the *maqāma* able to argue for the sultan to, as Ibn Lubb might say, abandon his subjects? ᶜUmar of Málaga saw the issue in a different light. He was merely trying to save his ruler's life, and for this purpose he cited the combined authorities of Ibn Rushd and ᶜAmr b. al-ᶜĀṣ:

> It is said to me, my lord, that you agree with the recorded tradition specifically concerning such as this sickness. In it there is a prohibition of leaving the houses and places of this sickness, and from advancing upon its fighting grounds and places of struggle. The tradition is sound and there is sound guidance in a true saying, yet the scholars have regarding it spoken in great detail, which has been summarized and explained by the Imam Ibn Rushd in his book *Al-Jāmiᶜ min al-Bayān wa-l-Taḥṣīl.* All agree upon the prohibition in this tradition not being one of forbidding but one in the manner of right guidance, *adab* and teaching. There is no sin or distress for one who stays or one who leaves. ᶜAmr b. al-ᶜĀṣ said that for people of intelligence it is better to leave, being on one's guard against the belief that leads to *fitna.*[86]

ᶜUmar does not say that the plague is contagious, and through his citation of ᶜAmr b. al-ᶜĀṣ he implies that the chief danger that one might incur from fleeing the plague is that one might believe that it possesses the ability to cause harm. The basis for his advocating flight is negative: Ibn Rushd had explained how the Prophet's words on not leaving a plague-struck country are merely advice, not a binding order. There was therefore nothing in the way of the sultan's leaving Granada in order to escape its corrupted air. Unfortunately, the historical record has not passed down to us whether ᶜUmar's advice was heeded or not. It can be assumed that some of the entourage at the sultan's court would have presented to him views opposing those of the legal scholar from Málaga, who, after all, was arguing for the ability of corrupted air to cause sickness—a proposition that had long been accepted medically but which was controversial in the legal sphere, where it could be seen to clash with Prophetic tradition.

In any event, the view of ᶜUmar of Málaga on the issue of contagion is seldom encountered in the historical record. Instead, roughly a half century after his poem was written, we find contagion being debated in a very different way by two of the most prominent jurists of the Muslim West in the late ninth/fifteenth century.

Continued Perplexity: Al-Mawwāq's Questions to al-Raṣṣāᶜ on Plague and Contagion

More than a century after Ibn Lubb wrote his fatwas on the plague, the disease continued to ravage both al-Andalus and North Africa, returning every decade or so. While the historical sources for the eighth/fourteenth–ninth/fifteenth centuries, especially for North Africa, are curiously reticent regarding the extent and the effects of the plague episodes, the proper response to the plague continued to be debated by jurists.[87] The most important and intriguing testimony that we have to a continued legal interest in the subject is found in a recently edited correspondence between two chief judges (*qāḍī al-jamāᶜa*) of their communities, the first a prominent Granadan scholar, al-Mawwāq (d. 897/1492), and the second a leading Tunisian jurist, al-Raṣṣāᶜ (d. 894/1489). In 886/1481, al-Mawwāq wrote to al-Raṣṣāᶜ, with whom he had previously corresponded, asking his opinion on twenty-five problematic issues, seven of which related directly to plague and contagion.[88] The exchange between the two scholars is of interest for many reasons, among them that both were intellectual descendants of scholars who had addressed the plague in previous generations, al-Mawwāq of Ibn Lubb and al-Raṣṣāᶜ of Ibn ᶜArafa.[89]

Beyond this, the exchange contains the most detailed discussion of contagion and the plague that we possess for the Muslim West during this period. What distinguishes the text from those previously discussed in this chapter is that we possess both questions and answers, and both scholars framed their contributions to the debate around contagion with a sophistication and concern for detail rarely seen previously.[90]

Al-Mawwāq's questions can be summarized as follows:[91]

1. With an eye to identifying the religiously permitted actions in time of plague, what can be said, according to reason, about its cause?
2. It is commonly said that the plague is caused by jinn. Could you comment on the nature and the reliability of the hadith upon which this belief is based?
3. Considering the recent views of Ibn Ṣafwān (d. 763/1362),[92] Ibn Khātima, and especially Ibn al-Khaṭīb, should one support their position of breaking off contact with the plague-stricken, or should instead contagion be denied outright?
4. Given that you can demonstrate the proper view on this matter, what scholarly precedents exist for this view, and, if the view of the aforementioned scholars is false, how does one interpret the empirical evidence to the contrary in a religiously appropriate fashion?
5. Taking into account the views of Ibn ᶜAbd al-Barr, Ibn Rushd, Ibn Nājī (d. 837/1434),[93] Tāj al-Din al-Subkī (d. 771/1370),[94] and al-Baghawī (d. 516/1122),[95] how should one give a fatwa on the issue of forbidding flight from the plague?
6. Is it mandated or permitted to congregate outside the city and pray for the plague to end, as one does when praying for rain?
7. What is the legal status of someone who is in a plague-stricken area? Is he to be treated as a sick person who is about to die, or does he have the status of a healthy person until the signs of sickness of illness are seen upon him? The Shāfiᶜīs have related that the Mālikīs speak of this, and al-Burzulī has expressed himself on the matter.

These questions reveal that a broad set of issues regarding the plague, though addressed by previous generations of jurists, continued to occupy scholars in the ninth/fifteenth century. They also reveal, and al-Raṣṣāᶜ's answers support this, an increased interest on the part of Mālikīs in the Maghrib in Shāfiᶜī scholarship in the ninth/fifteenth century, something that is intriguing because of the considerable amount of tension that existed between the two schools during the same period in Egypt and elsewhere.[96]

In the seventy-five pages of the edited edition of al-Raṣṣāᶜ's response to al-Mawwāq's queries, he relies heavily on Ibn Ḥajar's *Fatḥ al-Bārī* and *Badhl al-Māᶜūn*. Although his position on contagion is very similar to that of Ibn Lubb, he shows no sign of being aware of the latter's opinions, while he explicitly and repeatedly addresses the arguments of Ibn al-Khaṭīb and Ibn Khātima. Broadly speaking, al-Raṣṣāᶜ denies contagion, but he does so by emphasizing that the plague is etiologically distinct from other epidemics in that it is "caused" by jinn and not by the corruption of the air. Firmly situated within a traditional Ashᶜārī understanding that the natural world is determined by God's habit (*ᶜāda*), al-Raṣṣāᶜ links the fraudulent belief in contagion with the view that the (proximate) cause of the plague is corruption of the blood. True believers in God, he notes, hold that only God has any influence. Instead of merely reaffirming Ashᶜarī orthodoxy, al-Raṣṣāᶜ then connects a belief that the plague is caused by jinn with contemporary Galenic medical theory: "What is correct is in the hadith 'Verily God strikes whom He wills, raises up whom He wills, saves whom He wills, kills whom He wills according to what He has previously known and determined.' We are not denying the corruption of blood any influence, but [see it as] a habitual affair occurring with the pricking of jinn."[97] The etiology of the plague is known: it is the result of jinn sent by God to pierce mankind, an act that leads to the corruption of the blood and the resulting symptoms that are described by doctors. While this act is a mercy and can result in martyrdom for the enduring believer—in this as in many other facets of his argument, al-Raṣṣāᶜ follows Ibn Ḥajar's argument—it is permissible to protect oneself from the attack of the jinn as one would protect oneself when going into battle against unbelievers (which suggests that the jinn sent with the plague are also unbelievers).[98] This protection consists both of prayers and medicines that can strengthen the body and help ward off the efforts of the jinn.[99] Therefore, although al-Raṣṣāᶜ denies secondary causality, he presents a plague etiology that moves from God to jinn to a corruption of the blood of the victim and which can be affected or prevented by both physical and spiritual remedies.[100] All this takes place according to God's habit, which—though it can be interrupted at any time—would seem to be just as reliable in terms of predictive ability as an understanding based on secondary causality. At the same time, however, al-Raṣṣāᶜ argues in the following fashion against the authority of physicians in the matter of treating the plague:

> The stance of one who affirms that God is the only protector from illness is that the cause of the mentioned sickness was hidden from him, and a physician does not treat until after knowing the cause. If he does not know the cause, treatment is not appropriate. Because of this he said: No one wards off [disease] save God, and in this is an acknowledgment of our inability. Causes are in truth like ladles from which one consumes food or drink. On the authority of the physicians, it is said that it is not due to the pricking of jinn. If we knew that it was due to the pricking of jinn, we would know its cause, and if it were established that it was from the corruption of blood to the point that it became a deadly poison, then too its cause would be known. The inability to treat it is not due to an ignorance of the cause, but to the strength of its deadly poisonousness, so it is permitted to make reference to the cause (*fa-yajūzu istiᶜamal al-sabab*). Indeed, it is a sickness that isn't repelled save by God, and this creed does not exclude referring to the cause—because there is no efficient agent or creator save Him—and the cause can have an effect or not (*qad yukhṭī wa qad yuṣīb*) according to what God has decreed and desired. There is no doubt that God the Most High has made the helplessness of his creation clear and has broken the habit in the connection of the causes and their effects (*wa kharraqa al-ᶜāda fī irtibāṭ al-asbāb maᶜa musabbabāti-hā*). What is this but [the belief] of those of the scientists (*al-ḥukamā'*) and the physicians whose minds have been overcome by [a belief in] "cause" (*al-ᶜilla*) or "nature" (*al-ṭabīᶜa*). Their position has been invalidated by rational evidence, and [the fact] that the true action is that of the Chosen Actor who creates and chooses what He wishes.[101]

In support of his critique of physicians, al-Raṣṣāᶜ cites the opinion of Abū al-ᶜAbbās al-Ṣaqallī (d. ca. 820/1417), a Tunisian physician of some repute who acknowledged jinn as the causative factor in the plague.[102] This need to invoke the authority of the medical profession is not the only indication that al-Raṣṣāᶜ feels vulnerable in his strident defense of occasionalism. It is clear that in this passage the word "cause" (*sabab*) is better translated as "occasion," although its significance seems to fall between the two concepts, especially when al-Raṣṣāᶜ seems as much concerned with the nature of God's vehicle for causing plague—contagion or jinn—as he does with affirming the contingent nature of everything upon God.

It is when discussing the best way to *refer to* the phenomenon of the spread of the plague that al-Raṣṣāᶜ is at his most innovative: he argues strenuously against ever using the word *contagion* with reference to disease, but he does not see a problem with listing the occasions on which God habitually creates disease. He is familiar with the work of the Andalusian scholars cited by al-Mawwāq—Ibn al-Khaṭīb and Ibn Khātima—and he acknowledges their stature as thinkers, while disagreeing with their view of contagion.[103] Not only does al-Raṣṣāᶜ reject Ibn al-Khaṭīb's argument for the value of empirical evidence in proving contagion, but he also points out that ultimately the argument for contagion is based on the assumption that in the first case disease appears spontaneously, before being spread to others. This is, for al-Raṣṣāᶜ, a ridiculous notion, held only by philosophers who have been misled by the external appearance of God's habitual action into believing in the causative power of phenomena.[104] Contagion does not exist, neither in the case of the plague nor in that of leprosy. Perhaps, more importantly, the law does not consider proximity to the plague to lead to certain or even probable death. If it did, and al-Raṣṣāᶜ admits here that Ibn al-Khaṭīb was of the opinion that it would, then fleeing from it would have been mandatory. Instead, facing the plague is similar to facing an advancing army: one is forbidden from fleeing in such a situation because remaining leads to martyrdom, a great reliance upon God, raising the morale of those unable to leave, and an ability to tend to the sick or wounded.[105] On this issue he takes care to refute the exceptional view of Ibn Rushd, outlined at the beginning of this chapter, that it is in effect permissible to flee the plague. Here al-Raṣṣāᶜ follows very much the same view of Ibn Lubb: he argues that fleeing the plague constitutes failing to fulfill one's duty as a Muslim and to care for those who are old or sick and unable to flee.[106] In raising the subject of martyrdom, al-Raṣṣāᶜ is careful to follow the lead of Ibn Ḥajar, specifying that such a status is attained only by those who trust in God.[107]

Given al-Raṣṣāᶜ's comprehensive discussion of contagion and his coherent argument against an uncritical reliance upon empirical evidence, his willingness to have the habitual occasions associated with the occurrence of disease discussed in the open is all the more striking: "This is what appears correct to me (*hādhā alladhī ẓahara lī*) as an answer: that it is not forbidden to state the habitual occurrences (*al-asbāb al-ᶜādiyya*) as their significance is that the affair takes place with them and not due to them. So it is not correct to deny the existence of their connection, nor to forbid believing in it, nor to forbid applying the term occasionalism (*wa lā al-nahī ᶜan iṭlāq al-sabbabiyya fī-hā*). Rather it is forbidden to call it contagion as those who refer to it do."[108] This emphasis on the danger of using the term *contagion* speaks to al-Raṣṣāᶜ's awareness of the power of language and his fear that continued use of the term, however qualified, will lead the Muslim masses (*al-ᶜāmma*) astray.[109] In its thoroughness and sophistication, al-Raṣṣāᶜ's discussion of contagion expands upon the legal opinions of Ibn Lubb, while defending the same traditional Ashᶜarī position. Yet it did not put an end to the continued confusion that the issue of contagion caused for Muslim scholars. In the centuries following their correspondence, Ashᶜarī theology continued to influence the case against causality and contagion. Yet, even within the confines of Ashᶜarī thought, different views on the subject of causality were expressed. The next section of this chapter turns to causality and contagion in the thought of the North African jurist and mystic al-Yūsī (d. 1102/1691).

A Heretical Ashᶜarī View on Causality? Secondary Causation in the Work of al-Yūsī

Al-Ḥasan b. Mas'ūd al-Yūsī was born in ca. 1040/1630–31 and died in 1102/1691. He was a towering figure in the intellectual landscape of seventeenth-century Morocco; in recent scholarship he has been perhaps most famous for his long and admonishing letter to the Alawite sultan Moulay Ismāᶜīl (rl. 1672–1727).[110] In his *Discourses* (*Muḥāḍarāt*) he took the opportunity to comment on the issue of causality in the context of the Prophet's denial of evil omens and contagion. What distinguishes al-Yūsī from such Ashᶜarīs as al-Sanūsī is that he attempted to create a space for secondary causality within a framework in which God's will is explicitly credited with causing each and every act. He accomplished this by linking God's habitual action to his wisdom, arguing that while apparent causes have no power in and of themselves, their association with the results is reliable enough for the link to be taken seriously. Failing to understand this and denying that God does create things in association with each other is almost as great a sin as mistaking secondary for primary causes:

> Know that in the customary events (*al-umūr al-ᶜādiyya*) the common people and those of the elite who are deficient (*al-qāṣirūn min al-khāṣṣa*) are lost. Concerning the common people (*al-ᶜāmma*), if they see something (occurring) with something, they attribute it to that thing and ignore God the Most High. They don't know that God the Most High alone is the active agent (*al-fāᶜil*), and nothing of creation has any effect at all (*bi-ḥāl*). [Thus] they fall into polytheism and [the belief in] the unity [of God] leaves them. Concerning those of the elite who are deficient, they believe in the unity of the Lord Most High in the act, and that he has no partner. They follow it in this fashion and deny the wisdom of God (*ḥikmat Allah*) the Most High on his earth and in his heaven. If it were said to them that this thing causes the existence of another, they would say that

> this has not been determined (*hādhā lā mu'awwil ᶜalayhi*), for the cause has no effect and it is the same if it is present or not. This is also great ignorance, for if God the Most High is powerful, willing, and has no partner, He is also wise and makes things happen (in association) with things. He orders causes and effects (*asbāban wa-musabbabāt*) with wisdom from Him, the Most High, out of kindness for his worshippers, to put their souls at ease through perceived causes (*bi-l-asbāb al-mashhūda*).[111]

Reasoning in this fashion, al-Yūsī argued that medicines may be relied upon to cure people with regularity. He interpreted the traditions on fleeing from the leper and not watering healthy with sick animals in two ways: while acknowledging that the Prophet's words may be understood according to the legal principle of *sadd al-dharīᶜa,* he suggests that they may also be seen as a confirmation of God's habitual action.[112] Al-Yūsī is careful to emphasize God's ability to depart from his habitual action at any time—in the case of miracles, for example—but it is hard not to interpret his understanding of causality as one that would admit the existence of contagion. Yet, al-Yūsī's views may have been too subtle to have had much subsequent influence, and in the plague treatises of the eighteenth and nineteenth centuries, they are passed over.[113]

Conclusion

Causality was the cause of much confusion. For al-Qurṭubī, as for al-Sanūsī and the vast majority of Ashᶜarī and non-Ashᶜarī scholars examined in this chapter, no sensory evidence was sufficiently compelling to prove the existence of contagion. Indeed, they dismissed the reliability of sensory evidence altogether, forming part of a tradition of skepticism that has had adherents from the Greeks down to Hume and beyond.[114] Conversely, for al-Sanūsī, and for many other scholars as well, the existence of causality in the realm of medicine was tacitly or explicitly accepted. It is worth returning to the fact that in general, leprosy was often granted the status of effectively being contagious, whereas this was seldom the case with the plague.[115] Why was this the case? Prophetic tradition denies contagion in general, without making any reference to specific diseases. The doctrine, not given particular weight by Ibn Lubb, that dying by the plague leads to martyrdom, does not necessarily form a definite argument against contagion. The Prophet's admonition to avoid lepers may have played a role in its being considered dangerous, even though the hadith commentators and theologians did their best to explain that this tradition is for those believers who are unable to muster enough trust in God to withstand the trial of proximity to lepers. Yet lepers abounded, and the vast majority of people did not enjoy their company, whereas the plague occurred only intermittently, and its victims died quickly. The scholars were under much greater social pressure to isolate persons suffering from a long illness whose victims interacted with a community over years than they were to sequester those afflicted by the plague, the majority of whom died in a few days. Yet, at the same time that jurists argued for the exclusion of lepers from society, they took care to make sure that the rights of the lepers were not infringed upon. Their right to water, for example, takes precedence over their fellow Muslims' fear. They are still part of the *umma,* even if social interaction with them is not desired. The situation was different with the plague: here the rights of the individuals that Ibn Lubb sought to protect are also those of the sick, but this time there is no way to justify not remaining close to them.

As alluded to in the introduction, even if one did believe in the reliability of sensory perception, the evidence available to contemporary science regarding the plague was not strong enough to challenge the traditional interpretation of Prophetic Tradition as to the noncontagiousness of the plague. If one accepts the premise that Islamic law changes to accommodate the community's changing values and beliefs, one can posit that once a convincing enough argument for contagion has been made and acquires enough adherents, the traditional interpretation will undergo radical revision. How this happened in part in the nineteenth century is discussed in chapter 6.

Regardless of their stance on contagion, the writings of Ibn Lubb and al-Raṣṣāᶜ represent fascinating legal documents in their own right. Their authors took a body of received scholarly opinion regarding the plague and contagion and framed it in the language of Ashᶜarī *kalām,* the most advanced theoretical approach of their time. Their emphasis on how important it was for Muslims to help each other may be contrasted with the writings of Ibn Rushd, who was preoccupied with the issue of updating Mālikī law and justifying the school's opinions with Prophetic traditions. In their theology, there is no place for a disease that kills indiscriminately and destroys the social fabric of the Muslim community. Such a scenario threatens to make death random and thus meaningless. The disease cannot therefore be seen as contagious. Instead, God determines each and every death. The appropriate response to epidemic disease is to trust in God and not forget one's duty to one's fellow believer.

Contagion Revisited

Early Modern Maghribi Plague Treatises

This consideration demolishes at the same time what the ancients called the "Lazy Sophism" . . . which ended in a decision to do nothing: for (people) would say if what I ask is to happen it will happen even though I should do nothing; and if it is not to happen it will never happen, no matter what trouble I take to achieve it. This necessity, supposedly existent in events, and detached from their causes, might be termed *Fatum Mahometanum,* . . . because a similar line of reasoning, so it is said, causes the Turks not to shun places ravaged by the plague.

Leibniz, *Theodicy*

Thanks be to God, the arranger of the occasions and causes that determine death and life, and which have an effect in conjunction with illnesses and sicknesses.

Ḥamdān b. ʿUthmān, opening lines of *Itḥāf al-Munṣifīn*

NUMEROUS EUROPEANS and Muslims in the early modern period saw a firm division between European and Muslim attitudes toward epidemic disease—and used this difference to demonstrate the inherent "rationality" or "piety" of their respective religious or cultural traditions. In this chapter, I argue that Muslims have always held differing opinions as to the contagious nature of the plague and that the sea change that occurred in the nineteenth century, when the phenomenon of contagion became broadly accepted for the first time, drew on a rich history of debate between Muslim scholars on this subject as well as the "rational science" acquired from European colonial powers and their medical specialists. The argument over contagion takes place against the backdrop of one of the most vexing problems faced by historians of the early modern Muslim world, namely Europe's rise to political and intellectual prominence and the concurrent "decline" of Muslim nations. A related subject of contention is the portrayal of both "modernity" and "Enlightenment" as arriving in the Middle East for the first time at the hands of colonial powers in the eighteenth and nineteenth centuries. While these master narratives have been critiqued in many of their particulars, and various scholars have shown how local Muslim thinkers in the Middle East and elsewhere in the Muslim world were involved in a critical engagement with their heritage before they encountered either European colonialism or Enlightenment, the broad outlines of these narratives have yet to be replaced.[1] Here it is my aim to show how the understanding of science and even rationality as somehow intrinsically Western or European has influenced—I would argue distorted—our understanding of Muslim attitudes toward epidemic disease and the concept of contagion in the late medieval and early modern periods.

Before continuing, it is worth noting two of the historiographical preconceptions that have supported the traditional narrative that the Muslim world was in a superstitious and irrational stupor before the arrival of European modernity: (1) until recently (the past three decades or so), it was broadly accepted that after a highly innovative formative period, by the height of the Middle Ages, Islamic law and with it Islamic civilization as a whole entered into a period of stagnation that did not end until the imposition of European law codes under the colonial powers; and (2) similarly, it has been widely held—and was debated at length in the nineteenth century— that one of the chief reasons behind Muslims' difficulty in assimilating European knowledge and ways of thinking in the nineteenth century was Sufism, which, with its otherworldly focus, opposes the materialistic rationality promoted and exemplified by the colonial powers.[2] Without entering into an extensive discussion of the validity of these characterizations, I wish to note that they have facilitated an uncritical acceptance and privileging of some sources and epistemologies over others. Specifically, they have discouraged research into the precise ways in which Muslims during this period conceived of the plague and contagion and have prevented us from asking why and exactly how attitudes on these questions both varied and changed. Instead, historians have all too often accepted narratives in which Muslims who acted in what has been labeled a fatalistic manner were following Islam and Muslims who failed to behave in the same fashion were not following Islam. In the following analysis, building on previous chapters, I will show that there have been many differing understandings of what the correct Islamic practice is regarding contagion, all vying with each other for legitimacy and authority.

The two main sections of the chapter deal with (1) contagion in the North African plague treatises of the seventeenth to nineteenth centuries and (2) contagion and medical and legal change in the nineteenth century: the case of Ḥamdān Khoja. It is important to remember that the authors under consideration did not treat contagion as an isolated phenomenon but as a concept—accepted, rejected, or tolerated—that had, at various moments, medical, legal, social, and theological implications. It is likewise important to remember that these discourses were not practiced in isolation from each other: as demonstrated in chapter 5, theology influenced legal discussions of contagion, and as seen in chapter 3, so did medicine. The influence was not one-way.

Finally, and perhaps most difficult to assess clearly, there is the impact of colonialism and European political and economic prominence on the process of legal and medical change in North Africa. Although the Moroccan government doubtless resisted European attempts to control population flows during epidemics, seeing European interventions as affronts to its sovereignty, at times European states and their representatives rejected Muslim efforts to impose quarantines, because they would damage European trade interests. It should be understood that the precise policy on contagion advocated by a given ruler or scholar at a particular moment had less to do with Islam as an abstract religious system than with specific intellectual debates and political contexts.

The Plague Treatises of the Seventeenth–Nineteenth Centuries: Relying on God in Times of Plague

How, when, and why did attitudes in the Muslim world toward the existence of contagion in the case of plague change? The views on contagion explored so far in this book have shown a broad spectrum of opinions, and yet, when evidence from the hadith commentaries and Ashᶜarī theologians is added to the mix, the balance of opinion seems to weigh against the transmission of plague from one victim to another. In any case, when reading these treatises we must remember that conclusive empirical evidence for the transmission of the plague from one victim to another was not found until the end of the nineteenth century, when Alexandre Yersin (d. 1943) identified the bacteria later named after him, *Yersinia pestis*.[3] Previously, a lively debate existed among both Europeans and Muslims regarding the existence of disease transmission and contagion in the case of the plague.[4] In this section, I will give an overview of a series of plague treatises written in North Africa between the seventeenth and the nineteenth centuries, identifying the main attitudes toward contagion and the principal factors that shaped these attitudes. The texts surveyed here are, in chronological order:[5]

1. Muḥammad b. Aḥmad al-Ḥājj (d. 1128/1715), *Mas'ala fī Ḥukm al-ᶜAdwā*[6]
2. Aḥmad b. Mubārak al-Sijilmāsī al-Lamṭī (d. 1156/1743), *Jawāb ᶜamman Ḥalla bi-Bilādihim Ṭāᶜūn*[7]

3. Abū ^{c}Abd Allāh Muḥammad al-Shabbī al-Ḥāmidī al-Sūsī (d. 1163/1749), *Rāḥat al-Insān fī Ṭibb al-Abdān*[8]
4. Muḥammad b. al-Ḥasan al-Banānī (d. 1194/1780), *Risāla fī-l-Ṭa^{c}n wa-l-Ṭawā^{c}īn*[9]
5. Aḥmad Ibn ^{c}Ajība (d. 1224/1809), *Sulūk al-Durar fī Dhikr al-Qaḍā' wa-l-Qadar*[10]
6. Muḥammad b. Ahmad al-Rahūnī (d. 1230/1814), *Jawāb fī Aḥkām al-Ṭā^{c}ūn*[11]
7. Muḥammad b. Abī al-Qāsim al-Fīlālī (al-Filālī) (d. after 1252/1836), *Risāla fī-man Ḥalla bi-Arḍihim Ṭā^{c}ūn*[12]
8. Muḥammad b. al-Madanī b. ^{c}Alī Junūn (d. 1302/1884), *Kalām al-A'imma ^{c}alā Ḥadīth lā ^{c}Adwā*[13]
9. Al-^{c}Arabī al-Mashrafī al-Gharisī (d. 1313/1895), *Aqwāl al-Maṭā^{c}īn fī al-Ṭa^{c}n wa-l-Ṭawā^{c}īn*[14]

Why did these scholars feel compelled to add their thoughts on a subject on which so much effort had already been spent? The most straightforward answer is that the plague and other epidemic diseases maintained an ongoing presence. Despite the considerable amount of time and effort previous scholars had devoted to addressing the subject, the topic of contagion continued to be debated, indicating that later generations were not entirely satisfied with previous treatments of the topic. With a few exceptions, examined in the following pages, the authors of these treatises denied the existence of contagion and the transmission of disease in the case of the plague. In marshaling their arguments, they drew significantly on earlier authorities, including Ibn Rushd al-Jadd,[15] Ibn Lubb,[16] and especially Ibn Ḥajar.[17] Ibn Ḥajar's arguments against contagion and in favor of the agency of jinn were favorably cited by virtually every one of these authors. Other authorities cited just as often, whom I have not discussed previously, include Aḥmad b. Muḥammad b. ^{c}Abd Allāh al-Qalshānī (d. 863/1459), the Tunisian author of a famous commentary on the canonical *Al-Risāla fī Fiqh al-Imām Mālik* of Ibn Abī Zayd (d. 386/996); Aḥmad b. Aḥmad Zarrūq (d. 899/1493), a prominent Fāsī jurist and Sūfī; and Muḥammad b. Muḥammad al-Ḥaṭṭāb (d. 954/1547).[18] Judging by the ways in which they were cited, these three authors brought little that was new to the discussion; they had drawn largely on earlier sources.

Although these plague treatises uniformly denied the existence of contagion, they were far from unanimous on topics relating to contagion, such as entering or leaving a plague-struck area and whether the plague was transmissible. The denial of contagion by many of the authors can be linked to their adherence to Ashᶜarism.[19] As seen in chapter 5, Ashᶜarī theologians deny the existence of any actor save God, and they understand the concept of contagion to imply that the plague possesses an independent nature. As with al-Yūsī, this line of argumentation does not necessarily demand a denial of secondary causation, and two of our authors—al-Rahūnī and al-Filālī—explicitly advocate for the idea that God uses proximity to the plague as a cause for the transmission of disease. Both authors were writing at the same time as Ḥamdān Khoja, whose views are examined in the next section, but unlike him, they found a justification for precautions against the plague solely within the Islamic scholarly tradition.

Considering that many of the authors discussed here had some link to Sufism and made either explicit or implicit reference to the principle of trusting in God (*tawakkul*) in their treatises, the historical significance of the term *Sufism* should be briefly discussed. *Tawakkul* has at times been easily framed as passive fatalism on the part of Sufis, if not of Muslims in general.[20] It is certainly true that in some Muslim ascetic circles of the first/seventh and second/eighth centuries, *tawakkul* was understood to be inextricably interwoven with faith (*imān*), and its practice was held to be an essential part of the profession of the unity of God (*tawḥīd*).[21] At times, this understanding of *tawakkul* led to a rejection or "stripping" (*tajrīd*) of one's actions from a belief in intermediary means (*asbāb*): the ascetic would focus on God by refusing to wear armor into battle, by traveling into the desert without provisions, or by approaching dangerous beasts of prey, particularly lions.[22] In this context it is not surprising that prominent members of the early Muslim community, such as Abū ʻUbaydah b. al-Jarrāḥ (d. 17/638) and Shurayḥ al-Qāḍī (d. 76/695–96 or 78/697–98), were depicted as denying the efficacy of fleeing the plague.[23] Similarly, from the third/ninth century onward, many early ascetics, and others outside their circles as well, called for refraining from the use of medicine, either because sickness causes one to turn to God or because God will heal the afflicting disease in time.[24]

This extreme interpretation came under substantive attack by both nonascetically minded Muslims and some early Sufis of the third/ninth century. Within a few centuries, the dominant understanding of *tawakkul* shifted; it was no longer an imperative to demonstrate one's belief in God's unity by rejecting any secondary causes. It came to signify an interiorization of the concept to inform one's intention, not whether one relied on intermediary causes. This new understanding, which was clearly set down in the writings of such authorities as al-Muḥāsibī (d. 243/857), al-Makkī (d. 383/993 or 386/996), and al-Qushayrī (d. 465/1074), reflected a broader shift: no longer principally defined by ascetics, *tawakkul* was viewed by the Baghdadi Sufis of the third/ninth century as one of the interior spiritual states they sought to attain.[25] By the fourth/tenth century, Sufis such as al-Makkī had defined intermediary causes as sites of God's wisdom, and *tawakkul* was increasingly understood to be the purview of those spiritually elect who were able to carry out acts of asceticism without thereby damaging their own internal belief in God.[26] Further, authors as far back as al-Muḥāsibī in the third/ninth century criticized the belief that abstaining from medical treatment was a legitimate expression of *tawakkul* by equating such negligence with suicide.[27] By the time the renowned jurist, theologian, and mystic al-Ghazāli (d. 505/1111) discussed *tawakkul* in his influential *Revival of the Religious Sciences* (*Iḥyā' ʿUlūm al-Dīn*), he showed trusting in God to be compatible with the use of medicine, which was in fact mandatory in cases feared to be fatal.[28] Al-Ghazālī also argued that it was prohibited to flee the plague, both because it was one's duty to take care of those who are sick with the plague and out of fear of spreading the disease: "Muslims are like a building with one part supporting another, so the faithful are like a single body: when a complaint comes from one member it is communicated to the others."[29] Nonetheless, while al-Ghazālī accepted the contemporary medical orthodoxy that the plague was caused by miasma, he also allowed that if a plague-afflicted community needed assistance, one could approach them to alleviate their suffering.[30] With some circumspection, however, he refrained from addressing the issue of contagion itself. Speaking of the proper attitude toward the plague, he noted: "These are delicate matters, so whoever does not ponder them but looks only to the literal meaning of the reports and traditions will find many contradictions in what he hears. In fact, the servants [of God] and ascetics made many errors in this domain, so knowledge and the benefits flowing from it are especially noteworthy here."[31] While the proper understanding of *tawakkul* remained a matter of debate in the centuries following al-Ghazālī, his contribution to the issue of responding to the plague resonated with many of the authors of plague treatises in the early modern period.[32]

Two of the treatises written in this period warrant detailed attention. In a sequel of Abū ʿIsā Sīdī al-Mahdī al-Wazzānī (d. 1342/1923) to al-Wansharīsī's tenth/fifteenth-century collection of fatwas, *The New Proclaimed Standard Collection of Fatwās of Later Scholars of North Africa* (*Al-Miʿyār al-Jadīd al-Jāmiʿ al-Muʿrib ʿan Fatāwā al-Muta'akhkhirīn min ʿUlamā' al-Maghrib*), al-Rahūnī's treatise is placed immediately following that of Aḥmad b. Mubārak, a respected jurist and Sufi who is today best known for *Al-Ibrīz*, a work in which he summarizes the teachings of his spiritual instructor ᶜAbd al-ᶜAzīz al-Dabbāgh (d. 1131/1719). In his own plague treatise, Ibn Mubārak argued, referring in part back to Ibn Rushd, that within the Mālikī school, the majority held that it was permissible to leave a plague-struck area as long as one did not flee.[33] It is at this point that al-Wazzānī introduces the treatise of al-Rahūnī: "Al-Shaykh al-Rahūnī disagreed concerning what Aḥmad b. Mubārak said regarding not forbidding one's approaching from his country for purposes of trade and the like, and advised the permissibility of forbidding this. He said the following in his answer regarding diverse matters he was asked about: Regarding prohibiting one in whose area there is no plague from approaching from where he is, I know no one who addressed himself to this explicitly (*taᶜarraḍa lahu ṣarīḥan*), save what I have found in an opinion attributed to the teacher of our teachers, the renowned and knowledgeable (*mushārik*) Aḥmad b. Mubārak. He then quoted (*naṣṣa*) what I [al-Wazzānī] have summarized [of Aḥmad b. Mubārak's treatise]."[34]

Al-Rahūnī, a prominent mufti and legal scholar in early-nineteenth-century Morocco, devoted a significant part of his treatise to summarizing the large number of views on the subject of contagion, including whether it was permitted to enter or leave an area in which the plague was present.[35] Though stating that he was relying on previous authorities, including Ibn Rushd, Ibn Lubb, and Ibn Ḥajar, al-Rahūnī came to a conclusion markedly different from that of any of his predecessors. The center of his argument lies in refusing to accept the distinction between leprosy and plague made by many previous scholars. He begins expounding this view by advocating the fifth of the six opinions given by Ibn Ḥajar on the subject of contagion in his *Fatḥ al-Bārī:* The denial of contagion is meant to refute the pre-Islamic belief that sickness is contagious by its nature and to show that everything depends on the will of God. For this reason the Prophet ate with lepers, to show people that it is God who causes sickness and heals. Yet he also advised against being in proximity to lepers in order to make it clear that proximity is one of the causes through which the will of God operates.[36] Al-Rahūnī claims that this is the opinion of Mālik as found in the *ᶜUtbiyya,* which was followed by Ibn Rushd and approved by Ibn Zarrūq, and which must be followed by Mālikīs. He does not mention that Ibn Ḥajar himself did not approve of this opinion.[37] Since Mālik famously stated that he did not see any harm in entering or leaving a plague-struck area, and Ibn Rushd explained that this was due to the strength of Mālik's own trust in God, al-Rahūnī can justifiably be seen as, at the least, quoting previous authorities selectively.

The first thing we can deduce from this opinion, al-Rahūnī tells us, is that if one is in an area not affected by the plague, one should prevent anyone from a plague-struck area from entering.[38] Relying on an Abū al-ᶜAbbās b. Mubārak, al-Rahūnī emphasizes that it does not matter whether the person is sick with the plague; he should be prevented from entering.[39] He continues by citing al-Ghazālī's view, from the *Kitāb al-Tawakkul* in his *Iḥyā',* that the plague infects only after a long period of inhaling corrupted air, and thus it is permissible to admit those who have been in a plague area for only a short time. The true reason for forbidding people from leaving, al-Ghazālī continues, is to ensure that enough Muslims remain to take care of the sick.[40] There is benefit in this opinion, al-Rahūnī acknowledges, but he emphasizes that it does not decide the matter, being only an interpretation (*takhrīj*) on a controversial matter, without a definitive textual source (*naṣṣ*).[41] Nevertheless, al-Rahūnī goes on to cite with approval Ibn Lubb's rejection of Ibn Rushd's opinion that interacting with one who has left a plague-struck country is tantamount to suicide (with a reference to Q2:195). Still, one should not go so far as Ibn Ḥajar and claim that the safest course is to follow the Prophet's example and eat with the lepers. This hardly follows, al-Rahūnī notes, for, especially in a time "such as ours," those who are likely to be placed in a position of interacting with persons emerging from an area of the plague are common people, women, slaves, and children. These groups cannot be expected to show such a high level of trust in God as that described by Ibn Ḥajar.[42] Drawing on the understanding of *tawakkul* that was prevalent among many Sufis of the classical period, such as al-Makkī, in which such feats of spiritual athleticism were not expected of the broader Muslim community, al-Rahūnī, like al-Ghazālī, was able to argue for prohibiting anyone from leaving a plague-struck area.

What about entering such an area? There are two reasons one might not want to allow someone to do this. The first is that it is against the revealed law. Citing the opinions of Ibn Rushd and al-Qalshānī that entering is either not a sin or only reprehensible, al-Rahūnī declares that legally it is in fact permissible. The second reason is that one stops someone from entering such an area out of fear that he will bring the plague back with him when he returns. This too is not convincing, al-Rahūnī states, for the person might die or exit the country somewhere else. If he does return, he should be prevented from entering the nonafflicted area.[43] To support his position, al-Rahūnī cites the example of the famed Tunisian scholar Ibn ᶜArafa (d. 803/1401), who, when the plague first broke out near his usual teaching place, hesitated to approach the infected area until God strengthened him.[44] Al-Rahūnī ends his treatise by relating at length Ibn Lubb's view that one should stay in a plague-struck area to take care of one's Muslim brethren.[45]

If al-Rahūnī emphasized the importance of hindering people from leaving a country where the plague had broken out, his contemporary al-Fīlālī argued that one is permitted to leave such an area. Al-Fīlālī was a prominent jurist from Sijilmasa in the south of Morocco, who moved north to Rabat and settled there.[46] Drawing on Ibn Rushd's exposition of Mālik's opinion, according to which leaving a plague-struck country is disapproved of but not forbidden, and referring to Zarrūq, among other authorities, al-Fīlālī argues that the authorities of the Mālikī school agreed that this was a case of disapproval and not prohibition. Al-Fīlālī acknowledges that prominent scholars of other schools (he specifically mentions al-Qasṭallānī) understood this matter in a different fashion, but he emphasizes that it is important for Mālikīs to follow the scholars of their own legal tradition.[47] He apparently feels that this position was in need of explanation, for he spends some time explaining how every *mujtahid*'s opinion is correct so long as it does not explicitly contradict revelation.[48] As his treatise progresses, it becomes evident that al-Fīlālī is deeply invested in proving that there is no religious objection or impediment to believers who wish to leave a plague-affected area. He notes that there are three types of people who fail to leave when the plague appears: (1) those who are hindered from leaving by their poverty and lack of means, (2) those who are hindered by their fear for their children and all they have collected of the rubble of this world (*ḥuṭām al-dunyā*), (3) and those who are prevented from leaving by their ignorance and lack of knowledge of the legal permission (*al-rukhṣa al-sharᶜiyya*) to leave, along with their belief that anyone who leaves and dies will die an unbeliever.[49] Al-Fīlālī emphasizes the importance of knowing that one is allowed to leave such an area and asserts that those who flee thinking it forbidden are indeed sinning.[50] To explain exactly how knowledge of its permissibility helps protect those leaving from sin, he emphasizes that those leaving do not think that this act in itself guarantees them safety, but rather that God created a link between fleeing the plague and maintaining good health. In effect, al-Fīlālī notes, leaving such an area is tantamount to going to a doctor to receive medical treatment. If seeking medical aid is allowed—and here he cites a list of Prophetic traditions showing that it is allowed—then so too is distancing oneself from the plague.[51] Throughout his treatise al-Fīlālī walks a fine line between subscribing to the Ashᶜarī concept that God's habit (*ᶜāda*) produces the appearance that objects can influence each other, on the one hand, and saying that one can rely upon this habit and base one's actions upon it, on the other.[52] Like Ibn al-Khaṭīb, he finds the caliph ᶜUmar's claim that he was fleeing from the will of God to the will of God a useful example to cite. When he comes to the issue of contagion, al-Fīlālī states clearly that God has made interacting with sick people a cause of the transmission of disease.[53] To be sure, if one's faith in God is strong enough to stay near the plague, then one is certainly allowed to do so. Those weak in faith, however, should heed the Qur'anic injunction (also alluded to by Ibn al-Khaṭīb) not to play a role in their own destruction.[54]

Both al-Rahūnī and al-Fīlālī, like al-Yūsī, with their varying stances on contagion, disease transmission, and the plague, present themselves as adherents of Ashᶜarism even as they argue against a narrow understanding of occasionalism. Whereas al-Rahūnī advocates isolating the sick, al-Fīlālī is interested in justifying the behavior of those who, hearing of a plague outbreak, choose to flee. Both scholars draw on previous discussions, interpreting them with an implicit and at times explicit awareness of the flexibility of the legal, medical, and theological traditions. They also admit that a spiritual elect can legitimately choose to practice a more demanding form of *tawakkul* in the context of the plague, one not appropriate for the majority of believers.

The views of al-Rahūnī and al-Fīlālī, with their acceptance of some type of secondary causation, were hardly shared by all of their colleagues. Muḥammad b. al-Ḥasan al-Banānī (d. 1194/1780) and Aḥmad ibn ᶜAjība (d. 1224/1809)—both acclaimed scholars—rejected the transmission of disease in the case of the plague completely, and the former wholeheartedly embraced the agency of the jinn in its causation. The fact that both of these scholars were Sufis may have played a role in their opinion on causation, for the Sufi ideal of trusting in God (*tawakkul*) dovetails nicely with Ashᶜarī occasionalism.[55]

In his treatise, composed on the occasion of the plague's breaking out in Fez in 1156/1744, al-Banānī relates the anecdote reported by Ibn Ḥajar from Aḥmad b. ᶜAdnān on hearing two jinn discuss whether to pierce him, and he then quotes a similar story from al-Ḥaṭṭāb regarding an anonymous narrator: "[He was] in Cairo with his mother in 881 when the city was struck by the plague. One night his mother was awake; she was a virtuous (*ṣāliha*) woman. She said to him: I have just been pierced, for I saw men with arrows in their hands piercing people, and they pierced me in places on my body. She showed him the places and then she died of it, God have mercy upon her. I [al-Ḥaṭṭāb] said: We have seen much of this in this epidemic year. There was [the case] that a woman, after she was pierced, reported that one of the Jewish jinn struck [her], [and] another told her husband after being pierced that a jinn had pierced her. The matter was like this."[56] Writing more than a half century later in the northern Moroccan city of Tétouan, the prominent Sufi Ibn ᶜAjība objected when local authorities, including some religious scholars, decided to lock the city gates when they heard of the plague's approach, some of them advising the inhabitants to flee.[57] Ibn ᶜAjība's view, similar to al-Banānī's, was that the correct belief was to understand the plague to be due to the action of the jinn.[58] Yet, he went further, offering his personal observations regarding the plague that afflicted Morocco between 1798 and 1800:

> I have seen many of our companions perform the washing of the dead (*taqaddamū li-ghusl al-mawtā*) and tend to the sick in the cities of Tétouan, Tangier, Salé, and Rabat and the tribal areas. Indeed, nobody besides them did this. They washed and wrapped [the dead] and tended to the sick. Nothing happened to them. . . . I saw one of them who was given a piece of clothing (*qushāba*) whose owner had died of the plague. He put it on straightaway, nothing happened to him, and he lived a long time after the plague. I saw one of our Sufi companions (*ahl al-khabar*) approach the country where there was plague, and he remained there more than a month, washing, shrouding, and tending to the sick. Then he returned healthy and lived for a long time after the plague. Therefore, supporting contagion and transmission is without merit. I used to say (*kuntu naqūl*) to our companions: whoever wishes to train his certainty [in God] (*tarbiyat al-yaqīn*) and to learn strength and bravery, let him go to its place [i.e., that of plague], trusting in God, relying upon the words of Ibn Rushd along with the details we have relayed above. And regarding locking oneself in against it (*al-taḥaṣṣun min-hā*) by guarding (*ḥirṣ*) the doors and locking them, there is no benefit in it.[59]

Like al-Fīlālī and al-Rahūnī, Ibn ᶜAjība draws on the opinion of Ibn Rushd that it is permissible to enter or leave a plague-struck area. Yet, instead of worrying about the implementation of a quarantine or justifying people's leaving the plague's proximity, he, like Ibn Lubb and al-Ghazālī before him, is preoccupied with taking care of the dead and dying. Like Ibn Ḥajar and others, he cites empirical evidence to refute contagion and even advocates exposing oneself to the plague to strengthen one's faith in God, a demanding example of *tawakkul.* Admittedly, Ibn ᶜAjība may have believed that such behavior was appropriate only for Sufis like himself who were strong in faith and able to bear the plague patiently, achieving martyrdom.[60] If so, he may have found comfort in the fact that he and his sons, like the famous Companion of the Prophet Muᶜādh b. Jabal (d. 17/638) who asked for this honor, died of the plague themselves.[61]

These North African scholars framed their questions in largely legal and ethical terms, rather than within an administrative framework. How does their reading of the treatment of contagion in the plague treatises relate to the policies enforced by North African governments from the eighteenth to the twentieth century, and how, if at all, do they relate to the imposition of quarantines? More pointedly, was the choice to impose quarantines, to stop the movement of goods and people, exclusively a European innovation, and how did Muslim authorities in North Africa justify quarantines once they imposed them?

The Acceptance of Contagion within the Framework of Colonialism: Ḥamdān Khoja

In the second half of the eighteenth and the first half of the nineteenth centuries, European economic and political interests in North Africa and the Middle East expanded, leading in some cases—Aden and Algeria—to the European occupation and administration of these countries as colonies. In many other areas, including Tunis and Morocco, European states used political pressure and economic institutions to further their own national interests. While this is certainly not the place to consider the political and cultural aspects of this era in detail—they have been the subject of many excellent studies—this context shaped European portrayals of Muslim attitudes toward the plague and Muslim attitudes toward European institutions such as the quarantine.[62] Nancy Gallagher has shown how in Tunisia, during the same period when Ibn ᶜAjība, al-Fīlālī, and al-Rahūnī were writing their plague treatises, there was a similarly lively debate between scholars and administrators regarding whether one should protect oneself from the plague and other epidemics such as cholera.[63] Despite later claims to the contrary, she shows that the chief reason that Europeans took control of administering the quarantine during the 1830s was not that local authorities were reluctant to implement the procedure, but that they did so too stringently, thereby disturbing European commercial interests.[64] Although Muslim governments in North Africa did not always acknowledge the contagiousness of plague—consider the examples of Muḥammad Bey (rl. 1855–59) in Tunisia and Moulay Sulaymān (rl. 1792–1822) in Morocco—the work of Gallagher and others strongly suggests that Muslims were aware of the desire of the European powers to use quarantine procedures to further their control over North African ports.[65] From the 1860s onward in Tunisia and by the end of the century in much of the Middle East, Europeans controlled the licensing of doctors, ran the quarantine boards, and cast increasing doubt on the medical knowledge of Muslim doctors.[66] At the same time, religiously articulated views on the plague, contagion, and quarantine increasingly lost relevance for representatives of Middle Eastern states.[67] Yet, that the traditional religious discourse on the subject of the plague and contagion was still relevant to a broad popular audience in the nineteenth century is evidenced by the fact that in the 1830s both the Ottoman government and the ruler of Egypt, Muḥammad ᶜAlī, made explicit references to Prophetic tradition when they acknowledged the contagious nature of plague.[68] On May 9, 1838, an official statement was printed in the first official newspaper of the Ottoman Empire, *Takvīm-i Vekāyiᶜ*, in which strict Ashᶜarī occasionalism was denied, and, with an allusion to the "Flee from the leper as from the lion" tradition, the existence of contagion was defended and belief in it was demanded.[69] Muḥammad ᶜAlī quoted the same tradition during the cholera epidemic of 1831, when he wrote to his secretary demanding the enforcement of the quarantine.[70]

As the nineteenth century progressed, the plague treatise may have become an increasingly irrelevant genre in Muslim scholarship, but one of the last examples that we possess deserves mention, because it explicitly attempts to justify the European institution of the quarantine within the traditional framework of Islamic scholarship. Ḥamdān b. ᶜUthmān Khoja (d. ca. 1258/1842) was an Algerian scholar of Islamic law who visited France and advocated for the rights of Algeria in his *The Mirror* (*Al-Mir'āh*), which he translated into French in 1833.[71] He was also the author of a treatise on the necessity of implementing the quarantine and its compatibility with Islamic law, entitled *Presentation to the Just and the Cultured on Protecting Oneself from Epidemics* (*Itḥāf al-Munṣifīn wa-l-Udabā' fī al-Iḥtirāz ᶜan al-Wabā'*).[72] This treatise is exceptional in that its author advances an eloquent and well-informed argument for the permissibility of adopting foreign customs if they benefit the Muslim community. In addition, though stating his adherence to Ashᶜarism and acknowledging the necessity of trusting in God, he clearly defends secondary causation and is able to reconcile the plague's being caused by jinn with the effectiveness of the quarantine; this position is similar to that of al-Rahūnī and al-Filālī, whom he does not cite. Drawing on previous authorities, al-Ghazālī among them, he argues convincingly that avoiding the plague is in accordance with Islamic tradition and is obligatory.[73] Considering that he wrote the treatise during a time of political turmoil and French expansion in Algeria, it is not surprising that his treatise, with its call for the establishment of lazarettos and quarantine infrastructure, seems to have had little immediate effect in North Africa.[74]

Ḥamdān Khoja, who was a jurist by profession, was trained in the Ḥanīfī school of law, the official law school of both Algeria and the Ottoman Empire. In 1249/1833, against the backdrop of events that led to the Ottoman loss of control over Algeria and France's establishment of colonial rule, he was elected by fellow members of the Algerian elite to travel to Paris and argue there for the merits of

Algerian independence. In 1251/1835, having failed in his mission, he left Paris for Istanbul, where he spent his remaining years writing and translating. The *Itḥāf* was written in 1252/1836.[75]

Ḥamdān Khoja introduces his treatise by portraying himself as a devout Ashᶜarī who believes in secondary causation and who wishes for Muslims to adopt a European institution, the quarantine, that has served them well. At almost sixty years of age, he had witnessed the confusion and consternation caused by numerous epidemics in Algeria, all the while observing the manner in which Europeans (*al-faranj*) protected themselves.[76] To make his case, he structures his book in three chapters, preceded by nine principles (*maqālāt*), which summarize his argument:

1. God is the Creator of everything, both good and evil.[77]
2. God has created all causes (*asbāb*) and effects (*musabbabāt*), as well as the connections between them.[78]
3. God has decreed that death and danger are to avoided: the use of medicine does not conflict with trusting in God (*tawakkul*).[79]
4. Certain types of *tawakkul* are appropriate only for the spiritually elect.[80]
5. Not all knowledge of links between causes and effects is attained through revelation or inspiration; some also comes through experimental knowledge.[81]
6. All necessary causes are not sufficient: while interacting with a leper is necessary for the transmission of the disease, other factors can prevent this from happening.[82]
7. The Europeans have attained superior knowledge in the natural sciences, including medicine, while Muslims have focused on the literary and religious sciences.[83]
8. Those who are in positions of political power must protect those living under their rule while ignoring the fanaticism of the ignorant.[84]
9. The Europeans have protected themselves through the use of the quarantine for centuries. Simply because Muslims don't have a name for this institution does not mean it has no basis in Islam.[85]

The three chapters that follow expound upon these principles and demonstrate that Ḥamdān Khoja had read widely in Muslim legal and theological writings on the contagion debate. The first chapter is a summary discussion of relevant Qur'anic verses, Prophetic Traditions, and previous scholarly opinions. Much of this material has been discussed in chapters 1, 3, and 5; what is new in Ḥamdān Khoja's discussion is his emphasis on secondary causation alongside his insistence that God is the only causal agent. The error that needs to be avoided, he notes, citing the words of the Prophetic Companion Abū Mūsā al-Ashᶜarī (d. 82/701), is to think that one *necessarily* saved oneself from the plague by fleeing it. One's ultimate salvation, of course, depends upon God, who has, however, provided religious sanction for believing in secondary causation in the Prophetic tradition "Flee from the leper as from the lion." Here, Ḥamdān Khoja was following the lead of an earlier Algerian scholar, Muḥammad b. Aḥmad al-Sharīf al-Jazā'irī (d. 1139/1727), who argued in his *The Blessing and the Consolation* (*Al-Mann wa-l-Salwa*): "The order to flee was to make it clear that it [i.e., leprosy] is one of the occasions through which God makes His habit occur by it [proximity to the sick] leading to its effects [the disease's transmission] (*allatī ajrā Allāh al-ᶜāda bi-anna-hā tufdī ilā musabbabāt-hā*). For this reason, in the order to flee is proof of secondary causation (*thubūt al-asbāb*)."[86] Both here and in the citation of other works—most notably *The Rectification of False Beliefs concerning What Is Related regarding the Plague* (*Taḥqīq al-Ẓunūn bi Akhbār al-Ṭāᶜūn*) of Marᶜī b. Jamāl al-Dīn al-Maqdisī (d. 1033/1623), a Ḥanbalī jurist from Palestine—Ḥamdān Khoja argues for the permissibility of fleeing from the plague, provided one does so with the correct intention.[87] He is aware of those who oppose his views on the plague, such as Ibn Ḥajar, but argues that the latter's denial of contagion is but one opinion on the subject and that those who are fanatical on this issue will change their mind once made aware of the evidence he has presented. The source of the confusion, he observes, is that the Prophet addressed his words to different addressees, an interpretation found in the hadith commentaries as far back as the fifth/eleventh century.[88]

In the second chapter of the *Itḥāf,* Ḥamdān Khoja turns to the question of whether it is permissible to adopt an institution developed by unbelievers (*al-kuffār*). This is hardly only an academic question. Ḥamdān Khoja was writing only a few years after the death of the great Moroccan historian, traveler, and diplomat Abū al-Qāsim al-Zayyānī (d. 1249/1833), who studied with al-Bannānī and who claimed in his *Al-Turjumāna al-Kubra* that the quarantine is a heretical innovation (*bidᶜa*).[89] Since there is no scriptural basis in either the Qur'an or Prophetic Tradition for what one is to do when approached by someone coming from a plague-struck area, Ḥamdān Khoja argued that it is necessary to turn to legal theory (*al-uṣūl*) for an answer.[90] As shown in his book's first chapter, it is permissible to believe in secondary causation; thus, once one has established causality and knows, either from a textual source or through experience, how harm occurs, it is legitimate to take steps to ward off danger. With some exaggeration, Ḥamdān Khoja notes that Europeans have been using the quarantine for centuries, in areas including those inhabited by Muslims, such as Tunis, Libya, Tétouan, and Fez, and that, for the most part, these areas have been free of epidemics. He himself had followed the rules of quarantine for more than twenty years in Algeria, and while his insight into these rules was not as deep as that of the Europeans, he and his family had remained safe. Sensitive to the loaded significance of the word *contagion,* Ḥamdān Khoja observes that out of respect for the Prophet, one should not refer to the transmission of leprosy and epidemics as contagion per se; at the same time it is necessary to emphasize that the Prophet stressed that diseases are transmissible, and not only between animals.[91]

The heart of the second chapter is taken up with a point-by-point refutation of the objections raised by those "fanatics" who obstinately reject contagion. Many of Ḥamdān Khoja's points here are innovative. Taking up the Prophetic tradition "Who infected the first?" often used by past scholars to ridicule the theory of contagion for relying on an infinite regression of causes, he points out that when one observes that sexual intercourse produces children, one does not ask when the first child was born.[92] Further, he notes, epidemics are not caused only by contagion, but as we learn from the medical literature, poisonous air can affect an individual to the point of his becoming contagious.[93] Many have raised the question—I think here of Ibn Lubb and Ibn Ḥajar—how it could be that the plague is contagious, when many who interact with the sick or wash their bodies do not become infected. Ḥamdān Khoja answers by giving the examples that sailing leads to seasickness and intercourse to the birth of children, implying that both are necessary but not sufficient causes.[94] To the question of why, if as stated by the Prophet, the plague is a mercy and a martyrdom, one should seek to avoid it, he offers his imagined interlocutors two answers: (1) there is a difference between the reward of the next world and that of this one, and, more convincingly, (2) the martyrdom attained from dying of the plague is hardly less than that of dying in battle, and as Muslims are commanded to arm themselves before battle, so too they should take every precaution to protect themselves from the plague.[95] Against the objection that it is unthinkable for a new ruling to be discovered thirteen centuries after the revelation of a law, Ḥamdān Khoja explains that the case of the quarantine is similar to that of a poisonous plant that was recently discovered and against which one needs to protect oneself.[96] Admittedly, this argument has flaws: as the Muslim community had been struggling with epidemic disease since the life of the Prophet, so the opportunity had long existed to argue for the isolation of those approaching from plague-struck areas. Nonetheless, the statement bolsters Ḥamdān Khoja's larger argument for the need of revealed law to respond to new discoveries and situations. Finally, Ḥamdān Khoja takes up the question of plague etiology and whether it is the result of the pricking of jinn, as many scholars claimed. He agrees emphatically with the widely attested agency of the jinn, adding that, epidemics being the result of inhaling corrupted air, experts (*al-ḥukamā'*) have claimed jinn are composed of these vapors.[97] In this fashion he reconciles the two most widely held theories of how the plague originates. True, it is not entirely clear how sicknesses are transmitted, but that they are is without question.

In his third chapter, Ḥamdān Khoja describes the working of quarantines in detail, basing his observations on having experienced the quarantine four times: twice in Spain, once in France, and once in Italy.[98] The only criticism he has in this generally informative and glowing description of European administrative competence is that the unbelievers fail to treat the bodies of the dead with appropriate respect.

The conclusion to his treatise opens with practical recommendations for the Ottoman sultan. These include placing a doctor in every city and village in the Ottoman Empire, in accordance with al-Ghazālī's statement that medicine is a collective obligation; preparing quarantine areas at the borders of the empire; and consulting the Europeans for advice based on their experience in the matter.[99] The last pages of the treatise discuss the fact that he has heard, while composing his treatise, that someone had recently written a treatise arguing that anyone who observes the rules of quarantine is to be considered an unbeliever. Ḥamdān Khoja appears deeply troubled by this news and speculates that the author is affiliated with a fraudulent Sufi group or is trying to appeal to that group's fanaticism. He notes that the author is implying that a number of the Prophet's Companions who advocated fleeing from the plague were unbelievers. Ḥamdān Khoja is notably not criticizing Sufism per se, and he has in fact previously in his treatise expressed openness to some Muslims engaging in *tawakkul* to a much greater degree than others, but he does believe that the unknown author has engaged in willful misconstruction of selected Qur'anic verses and weak hadith, transgressing the limits of proper religious conduct, contrary to Qur'anic precept (Q5:77). The whole affair reminds him of al-Ghazālī's tripartite division of mankind in the *Revival of the Religious Sciences:* "A man who knows and knows that he knows, he is a scholar: follow him. A man who doesn't know and knows that he doesn't know, he is ignorant: teach him. A man who doesn't know and doesn't know that he doesn't know, he is a devil: avoid him."[100] For our author, the quarantine opponent is clearly among the last group.

Ḥamdān Khoja recognizes, however, that his unnamed critic may well have a sympathetic audience, for he spends the last ten pages of his treatise marshaling a series of arguments against those who have misunderstood the Prophetic tradition "Whoever imitates a people becomes one of them." This tradition should hardly be understood, he notes, to signify that simply because unbelievers preceded Muslims in wearing "pants," or in calling them such, that they are forbidden. These extremists have confused imitation (*tashabbuh*) with similarity (*mushābaha*): after all, the fact that both water and wine are drunk out of crystal glasses does not mean that drinking water is prohibited. The issue is one of intention, and it is permitted to imitate the unbelievers insofar as one is not imitating their unbelief, although Ḥamdān Khoja stresses the difficulty of knowing the actual intention of another and the importance of thinking well of one's fellow Muslims.[101] In final refutation of the arguments of this group, Ḥamdān Khoja summarizes a treatise he has just stumbled upon by Idrīs b. Ḥisām al-Dīn al-Bidlīsī (d. 930/1524), entitled *Rejecting Epidemic-Struck Areas* (*Al-Ibā' ᶜan Mawāqiᶜ al-Wabā'*). Al-Bidlīsī was traveling from Istanbul to Alexandria when he heard that an epidemic had broken out in Egypt and decided to return to Istanbul. Criticized by the scholars of Damascus and Aleppo, he wrote this treatise to justify his decision and to describe how to protect oneself from epidemic diseases.[102] Ḥamdān Khoja approves of this treatise, but he was at first disturbed by the ending of it; al-Bidlīsī advised what Qur'anic verses one should recite into the ear of a sheep, to protect oneself from the plague before slaughtering it and eating it. This is little more than putting faith in spells, Ḥamdān Khoja notes, and is beneath the stature of a respected scholar like al-Bidlīsī. He relents, however, and observes that the Prophet did—as we saw in chapter 1—approve of good omens and that al-Bidlīsī's advice was little more than Prophetic precedent.[103] Ḥamdān Khoja ends his treatise with a plea for all his readers to consider its content and to address in writing any mistake that they find in it. Unfortunately, we do not know how the work was received or how widely it was read in Istanbul, though Ḥamdān Khoja's editor Muḥammad b. ᶜAbd al-Karīm claims that upon its completion, the author translated the *Itḥaf* into Turkish.[104]

Conclusion

In 1831, as cholera ravaged Istanbul for the first time, the Ottoman sultan Maḥmūd II, still on the defensive after the military defeats suffered in the 1820s, undertook a review of Anatolia and the Ottoman-controlled portions of the Balkans in order to estimate how many troops he might be able to assemble as he reorganized his army.[105] It emerged clearly from this study that the central part of the Ottoman Empire had suffered substantial demographic losses due to both cholera and the plague. While initial attempts were made to impose quarantines during the early 1830s—at the very time that Ḥamdān Ibn ᶜUthmān was writing his treatise—these were largely ineffective, because they took place in the absence of necessary infrastructure and organization. In 1839, following the 1838 public statement that plague was contagious and that the highest religious scholars of the empire sanctioned fleeing from it, Mahmūd II established the Imperial Council of Health. During the following decade, a quarantine system was established throughout the empire, which included—much as Ḥamdān Khoja had advised—the establishment of local sanitation offices and lazarettos. By 1850 these numbered more than sixty sites, employing several hundred health workers, and in 1853 the entire system was seen as highly effective by the French representative to the Council of Health.[106] Debates over the best way to control epidemics did, however, remain a central tension between the Ottoman Empire and European powers—especially Britain—throughout the remainder of the nineteenth century and well into the twentieth.[107]

The situation played itself out in a strikingly different fashion in the semi-independent Ottoman province of Egypt, where the Egyptian Pasha Muḥammad ᶜAlī was a firm believer in the implementation of quarantines and lazarettos, while the French doctor who directed the first Egyptian medical school, Antoine Clot, was an avid anticontagionist.[108] Despite Muḥammad ᶜAlī's respect for European medical knowledge, Clot Bey had to bow to the ruler's belief in contagion and support the work of the Sanitary Board, which regulated the quarantine. The sultan further distinguished his sanitary regime by having it administered by an Egyptian official from 1840 onward, much to the dismay of the European powers, who were used to having their diplomats play a pivotal role on the sanitary boards and who saw this as an infringement upon their trade interests.[109]

A half century later, in Morocco, where the ruler was more vulnerable to colonial influence, the implementation of the quarantine received much less support; it appears to have been implemented in a limited fashion in Tangiers and other ports by sanitary boards that were run by European delegates. In 1878, the prominent historian and jurist al-Nāṣirī (d. 1315/1897) wrote a legal opinion in which he argued not only that the quarantine was against revealed law, but also that its potential benefits paled before the harm it caused. Similarly, in his famed historical work *Al-Istiqṣā,* he sharply criticized the Saᶜidian sultan Aḥmad al-Manṣūr (rl. 1578–1603) for advising his son to flee Marrakesh upon the outbreak of an epidemic and for following European rules of the quarantine to dip letters originating in epidemic-struck areas in vinegar before reading them.[110] Al-Nāṣīrī's opposition to the implementation of the quarantine in Morocco was doubtless in part a reaction to the expansion of European control over Moroccan borders and politics. The Moroccan state, after military defeats by the French and the Spanish in 1844 and 1860, had begun to look to European countries for military as well as medical expertise.[111] Hardly naive, the Moroccan sultans of the late nineteenth and early twentieth centuries attempted to benefit from (largely) French medical knowledge without losing political capital among their people, while at the same time preventing French doctors from functioning as spies and aiding France in its colonial designs on Morocco.[112] Ellen Amster has shown eloquently how it was precisely as a result of this tense environment, in which many Moroccans looked at the Moroccan state's reliance on European doctors with suspicion, that the murder of the French doctor Emile Mauchamp led to the French invasion of the Moroccan city of Oujda in 1907, with the result that France took control of the entire country in 1912.[113] Al-Nāṣirī was then rightfully wary of the Moroccan state's motives in assenting to or promoting European sanitary procedures, although he himself presented at best a truncated understanding of the richness of Muslim writings on the subject of contagion and showed no awareness of the treatise of Ḥamdān Khoja.

Against this backdrop of politicized public debate over the proper response to contagious diseases and epidemics, what are we to make of the plague treatises examined here? Previous scholarship has depicted this tradition of scholarship as largely static or representative of a stifling orthodoxy that is variously seen to have been informed by an unchanging legal system, fatalistic Sufism, or rigid Ashʿarī theology. In this chapter I have shown that Muslim scholars discussed both plague and contagion with a wide variety of approaches and drew on all three of these discourses in often highly nuanced fashions. Naturally, the views of the authors discussed here should not be taken as representative of the inhabitants of the Middle East and North Africa as a whole, a population with whom charms and incantations were often widely popular.[114] But a consideration of the variety of approaches explored by these authors should move us, yet again, to consider the richness and depth of the Muslim scholarly tradition on an issue such as contagion, the existence of which was far from generally accepted by scholars in either the Middle East or Europe well into the nineteenth century.

Reframing Muslim and Christian Views on Contagion

IN THE NINTH/FIFTEENTH century, Ibn Marzūq al-Ḥafīd (d. 842/1438) wrote the following of being sent to the sultan of Fez in 803/1400 by the sultan of Tlemcen:

> That year there was a great epidemic in the Maghrib, and when I set off for Fez, he sent with us messengers of his, accompanied by a Christian who was with them. . . . Their intention in doing what they did was not to approach the epidemic by entering the castle [whose inhabitants had the plague]. This was their choice and I was in agreement with them. The Christian asked: "What's with these people who don't enter this place? His translator—as he didn't speak Arabic well—said to him: "They have fled from the epidemic." Then the Christian said what we were told had the following meaning: "Fleeing will not save them. There is no doubt that what God has decreed is what will be." When I heard these words, I was dismayed and confused about what I was doing, as it is well known that according to Prophetic Tradition one shouldn't approach such an area. I rejected completely that it should seem that one who had no knowledge [of hadith] and who was an unbeliever should be greater in entrusting himself to God's order and more believing in what had been decreed. I knew that it was a trial, so I advised advancing and entered [the castle], though I didn't order the others what to do.[1]

The dramatic juxtaposition of Muslim and Christian responses to the plague that Ibn Marzūq portrays in this passage would have made little sense to an earlier generation of scholars working on religious reactions to the plague, in large part due to the influence of the work of historian Michael Dols.

In 1974, while working on what became recognized as a groundbreaking book on the Black Death in the Middle East, Dols published a short article entitled "The Comparative Communal Responses to the Black Death in Muslim and Christian Societies."[2] In this article he set out a remarkably clear opposition between Christian and Muslim responses to the Black Death, discussing both the intellectual reactions and those of the respective societies in general. For Dols, Christian medical responses were characterized by a belief that miasma was the causal agent and a clear commitment to the concept of contagion.[3] Drawing primarily on secondary scholarship, Dols argued that Christians in Europe saw the plague as a punishment for their sins. As a consequence, they were increasingly attracted to millennial movements and the contemplation of the collapse of the social order. The flagellant movement attracted increased membership, and religious minorities—especially the Jews—suffered renewed and intense persecution because of the belief that they had poisoned Europe's wells.[4]

Whereas the very structure of European society was threatened by the Black Death, Dols argues that Muslim society accepted the plague as part of God's will: "For the Muslim the Black Death was part of a God-ordered, natural universe; for the Christian it was an irruption of the profane world of sin and misery."[5] The Muslim response may be characterized by the Prophetic traditions that equate the plague with martyrdom, prohibit either entering or leaving a plague-struck area, and deny contagion unconditionally. All of these tendencies were given their canonical form in Ibn Ḥajar al-ᶜAsqalānī's *Badhl al-Māᶜūn.*[6] Dols notes that Muslims "did not declare that plague was God's punishment; they did not encourage flight; and they did not support a belief in the contagious nature of plague—all of which were prevalent in Christian Europe."[7] Instead, Muslims gathered communally to pray and carried out organized processions through the streets. Traditional religious and secular authorities were not challenged, the end of time was not heralded, and religious minorities were not persecuted more than usual.[8] Seeing in the plague the will of God, Muslims did not see the disaster as a result of their own sins, and the *ᶜulamā',* as both intellectual and social elite, were able to shape and direct broader, public responses to the Black Death.[9]

For many years Dols's article, which was exceptional in its scope, remained the only reference directly addressing the topic of comparative religious responses to the Black Death. But it suffered from conceptual flaws. The greatest of these is Dols's easy equation of religion with culture, along with his claim that a comparison between Christian and Muslim reactions to the Black Death reveals "what is essential to the identity of each culture."[10] Understandably, Dols picked examples of communal behavior that strengthened his thesis, such as juxtaposing the flagellant movement in Christian Europe with processions and public prayer in the Muslim Middle East. Yet the flagellant movement was restricted to certain parts of Europe—it never appeared in Iberia—and the examples of public prayer and processions mentioned by Dols are solely from the Mashriq, specifically Cairo and Damascus. But the emphasis of Dols is on the differences between Muslim and Christian intellectual traditions and the respective behaviors that these traditions produced: Christians viewed the plague as "an individual trial," believed in contagion, and fled the plague; while Muslims emphasized social responsibility, denied contagion, and took solace in death from the plague as a form of martyrdom.[11] In order to evaluate Dols's argument and the role played by contagion within it, we need to turn to the broader question of how Christians, Muslims, and to a lesser extent, Jews, responded to the Black Death.[12]

A Misdiagnosis?

The historiographical stakes in comparing the responses of religious communities to epidemic disease are high. Before examining more general observations regarding the ways in which these three groups drew on religious sources to make sense of the plague, it is worth reiterating a theme that has run through this book. In the sixteenth and seventeenth centuries, Protestant authors argued about whether or not one had a duty to stay and tend to one's afflicted Christian brethren, and those who advocated fleeing the plague compared their opponents on occasion to Turkish Muslims.[13] Similarly, the German philosopher Leibniz (d. 1716) argued against fatalism by comparing its adherents to the Turks who failed to avoid areas struck by the plague.[14] While the views of these authors can certainly be explained in part by the ideological exigencies of the period, historians of the Black Death today have similarly differentiated between Christian and Muslim responses to the Black Death, arguing that the former accepted contagion theory and flight from the plague, while the latter did not, believing that the epidemic was decreed by God and that it was not contagious.[15] The assertion that Muslims accepted the Black Death and (more generally) the plague fatalistically and denied the plague's contagion is hardly a neutral one: it has often been taken to imply that there were scriptural or theological reasons why Muslims in general were not as open as Christians to fleeing from the plague or as willing to accept the (presumably) overwhelming empirical evidence for the plague's contagious nature. As a corollary, it is argued that any Muslim fleeing the plague and accepting its contagious nature must have been treated as a heretic and punished by the Muslim community. Here the example of Lisān al-Dīn Ibn al-Khaṭīb, the prolific and rightly celebrated Granadan vizier and scholar whose views on contagion are discussed in chapter 3, is relevant. In a plague treatise written in the aftermath of the Black Death, Ibn al-Khaṭīb argued that, despite sayings attributed to the Prophet Muhammad, the plague was in fact contagious and there was ample empirical evidence to prove it. Ibn al-Khaṭīb's conviction for heresy and his murder twenty-five years after the

Black Death is widely construed by students of medieval European history as a product of the rigid and intolerant nature of Islamic orthodoxy; and, I suspect, it encourages a general impression that scientific thought in the Muslim world was in decline.[16]

In chapter 3, I argued that Ibn al-Khaṭīb's views, far from unique, were merely a particularly strident expression of a minority view advocated openly by many Muslim jurists who believed in the transmission of disease, whether under the rubric of contagion or not.[17] Far from being considered heretical, Ibn al-Khaṭīb's opinions on the plague were debated by succeeding generations of scholars, as was seen in chapter 5 in the exchange between al-Raṣṣāᶜ and al-Mawwāq.[18] I have returned to the example of Ibn al-Khaṭīb because his case reveals that, while general views and practices relating to the Black Death can be identified with specific religious communities with some accuracy, the degree of variability of these beliefs needs to be emphasized. In addition, as will be seen below, Muslims, Christians, and Jews shared a considerable number of attitudes toward the plague.

Prayer, Procession, and Persecution

Our sources for explicitly Muslim and Jewish religious, as opposed to medical, responses to the Black Death are chiefly chronicles and plague treatises, whereas on the Christian side, we can also refer to a large number of ecclesiastical and administrative materials.[19] Broadly speaking, Christians, Muslims, and Jews believed that the Black Death was a punishment from God, sent down to punish those of them who had sinned.[20] In Christian circles, possible candidates for the sins that brought on the plague included pride, lust, impiety, simony, and licentiousness, not to mention indecent clothing and filial disobedience—though their exact nature was often left unspecified, as was the case in most Jewish writings.[21] Since the plague was indiscriminate in its victims, the massive death it brought about raised the question of theodicy: why would God cause the death of so many potential innocents? Some Christian scholars, for example, explained the death of children to the plague by referring to their failing to honor their parents or, conversely, considered their death a punishment for the sins of their parents.[22]

As for the cause of the plague, the problem for Muslims was admittedly different than for Christians, for the Prophet's Companions experienced the first pandemic in Syria in the seventh century, during the initial expansion of the early caliphate. Josef van Ess has shown how this initial encounter with the plague by

Muslim troops who were undertaking *jihād* to spread Islamic rule, and who believed that martyrdom was their reward if they died doing so, led to the equation of death from the plague with martyrdom in traditions attributed to the Prophet himself. Comparing the Muslim with the Christian response to the plague, van Ess notes that early Christian belief that the plague would result in martyrdom—as in the writings of Cyprian (d. 258)—was exceptional, whereas the early encounter with the plague in the history of Islam caused the equation of death by the plague with martyrdom to have a much more profound resonance for later generations of Muslims.[23] To be sure, the nascent Muslim community's early encounter with the plague also produced a body of Prophetic traditions that prohibited either entering or exiting a plague-afflicted area, leaving later Muslim jurists and theologians to explain how the plague should be avoided, even though death from the plague was martyrdom. Depending on the jurist, the authority of one or another part of the Prophet's legacy was emphasized, with some prominent jurists emphasizing the need to flee the plague and barely mentioning the doctrine of martyrdom, if at all.

Both Muslim and Christian communities around the Mediterranean responded to the Black Death with processions, public gatherings, and prayer. Christian communities in Europe had held penitential processions to end and ward off natural catastrophes since the ninth century, and with the arrival of the Black Death, they continued to do so, while also listening to "catastrophe sermons" given by the clergy.[24] For even though within Christian circles it was widely held that the plague was contagious, God's ability to intervene and protect the Christian community was believed to be greater than the risk posed by public gatherings.[25] In any case, the contemporary understanding of contagion was quite different from that professed by modern medicine.

For their part, Muslim communities throughout the Middle East withdrew outside their cities to fast and pray together in hopes of ending the plague. Here too, such behavior parallels ritual actions taken during other natural disasters, such as drought, when Muslim populations would gather to pray for rain.[26] Though at times debated, this action was approved by prominent supporters of the idea that the plague leads to martyrdom such as Ibn Ḥajar al-'Asqalānī (d. 1448), who noted that belief in God's decree did not imply refraining from using medicines to cure disease and that the plague was in this sense a sickness like any other.[27] In addition to listening to sermons, Muslims preferred to demonstrate their piety and penitence by listening to the recitation of the Qur'an and the public reading of the canonical collections of Prophetic Tradition, particularly that of al-Bukhārī.[28]

Believing Doctors: Medicine, Faith, and the Plague

During and following the Black Death, Christian, Muslim, and Jewish doctors and scholars wrote hundreds of treatises on the plague, drawing principally on Galenic medicine.[29] While most of these treatises are chiefly concerned with describing the plague and suggesting preventive measures and remedies, they also offer insights into the authors' understandings of the religious significance of the plague. This is of special importance for the Jewish plague treatises, to which Ron Barkai has devoted a number of articles, demonstrating not only that Jews in France and Iberia translated into Hebrew plague treatises written by Christians, but also that they composed numerous original treatises after the Black Death. Barkai shows that the majority of the Jewish treatises examined by him clearly place the origin of the plague with God, and he notes that none of these treatises describe the plague as contagious.[30] More recently, Susan Einbinder has emphasized that there were a variety of Jewish views on the plague; she believes she has found at least one reference to Jewish scholars who thought the Black Death was contagious.[31]

Jewish authors framed and introduced their discussion of the plague with biblical quotations, similar to the manner in which Muslim plague treatises make reference to both Qur'an and hadith before entering onto a description of treatment and remedies. One irony deserves to be mentioned in this context, namely that whereas Jewish authors at times refer to the plagues God sent upon Pharaoh and the Egyptians as a sign of God's ability to punish sinners, Muslim scholars at times cite a Prophetic tradition explaining that the origin of plague lies in a punishment that God sent down upon the Jews themselves long ago. Similarly, Pope Clement VI (d. 1352) noted in a mass the example of David's sin that resulted in the punishment of the people of Israel by plague (2 Sam. 24:15–17).[32]

In addition to Jewish plague treatises that are still coming to light, as we saw in chapter 6, many Muslim plague treatises continue to languish in manuscript. Considering the degree to which the foundational sources for any evaluation of religious attitudes to the plague, especially for Muslim and Jewish communities, have yet to be made available to more than a few scholars, it seems precipitous to offer any blanket generalizations regarding the attitudes of these communities.

Conclusion

The anecdote quoted at the beginning of this chapter, taken from an as-yet-unedited manuscript, is quoted by the Tunisian scholar Muḥammad Ḥasan in his extensive introduction to his 2007 critical edition of a correspondence—examined in chapter 5—between the Granadan al-Mawwāq (d. 1492) and the Tunisian al-Raṣṣā' (d. 1489).[33] Ḥasan uses this anecdote, and another one similar to it, to argue that Christians were generally fatalistic in the matter of the Black Death, whereas Muslims, while holding a diversity of views, argued for fleeing the plague and had begun instituting quarantines as early as the time of Ibn Khātima in the fourteenth century.[34] Hasan has in some ways established a mirror image of the argument made by Dols, although he draws on significantly fewer sources and ignores a substantial body of secondary scholarship that contradicts his argument. The danger of being led by a comparative framework to make broad and inaccurate generalizations is apparent in both cases.

In order to circumvent this danger, and to achieve a more nuanced approach to understanding religious responses to the Black Death, more comparative work is desirable. Stuart Borsch's 2001 work *The Black Death in Egypt and England: A Comparative Study,* which deals with the economic effects of the pandemic on both countries and offers a nuanced and detailed explanation for why Egypt emerged from it weakened and England emerged strengthened, is a model in this regard. Another example, and a promising beginning to a comparison of Byzantine and Muslim religious attitudes to the Black Death, is found in the collaborative work of Marie-Helène Congourdeau and Mohamed Melhaoui.[35] The reframing of how we approach the study of the religious and cultural history of the Black Death should not, of course, be restricted to interreligious investigations. Jussi Hanska's comparative study of how Christian communities responded to natural disasters is an excellent example of how the Black Death, a subject that doubtless will continue to fascinate students of history, can gain new life when placed into a new context.[36]

Dols's overall intention in his article was laudable. By emphasizing the differences between Christian and Muslim responses to the plague, while acknowledging that medical scholars in both Christendom and Islam shared similar understandings of the disease, he aimed to emphasize the degree to which religion is able to shape and give significance to communal responses to the Black Death.[37] In doing so, however, he minimized the wide variety of views held by both Christian and Muslim scholars and, uncharacteristically, treated the concept of contagion ahistorically, failing to note that many Muslim scholars, while avoiding the term *contagion,* supported the notion that disease may be transmitted. In recent studies, European medievalists have begun to reassess responses to the Black Death, noting that established sources of authority, both medical and spiritual, continued unchallenged following the plague.[38] In my own research on Christian Iberian responses to the plague, especially in Castile in the fourteenth century, I have found no indication of the prevalence of millennial expectations or of the breakdown of social order. In addition, it remains unclear exactly what occurred in Iberia between 1348 and 1391 to cause the change in social relations and perspectives that brought about the dramatic persecution of Jews in the latter year.[39]

In this book I have attempted to offer a more nuanced, but also qualitatively different, approach to comparative history than that offered by Dols in his article. Although there are clear differences between the discussions of contagion found in Christian and Muslim sources, with Christian scholars paying much more attention to the metaphoric implications and uses of contagion and Muslim scholars struggling with the theological implications of disease transmission, I am reluctant to characterize these two bodies of scholarship as generating or reflecting completely distinct social responses to the plague. With respect to contagion, at least, we find in both traditions an acceptance of disease transmission, while in neither is there agreement as to exactly how it occurs. In both, disease transmission is sometimes referred to as contagion (admittedly much more so in Christian sources), although the meaning of the term varies significantly and can include phenomena as discrete as the evil eye, the effects of pornography (Ibn Lūqā), and the transmission of disease from one individual to another.

Instead of attempting to extract from scholarly traditions a religious, cultural, or even civilizational identity or character, it is more useful and more accurate, I believe, to focus on the parameters within which these traditions debate and define ideas and concepts. I have here aimed to show how Muslims and Christians discussed the subject of contagion, looking at the texts they considered authoritative references, the choices they debated, the conclusions they reached, and some of the consequences of those conclusions. These two scholarly traditions are difficult to characterize definitively, for each one contained a wide variety of views and was constantly changing. Their evolving nature can be linked to their reflecting the interactions of scholars with a broader public. Both Saint Vincent Ferrer and Ibn Lubb, for example, referred to contagion and defined its significance because they understood themselves to be responsible for the public good and the nature of communal interactions. It may well be sufficient to attempt to understand the intellectual circumstances that made specific conceptions of contagion possible as well as the reasons why these conceptions remained malleable and open to change, without establishing a larger significance of the difference between Muslim and Christian views. That task, if at least partially accomplished in this book, would represent one further step in our understanding of disease in the premodern period.

Contagion in the Christian Exegetical Tradition

Given the extent to which contagion was employed as a metaphor by Christian authors in the Middle Ages, these comments can hardly constitute an exhaustive documentation of the role contagion played in the Christian tradition of biblical exegesis. Instead, this brief survey offers an impression of how the concept fulfilled varying roles in the hands of different authors. The first passage with relevance to contagion that attracted the exegetes' attention was the discussion of leprosy in Leviticus, chapters 13 and 14. For Christians in the later Middle Ages, like the Muslim authors discussed in chapter 1, leprosy was the contagious disease par excellence. Yet, readings of the biblical text have shown that the authors of Leviticus were principally concerned with issues of ritual purity and not contagion; furthermore, the disease designated by the Hebrew *ṣara'at* was not leprosy at all, but another skin disease.[1] The enforced removal of the leper from the camp for a period of at least seven days was not out of fear that the leper was contagious, nor did it have moral significance—the leper was not removed for having committed a sin. Instead, the leper, like the menstruating woman, was ritually impure and thus not allowed to rejoin the community until after being declared pure once again.

While leprosy was not described as contagious in the Bible, and neither was it linked explicitly to sin, exegetes soon saw it as signifying a punishment for transgression. This was not a tendentious interpretation. In Numbers 12, Moses's sister Miriam is struck with leprosy after criticizing her brother for having married an Ethiopian woman and subsequently, along with Aaron, claiming prophet-hood for herself. In 2 Kings 5, Gehazi, a servant of the prophet Elisha, is struck down with leprosy after engaging in simony with Naaman, a Syrian captain whom Elisha had cured of his own leprosy. In 2 Chronicles 26, the king Uzziah is afflicted with leprosy after arguing with a priest about his right to burn incense in the temple. Finally, a popular legend included in Midrashic texts said that the Jews who worshipped the Golden Calf were punished with leprosy.[2] Brody has noted that in the Midrash, Jewish commentators of the second century CE linked leprosy to sin, designating specific sins—sometimes seven, sometimes ten—as causes of the onset of the disease.[3] The degree of influence their exegesis had on later Christian authors is unclear, yet Brody points to a more immediate fashion in which Christians may have come to see leprosy as inherently connected to sin: "Of course, Christian commentators had an additional reason for linking leprosy and sin. When the Hebrew came to be translated into Greek and the Latin, the words used to translate *tameh* ("unclean") were the Greek *akathartos* and the Latin *immundus*, words which in the Middle Ages have no cultic sense, but which did have distinct moral connotations."[4] In a discussion of contagion, the relevance of equating leprosy with a state of sin, of its constituting a physical marking of sin upon the body, lies in the easy conflation of disease and immorality. Where one can be transmitted, so can the other, and perhaps both together. In the writings of the Christian authorities of late antiquity, the link between the disease and the most pressing if not most dangerous sin—heresy—was promptly made: Gregory the Great (d. 604), in his *Moralia,* saw in Jesus's healing of the ten lepers in Luke 17 a representation of heretics being brought back into the body of the Church. Their sin was for him visible upon their body, the patchiness of their skin equivalent to the mixture of good with evil within them.[5]

The second biblical passage that was later cited in considerations of contagion was 1 Corinthians 5:6–8, in which Paul warns the Corinthians of the danger of allowing those guilty of fornication to remain among them. Here, not only the dangers of tolerating sin, but also of interacting with those who have sinned, are emphasized. The verses received substantial exegetical attention during the Middle Ages and deserve to be considered in their own right. In the Vulgate they read:

> Non bona gloriatio vestra. Nescitis quia modicum fermentum totam massam corrumpit? Expurgate vetus fermentum, ut sitis nova conspersio. Sicut estis azymi. Etenim pascha nostrum immolatus est Christus. Itaque epulemur non in fermento veteri neque in fermento malitiae et nequitiae sed in azymis sinceritatis et veritatis.
>
> (Your glorying is not good. Know ye not that a little leaven leaveneth the whole lump? Purge out therefore the old leaven, that ye may be a new lump, as ye are unleavened. For even Christ our Passover is sacrificed for us: Therefore let us keep the feast, not with old leaven, neither with the leaven of malice and wickedness; but with the unleavened [bread] of sincerity and truth.)[6]

There is not here, nor is there but rarely in later exegetical texts, any explicit mention of contagion. Yet, as the exegetes explained, Paul's use of the image of flour being mixed with leaven expressed an intense concern with the danger that moral corruption would occur because of proximity to a corrupted or diseased substance. Paul had chosen the image of leaven from the Gospels, where Jesus had patiently explained to his disciples that in warning them of the leaven of the Pharisees he was not speaking literally but was referring to their doctrine (Matt. 16:6–12). Despite this reference, leaven was not depicted as inherently evil throughout the Gospels. Jesus also compared the kingdom of heaven with leaven in the case of a woman who, hiding leaven in her flour, found all of it to be leavened (Matt. 13:33; Luke 13:21).

Ambrosiaster's fourth-century commentary on the letters of Paul contains an early comment on 1 Corinthians 5:6–7.[7] There is little mention here of fornication, the sin that Paul was explicitly addressing in his letter. Instead, the passage is related to sin in a more general fashion. The author stresses that the principal danger lies in not exposing a known sin, for then it spreads to others, infecting (*contaminat*) all those who do not avoid it or reveal its existence. Hypocrites are particularly at risk, since the sin cannot infect those who do not know of its existence, only those who pretend not to know.[8] Citing Matthew 16:11, the author defines "leaven" as wrong or evil doctrine. Christians are unleavened (*azymi*), or free of the old beliefs of the pagans and the Egyptians.[9] Being unleavened is, following 1 Corinthians 5:8, likened to living in truth and sincerity.[10]

This image is more fully developed in the writings of Saint Jerome (d. 420) in his commentary on Paul's letter to the Galatians. His exegesis of Galatians 5:9, *Modicum fermentum totam conspersionem fermentat,* is worth quoting at length. After citing 1 Corinthians 5:6–8, he writes:

> Now by these words he teaches that the spiritual bread of the Church that descends from Heaven should not be violated by the interpretation of the Jews (John 6:32–41). And the Lord had warned his disciples of the same, that they should beware the leaven of the Pharisees. Which the Evangelist had clarified, adding: *But he had spoken to them of the doctrine of the Pharisees* (Matthew 16:12). Why is this another doctrine of the Pharisees, if not [because it is] following the flesh in the observation of the Law? The meaning of this is therefore: You cannot believe the few men who come from Judaea, teaching something that should be condemned as a trap. The spark of the matter is small, and can hardly be discerned, not being apparent. But if it reaches tinder (*fomitem*), and the fire acquires however little fuel, it will consume fortifications, cities, extensive fields, and (whole) regions. This leaven is also a moderate parable in a different part in the Gospel (Luke 13:21). It seems nothing, an ordinary thing. But mixed with flour it corrupts the whole dough with its power. It carries this power with it in everything with which it is mixed: and so the perverse doctrine

> through one fool soon obtains two or three in the beginning, but gradually, like a cancer, it creeps in the body and as in the proverb of the common people, the scabies of one of the flock pollutes the whole herd. Therefore the spark, as soon as it has appeared, is to be extinguished, leaven is to be moved from the vicinity of dough, rotten meat is to be cut off, and the animal with scabies is to be prevented from the pens of the sheep, so that the whole house, dough, body, and heart is not burned, corrupted, made rotten, or killed. Arius was just a spark in Alexandria. Yet because he was not immediately suppressed, the whole world is populated with his flame.[11]

Jerome eloquently uses the image of the leaven, multiplied with other examples of the transmission of corruption, to draw attention to two dangers not mentioned by Paul. The first is that of the Jews, who reject Jesus's claim to be the bread of God come down from heaven and who try to refute this through duplicitous arguments. The second is heresy, specifically that of Arius, whose error had spread throughout Christendom. There is no mention of fornication, and the sin so generally described by Ambrosiaster is defined here as entirely doctrinal, an issue of violating orthodox belief. In this, the external danger (the Jew) and the internal danger (the heretic) are conflated into one. It is dangerous to be in the proximity of either.

Judging by the images chosen by Jerome—fire, leaven, rot, disease—he believed the transmission of false beliefs occurred through proximity, without explaining exactly how this transmission came about. There is no difference here between a fire spreading and—an example that would have been familiar to Muslim scholars—transmission of scabies from one animal to another.[12] The one hint that he offers for the nature of the transmission refers to how it takes place once within the victim's body: it creeps like a cancer.[13] The same image had been used by Paul in his second letter to Timothy (2 Tim. 2:16–18), warning Timothy of the speech of two men who erred in maintaining that the resurrection had already occurred.[14] Jerome may well have also been thinking of the writings of Cyprian (d. 258), who in his *Liber de lapsis* had described the danger of speaking with men who do not believe in God: "As much as you can, flee from this type of men; with healthy caution avoid contact with the ruinous adherents [of this belief]. Their speech creeps like a cancer, their conversation leaps across like a contagion, and worse yet, subsequently this noxious and poisonous conviction kills."[15] As noted above, references abound in classical sources to the danger of proximity to those who profess unorthodox beliefs, and this danger was often glossed as a "contagion."[16] It is not surprising to find such images in the letters of Paul and the writings of Cyprian and Jerome. Of greater interest is Jerome's reading of Paul's text to bring together the danger of the Jews with that of the contemporary heresy of Arianism. Interaction with both groups was spiritually perilous and should be avoided.

Also worth noting is Jerome's choice of the word tinder (*fomes*). Writing about the sixteenth-century Italian doctor and scholar Fracastoro, Vivian Nutton has argued that he was the first to use the word *fomes* as a technical one for the intermediary substance that passed from one subject to another and thereby caused contagion.[17] While Jerome is using the word as a metaphor and not a technical term, Nutton supplies the context for the way in which the shift from one to the other may have taken place: "Equally distinctive is his term for the intermediary in the transmission of an infected substance from a sufferer to a previously healthy host—*fomes.* This choice word was a technical term in theology for the minute portion of original sin left behind after baptism, which might, at any moment, burst into the fire of concupiscence when presented with a suitably desirable object. In this context *fomes,* whose literal meaning is woodchip or tinder, is an apt metaphor."[18] Whereas Jerome had used *fomes* and *fermentum* as synonyms, here we see how later authors differentiated them. The distinction was located at the moment of baptism, when original sin was—almost—washed away. Commenting on Paul in the ninth century, the French monk Haymo Halberstatensis (d. 850) glossed the Greek word *azymi,* explaining that it meant without leaven (*zyma*) and thus without sin.[19] Christians were able to attain this state through the act of baptism and, more generally, Christ's sacrifice of himself for them. Haymo does not mention *fomes* in connection with baptism in this passage, although elsewhere he uses it metaphorically to refer to sin.[20] Demonstrating that *fermentum* did not exclusively refer to sin, he also offered an allegorical interpretation of Matthew 13:33 (and Luke 13:21): the woman Christ spoke of represented the Church, who out of a love of God and a knowledge of the Holy Trinity, preached in Asia, Europe, and Africa (the three measures of meal), so that people in all three were drawn to a faith in Christ.[21]

Underlying the exegetical discussions around the meaning of 1 Corinthians 5 was the extensive and varied symbolical importance of bread and its equivalence to the body of Christ. To understand the continued importance for Christians to be "unleavened" (*azymi*), one has to look no further than the Host and the sacrament of Communion. Exegetes following Haymo continued to refine the metaphor of leaven. In the twelfth century, the Benedictine abbot Rupert of Deutz (d. ca. 1130–35) wrote: "He teaches the baptized with a clear likeness, encouraging us to be a new dough (*conspersionem*), without leaven, through which, just as out of many grains one loaf (*panis*), out of many men one body of the Church can be made."[22] Could those who had sinned become part of this bread? Rupert was doubtful. After all, one had to be pure to be baptized. While this might seem like a paradox, needing to be without stain in order to be purified, two different sins were in fact being addressed: original sin, with which you were born, and sins you committed in your life, such the fornication against which Paul had railed. Both seem here to be glossed with *vetus fermentum,* the old leaven that one should cast out in order to begin a new life. Rupert's position on this issue becomes clearer when his stance on the Eucharist, the unleavened body of Christ, is examined. An influential figure in his time, Rupert believed sinners should not be allowed to take the Eucharist; this position was controversial and nearly resulted in his being censured.[23]

It is in the writing of a contemporary of Rupert, Hervé de Bourg Dieu (d. 1150), that we find an explicit, if vague, reference to sin as contagion. Commenting on 1 Corinthians 5 and drawing on both Jerome and Ambrosiaster, he emphasizes that one should mourn for a sinning brother and remove him from the others in order not to be polluted with his contagion.[24] Unlike Rupert, he places no restrictions on those who can be admitted to baptism or on its power to purify of sin.[25]

That the passage in Corinthians continued to have relevance for the exegetes of the twelfth century is also seen in the writings of Richard of Saint Victor (d. 1173), who argued that it took only a venial sin for the entire body to be corrupted. He compares such a venial sin to the case of a spark that causes a fire while the father of the household is sleeping, destroying all that is in the house in a matter of an hour. One must be constantly vigilant, ready to expel the least bit of sin from oneself in order to stay pure. Otherwise one would be infected, and thus corrupted.[26] Richard was similarly exacting in his discussion of the meanings of "pure" (*azymi*): many were pure in faith but not in act, and many who seemed to be pure in act were not so in intention, being hypocrites; and then there were those who were pure in intention but not of a pure state.[27]

This survey of the exegetes of 1 Corinthians 5 suggests that since the time of Ambrosiaster the subject of contagion had attracted not only continuous but also growing attention. While in the many commentaries and comments on Paul's words, it may have appeared that contagion itself had been lost in a variety of metaphors, the exegetical discussion sketched here provides a helpful basis for understanding the later elucidation of contagion in the Iberian texts examined in chapter 2.

The Presence of Ashᶜarism in the Maghrib

The Ashᶜarī school of theology (*kalām*) plays a central role in the discussions of contagion in chapters 5 and 6, but little or no background is given there on how and when this school became important for the thinkers discussed in those chapters. Before turning to the thorny issue of causality and its place in Ashᶜarī theology, I will sketch here the prevalence of Ashᶜarism in North Africa and al-Andalus in order to establish the potential influence of theology on the legal question of contagion. We can safely assume that the fatwas collected by al-Wansharīsī, such as that of Ibn Lubb, represent only a fraction of those actually handed down by the scholars of the Maghrib during this period. If it can be shown that Ashᶜarism was widely studied and taught, then it is also possible to assume that the issue of contagion was conceptualized in theological terms in fatwas that are not extant. While some scholars have argued that Ashᶜarism was a marginalized movement and that those who practiced theology were discriminated against, others have recently rejected this opinion and have shown that Ashᶜarism was widely taught and practiced in the Islamic West through the end of the Almohad period in the first half of the thirteenth century.[1] As is apparent from the discussion of the scholars examined in chapters 5 and 6, Ashᶜarism continued to offer arguments that Muslim scholars considered authoritative well into the nineteenth century.[2]

Although the great nineteenth-century Orientalist Ignaz Goldziher believed that Ashᶜarism was not studied or taught in al-Andalus until the sixth/twelfth century—perhaps following al-Maqrīzī (d. 845/1441) in crediting Ibn Tūmart (d. 524/1130) for its introduction—recent scholars have argued that the date was as much as a century earlier.[3] Early proponents of Ashᶜarism in North Africa included a teacher of the great Mālikī scholar Ibn Abī Zayd al-Qayrawānī (d. 386/996), Abū Maymūna Darrās b. Ismaᶜīl al-Fāsī (d. 357/967), as well as Abū Isḥāq b. ᶜAbd Allāh al-Qalānisī (d. 361/969) and Abū al-Ḥasan al-Qābisī (d. 403/1012). By the middle of the fifth/eleventh century, according to al-Māzarī (d. 536/1141), Ashᶜarism had become widespread in both North Africa and al-Andalus.[4] The transmission of Ashᶜarism from North Africa to al-Andalus may have been carried out by the students of Abū ᶜImrān al-Fāsī (d. 430/1038), who, in 399/1008, traveled to Baghdad, where he studied with al-Bāqillānī (d. 403/1013), the prominent Mālikī Ashᶜarī scholar. Vincent Lagardère has identified eighteen students of Abū ᶜImrān's who were from al-Andalus, some of whom played a role in the transmission of Ashᶜarism.[5] Through one of his students, Abū ᶜImrān is linked to the formation of the Berber Almoravid movement, and the chronicler Ibn ᶜIdhārī (d. 712/1312) went so far as to describe his ordering the Almoravids to leave the desert and found an empire.[6] In addition, the once prevalent view that the Almoravids discouraged and even forbade Ashᶜarism has been shown to be erroneous. While the historian al-Marrākushī (d. 668/1270) states in his *Muᶜjib* that the Almoravid ruler ᶜAlī b. Yūsuf (rl. 500/538–1106/1143) denounced *kalām* after being pressured to do so by his jurists, this claim is not supported by any other source. Al-Marrākushī seems to have conflated the caliph's supposed opposition to *kalām* with his order that al-Ghazālī's books be burned, two distinct phenomena.[7] The Almoravid political and juridical elite may well have viewed Ashᶜarism with some suspicion, but this attitude was based on the fear that *kalām* could have a detrimental effect on the general populace, not on disapproval of the discipline itself. This can be seen most clearly in the stance of Ibn Rushd al-Jadd, whom ᶜAlī b. Yūsuf queried regarding the legal status of Ashᶜarism.[8] Ibn Rushd was named "Qāḍī of the community" (*qāḍī al-jamāᶜa*) by the Almoravid ruler in 1117, and he possessed great authority within the Almoravid Empire.[9] He himself did not practice *kalām*, and in his *Muqaddimāt* he had expressed his worry about exposing the common people to the arguments of theology.[10] In the fatwa in which he responded to ᶜAlī b. Yūsuf, however, he affirmed the legitimacy of *kalām* and of those who practiced it.[11] Having been asked whether all Mālikīs were Ashᶜarīs and whether al-Bāqillānī was Mālikī, Ibn Rushd differentiated between theological belief and juridical adherence, noting that what is important when considering a scholar's legitimacy is his command of the religious sciences and the methods recognized in the *sunna*.[12] In the case of al-Bāqillānī, Ibn Abī Zayd al-Qayrawānī, and other scholars mentioned by ᶜAlī b. Yūsuf, they no doubt had mastered these foundations, and their practice of *kalām* was therefore legitimate. Here, showing characteristic juridical astuteness, Ibn Rushd went beyond labels to address what he believed to be the final criteria for membership within the *umma*.[13]

While the judgment of the empire's highest juridical authority in favor of *kalām* indicates its legitimacy in the Maghrib in the sixth/twelfth century, of even greater importance is the degree to which *kalām* can be shown to have been practiced by scholars of the period. Delfina Serrano has noted that a review of the biographies of scholars from the late fifth/eleventh century to the third quarter of the sixth/twelfth century shows that those scholars who studied *kalām* were not punished; indeed, they were entrusted with posts of responsibility.[14] Among the other proofs of the widespread acceptance of Ashᶜarism advanced by Serrano are the absence of any opposition to *kalām* in the credos of faith written by Qāḍī ᶜIyāḍ and Ibn Abī Zayd al-Qayrawānī and the popularity of the greatest practitioner of *kalām* of the age, Abū Bakr b. al-ᶜArabī (he had more than 250 students).[15] From 485/1092 to 493/1100, Ibn al-ᶜArabī had studied in the East with, among others, al-Ghazālī, author of the famed refutation of philosophy *Tahāfut al-Falāsifa.*

Before turning to the relationship between Ibn al-ᶜArabī and other Western scholars to the work of al-Ghazālī, we should remember that the study of *kalām* advanced under the Almohads. Not only did practitioners of *kalām* weather the transition from Almoravid to Almohad rule better than their colleagues, but their numbers increased as well.[16] In the past this positive shift in the diffusion of *kalām* has at times been linked to the story of Ibn Tūmart, the founder of the Almohad movement who, after studying with al-Ghazālī, was sent back to the West to spread Ashᶜarism.[17] Scholars have recently reread the relationship between al-Ghazālī, Ibn Tūmart, and Averroes and the relationship of all three thinkers to Ashᶜarism. Yet, that Ashᶜarism fared better under the Almohads than under the Almoravids remains widely accepted. The importance of al-Ghazālī here lies in his discussion of causality and in the reception of his work in the Muslim West. Al-Ghazālī's works, especially his magnum opus, *Iḥyā' ᶜUlūm al-Dīn,* had an undeniable influence on followers of Ashᶜarism in the Maghrib as well as in the Mashriq.

Al-Ghazālī's works were burned by the Almoravids in al-Andalus in 1109 at the urgings of the renowned Cordoban judge Ibn Ḥamdīn (d. 508/1114), who taught Ibn Tūmart in Cordoba before the latter journeyed east and reportedly met al-Ghazālī.[18] As with the later burning of the works of Averroes, the reasons for the burning are not entirely clear. Delfina Serrano has argued convincingly that Andalusi scholars thought al-Ghazālī was privileging mystical over legal knowledge; they felt that his writings attacked their own authority.[19] However, if he erred in his theological views, it was not because he was an Ashᶜarī, but rather because he was not enough of one.[20] Almost a century ago, Asín Palacios described the virulent criticism by al-Māzarī (d. 563/1141) of al-Ghazālī and the later refutation by al-Subkī (d. 756/1355) of al-Māzarī's objections.[21] Al-Māzarī, whose commentary on Muslim's hadith collection we encountered in chapter 1, was a Mālikī scholar whose family was originally from Sicily and who lived in Mahdiyya, in Ifrīqiya.[22] He admitted that he had not actually had the opportunity to read any of al-Ghazālī's books, but he had heard much about their contents and advanced the following criticisms: first, al-Ghazālī was guilty of methodological errors in that he cited hadiths without their *isnād*s, and in one case he claimed that *ijmā*ᶜ existed on a subject when scholarly consensus was the opposite of what he claimed. More importantly, al-Ghazālī had himself admitted that he had placed things in his books that he should have omitted and that he had drawn too much on philosophy, privileging reason over revelation.[23] As Subkī noted two centuries later, however, al-Māzarī did not count al-Ghazālī as one of the philosophers. Subkī identified the core of al-Māzarī's objections to al-Ghazālī in al-Māzarī's own adherence to Ashᶜarism and the perception that al-Ghazālī was too close to the philosophers. In al-Ghazālī's defense, Subkī stressed that al-Ghazālī had studied *kalām* before he studied philosophy and that instead of imitating the arch-philosopher Ibn Sīnā, he had condemned him as impious.[24] In closing, Subkī offered a vivid portrayal of why al-Māzarī misunderstood al-Ghazālī:

> This group [al-Māzarī and others like him], may God have mercy upon them, is nothing so much like a pious people, pure of heart, who, while inclining to leisure (*qad rakanū ilā alhuwaynā*), saw a great Muslim knight, who had taken note of a large number [of opponents] of the people of Islam. He set upon them and plunged into their ranks, surrounded by them (*fī ghamrati-him*), until he blunted their spirit, routing them, so that their group scattered in all directions, as he split the heads of many of them. It happened that a little of their blood soiled him, and when he returned untouched, they saw him wash the blood from himself. He then went with them to pray and undertake the devotions, and they imagined that he still had blood on him and denied him [their company]. This was what occurred with them and al-Ghazālī.[25]

Whereas al-Māzarī objected to al-Ghazālī's closeness to the philosophers, his Andalusian contemporary Ibn al-ᶜArabī (d. 543/1148) was suspicious of his turning to Sufism in his later years.[26] In Ibn al-ᶜArabī's view, his former teacher had given up his previous goals and aims and had committed a cardinal methodological error by choosing to read texts nonliterally. Ibn al-ᶜArabī connected al-Ghazālī's Sufism to the political danger of the Bāṭinīs in the Mashriq and various rebellious groups in al-Andalus.[27] For Ibn al-ᶜArabī, then, al-Ghazālī's books were not burned by the Almoravids because of their author's Sufism per se, but because of the political danger associated with their methodology.[28] In taking this line, Ibn al-ᶜArabī prepared the way for later critics of al-Ghazālī, such as al-Ṭurṭūshī (d. 520/1126), Ibn Sabᶜīn (d. ca. 668/1270), Ibn Taymiyya (d. 728/1328), al-Shāṭibī (d. 790/1388), and Ibn Khaldūn (d. 808/1406), in his criticisms of Sufism and Ismāᶜīlism. Of specific interest here is Ibn al-ᶜArabī's belief that al-Ghazālī had slipped into the fallacy of believing in secondary causation. Admittedly, Ibn al-ᶜArabī came to this conclusion through a circuitous route: al-Ghazālī had stated that it was possible to know what is hidden (*al-ghayb*) by reaching a state of obliteration of the self (*al-fanā'*). For Ibn al-ᶜArabī this was too similar to the philosopher's theory of prophet-hood and the posited influence of the soul and the heavenly bodies. Al-Ghazālī, according to his Andalusī student, had taken up the theory of causation (*naẓariyyat al-sababiyya*) that Ibn al-ᶜArabī himself had, in accordance with traditional Ashᶜarī doctrine, denied.[29] Following Ibn al-ᶜArabī, whose death coincided with the fall of the Almoravid Empire, the writings of al-Ghazālī found greater favor under the Almohads.[30] The issue of causality, however, is particularly vexing and continued to be the subject of much discussion following both al-Ghazālī and Ibn al-ᶜArabī.

Causality from al-Ashᶜarī to Averroes

The issue of causality was a recurring one in Ashᶜarī theology and was subject to repeated discussion and reformulation well into the early modern period. In recent decades a great deal has been written on both Ashᶜarism and the nature of causality in the writings of various Ashᶜarī thinkers, especially al-Ghazālī.[31] Much of the confusion that has surrounded the issue of causation may stem from the fact that many thinkers seem to have admitted secondary causation in some scenarios while not in others. Indeed, no Ashᶜarī thinker offered an absolute denial of all causation, though some may have come close to doing so. One way to understand the Ashᶜarī stance on causality is to compare it to Ashᶜarī thinkers' better-known doctrine of *kasb,* or the degree to which man shares with God the responsibility for his actions. As in the case of causality, the issue for Ashᶜarī theologians was to preserve the doctrine of the unity of God, who in all cases must be seen as the cause of each and every action. In order to accomplish this while at the same time not denying man's responsibility for his acts, al-Ashᶜarī stressed that God created man's ability to cause acts, but not the acts themselves.[32] In this manner man can be seen to share in his actions through the power that God created in him, and to a limited degree at least, man represents here a case of secondary causality: for al-Ashᶜarī, man's generated causality (*qudra muḥdatha*) is the attribute that God creates in him at the moment that a given act takes place.[33] For a brief instant, then, man is able to use this attribute to take an action that is not the direct result of God's intervention but instead passes through man.[34] Nevertheless, there is an important distinction to be made between secondary causes in the case of man and in the rest of nature: "For the kalâm, the only true efficient causality is that of the agent who knowingly intends and wills his act and *kasb/iktisâb* is thus used to describe the relationship of such a created agent to his act, as opposed to those events which belong to no such agent."[35] The existence of secondary causality, understood as God's giving something the power of causation, is not applicable to nonhuman actors, including, for example, disease.

Ashᶜarism's solution to the perceived problem of causality in the natural world is the concept of custom (*al-ᶜāda*). It is God's custom to have wool burn when brought near flame, or to have some animals become sick when brought near other animals, but the perceived effect has nothing to do with the properties of flame or the ability of a disease to transmit itself. Instead, it is merely God's habit to cause these things to occur in this fashion. This concept is ascribed to the Ashᶜarites as early as Ibn Ḥazm (d. 456/1064), although it was later attributed to them as far back as al-Ashᶜarī himself.[36] Custom in itself does not, of course, completely rule out secondary causation. It may, after all, be possible for God's habit of causing sickness to occur in the vicinity of sick animals to be construed as his working through these animals and thus having them function as intermediate causes.[37] Yet this line of argumentation ran against the impulse behind the introduction of the concept: a desire to preserve the unity of God while denying any validity to the arguments of natural philosophers, or believers in natural law. God's custom rests at the heart of what has come to be known as Ashᶜarī occasionalism: in its fully developed form, the belief that God creates each event and object every instant and that there is no causal relation between one moment and the next. Central to occasionalism is a deep skepticism regarding sensory perception and a conviction that the real cause of an event is unseen and can be arrived at only through an understanding of how God structures existence. Scholars have struggled with exactly what Ashᶜarī authors meant by the term *ᶜāda,* especially in the influential work of al-Ghazālī, from whose writings the example of the wool and the flame was taken.

For many modern scholars, al-Ghazālī is the proponent par excellence of Ashᶜarism's rejection of secondary causation. In his study of al-Ghazālī's doctrine that ours is the best of all possible worlds, Eric Ormsby writes: "Whereas Muslim theologians virtually unanimously deny that there is any necessary connection between cause and effect—'the connection between what is deemed a cause in the habitual course of events (*fi-l-ᶜādah*) and what is deemed an effect is not necessary (*ḍarūrī*) in our opinion,' states al-Ghazālī—they do not thereby accept a universe surrendered to blind chance. Rather, the universe is the direct effect of the divine will. Whatever exists is created by God without any intermediary agency, and it is created instant by instant. What to us appears to be continuity and continuance in the course of things is in actuality the result of God's continuous creation, atom by atom, and instant by instant, of all existing things."[38] Even before Ormsby wrote these lines in 1984, scholars had questioned whether al-Ghazālī had been fairly interpreted on the issue of causality, and others have more recently seconded their doubts.[39] The passages of al-Ghazālī advanced by various authors to make their case differ from each other, although for the most part the debate has centered on the seventeenth chapter of al-Ghazālī's *Tahāfut al-Falāsifa,* in which he takes Aristotelian philosophy to task for failing to understand causality. For Courtenay, al-Ghazālī posited two theories of causality, in the second of which God creates in each cause a quality that leads to an effect and which, if not impeded, will regularly cause this effect.[40] This is not to be understood as a necessary relationship: it is one chosen by God and could be changed at any moment. Still, according to Courtenay, we have here the basis for claiming that, with caveats, al-Ghazālī was open to the idea of a natural order that possesses a limited capability for secondary causation. Focusing on the *Tahāfut,* but drawing also on several other works of al-Ghazālī, including the *Iḥyā',* Goodman has argued that while al-Ghazālī was critical of the philosophers, he rejected the atomism of classic Ashᶜarī occasionalism. Instead of accepting the notion of eternal Aristotelian natures (*ṭabīᶜa*) that define forms, he posits created natures (*khalqa*) that have effects on each other as long as one remembers that the first and true cause of each effect is God.[41] Following Goodman—and this is a point to which I will return—if al-Ghazālī is to be understood as an Ashᶜarī, we need to understand Ashᶜarism far more broadly that we have to date, and to separate it from a narrowly defined occasionalism.[42]

With a different emphasis, Alon has shown that al-Ghazālī accepted the existence of nonnatural intermediary factors such as angels, while at the same time saying that God created miracles though a manipulation of natural attributes: a prophet thrown into a fire is protected by God's changing the physical qualities of the fire so that it is no longer hot or by making the body of the prophet resistant to fire.[43] Here al-Ghazālī seems to be preserving the concept of a being's "nature" under a different name: quality (*ṣifa*), which is changed by God when he wishes but which normally behaves according to the attributes given to it by God. Similarly, Wolfson has shown how al-Ghazālī at times uses the concept "condition" (*sharṭ*) instead of "cause" (*sabab*, *ᶜilla*).[44] Drawing on Goodman's article, Perler and Rudolph, in their extensive survey of occasionalism in Muslim and European thought, have argued that al-Ghazālī denied the atomistic aspects of occasionalism and accepted the Aristotelian notion that forms possess natures, in a synthesis of Ashᶜarism and philosophy.[45] Halevi has described a broad acceptance of causality on al-Ghazālī's part, arguing that he accepted a form of natural causality in all but three topics: the world's creation, God's attributes, and the resurrection of bodies.[46] Even in these cases, Halevi notes, al-Ghazālī did not rule out God's working through intermediaries.[47] Similarly, Griffel, drawing on Frank's more recent work, has shown how al-Ghazālī understood that phenomena such as a person's belief were the result of a series of secondary causes.[48] Finally, looking beyond the *Tahāfut* to *Al-Maqṣad al-Asna* and *Al-Iqtiṣād fī l-Iᶜtiqād,* McGinnis has emphasized that al-Ghazālī advocated a modified occasionalism and differentiated between created forms possessing active and passive powers, denying the former and affirming the latter in order to maintain the possibility of scientific knowledge alongside God's actualization of each form's potential to affect others.[49] Most recently, Griffel returned at length to the subject of causality in al-Ghazālī's thought in his monograph on the scholar, *Al-Ghazālī's Philosophical Theology.* Here, he gives a useful overview of the debate on the subject of al-Ghazālī's views on cosmology and offers an rewarding examination of al-Ghazālī's use of the simile of the water clock to explain his understanding and support of secondary causality.[50]

The fact that these authors advance different proof texts and rationales to prove al-Ghazālī's belief in causality testifies that al-Ghazālī never clearly expressed a comprehensive view favoring secondary causality—at least, not as most understand it today.[51] If he had, it would be hard to understand why his works were—and for some scholars continue to be—connected to traditional understanding of occasionalism. One explanation for why al-Ghazālī expressed himself in such an equivocal fashion was noted and criticized by al-Māzarī, as mentioned above: al-Ghazālī acknowledged that he had included things in his writings (in this case the *Iḥyā' ᶜUlūm al-Dīn*) that he should not have. Al-Ghazālī's admission was perhaps connected to his writing for multiple audiences, in a similar style to his later exponent and critic Averroes.[52]

Writing in the decades following al-Ghazālī's death, his former student Ibn al-ᶜArabī took a decidedly clearer stance on the issue of secondary causation.[53] Using al-Ghazālī's example of an object that burns when brought near a fire, Ibn al-ᶜArabī admitted that there were observable habitual occurrences, but he denied that the perceived causes had any real effect. For him, as for many Ashᶜarīs, if something does not possess knowledge and will, it can not be considered able to cause anything. What our senses convey to us is only the perception of association (*iqtirān*), not a series of causal links. Those who believe in the connection of individual events are either ignorant, in the case of the masses, or unbelievers, like the philosophers and the astrologers.[54] In this classification, we may have a brief glimpse of the noneducated elites' belief in causality. Whereas the mistake of the masses is to give all too easy credence to their perceptions, the error of the natural philosophers and the philosophers is a belief in the character (*al-ṭabᶜ*) or nature (*al-ṭabᶜiyya*) of things.

In denying the independent existence of the natures of objects, Ibn al-ᶜArabī was drawing on a series of discussions in Islamic theology that extended as far back as the third/ninth-century debates between the Muᶜtazilīs and their opponents. As Marie Bernard has observed, "La notion de nature est en réalité une certain manière de concevoir et de résoudre le problème de la causalité."[55] Although varied understandings of the concept of nature did help many Muᶜtazilīs to explain the relationship between acts, their approaches were rejected by Ashᶜarism in the fourth/tenth century.[56] While each Ashᶜarī thinker presented his own critique of "those who believe in natures" (*aṣḥāb al-ṭabāʾīᶜ*), it is worth describing that of al-Bāqillānī (d. 403/1013), whose rejection of the natural philosophers was cited by Ibn al-ᶜArabī and whose writings were among the first Ashᶜarī works to reach al-Andalus and the Maghrib. In his *Kitāb al-Tamhīd,* al-Bāqillānī argued as follows against the power of the concept of nature to explain causality:[57]

- A determining cause (*maᶜnā*) is either existent or nonexistent.
- If it is nonexistent, it cannot produce existents.
- If it is existent, it is either created or uncreated.
  - If it is uncreated, it can cause only uncreated, that is eternal, effects; the world would then be eternal, coexistent with the nature that created it; since this is impossible, the nature that created effects cannot have been uncreated.
  - Therefore we understand that God is the eternal determining cause but that his acts have a place in time.
- This does not mean that God is the determining cause of men's acts (to avoid this problem, Bāqillānī relies on the doctrine of *kasb*).
- If you say that the creating eternal nature is alive, knowing, and powerful, then you are right, for it is God, the creator of the world, and while the law (*sharᶜ*) forbids one from calling God nature, reason does not.
- If you argue that it is a created nature that causes things, you invoke an infinite series of created natures, which is impossible because this will never reach an uncreated nature.

In al-Bāqillānī's refutation of the existence of other natures besides God, we can see the results of the previous two centuries of theological debate in the Muslim world: whereas the Muᶜtazilīs and the philosophers proposed that the world is eternal, the traditionists and later the Ashᶜarīs argued forcefully that only God was eternal, thereby emphasizing the radical difference between the Creator and his Creation. Part of this differentiation lies in the ability to be a true agent, for this role is limited to God. Only he is beyond contingency and thus capable of true knowledge and the ability to manifest an independent will. Any attempt to challenge this view by introducing an understanding of natures that can function as intermediary or secondary causes needs either to be quite subtle or to propose an acceptable alternative that does not threaten the unity of God.[58] Both of these conditions were fulfilled in the writings of Averroes (d. 595/1198), whose observations on the subject of causality, however, had little if any effect on his contemporaries or on subsequent generations of scholars.[59]

Despite Averroes's stinging criticism of al-Ghazālī's and Ashᶜarism's views of causality, Frank Griffel has recently stressed the similarities between the two thinkers.[60] In part, the similarities are explained by political context. Averroes was twenty-three in 1149, when the Almohads took Cordoba from the Almoravids, and he quickly sought out a place in the new order, aligning himself with Almohad ideology. During his scholarly career, he wrote several works, none of them extant, on the writings of the Almohad founder Ibn Tūmart; and in his commentary on Plato's *Republic,* he condemned the Almohads' predecessors, the Almoravids.[61] During his lifetime, Averroes served the Almohads both as judge (*qāḍī*) in Seville (1169–71) and as doctor to the Almohad caliph Abū Yaᶜqūb Yūsuf from 1182 to the latter's death in 1184. While it is still unclear why he fell out of favor in 1195, when his books were burned in Cordoba and he was exiled to Lucena, the episode is now considered as more an aberration than an indicator of a contemporary evaluation of his scholarship.[62] In the event, he was restored to a position of respect and authority before his death in Marrakesh in 1198.

In his study of Averroes's life, Urvoy has downplayed the link between Ibn Tūmart, the founder of the Almohad movement, and al-Ghazālī, emphasizing instead the similarities between Ibn Tūmart and Averroes.[63] A different scenario is presented by Griffel, who links Ibn Tūmart to, if not al-Ghazālī, then the intellectual environment of the Niẓāmiyya *madrasa* in Baghdad, where al-Ghazālī taught.[64] Although Griffel comments on notable differences between Ibn Tūmart's writings and the Ashᶜarism he encountered during his time in Baghdad, he shows a clear connection between the Ashᶜarism taught by al-Ghazālī, Ibn Tūmart's indebtedness to Ashᶜarī theology, and the promulgation of al-Ghazālī's works under the Almohads. Regardless of the general climate of the time, however, there is little doubt that Averroes held a low opinion of Ashᶜarīs in general and of their rejection of causality in particular.

Whereas the occasionalism propounded by many Ashᶜarīs sees God intervening at each and every moment, Averroes linked his belief in the eternal nature of the world to the eternal nature of the secondary causes used by God, each of which possesses its own nature.[65] The extent to which Averroes parted company with Ashᶜarī theology can be seen in his emphasis on how a denial of secondary causation would signify a denial of the possibility of knowledge itself: for how can one know anything if not through its causes? Here Averroes is rejecting the skepticism expressed by Ashᶜarism regarding sensory perception; he is affirming instead a remarkable optimism regarding the possibility of human knowledge. In the *Faṣl al-Maqāl,* a fatwa on the legal status of philosophy, he showed the extent of this optimism in his understanding of Q3:7, which reads as follows: "It is He who sent down to thee the Book; In it are verses basic or fundamental (Of established meaning); They are the foundation of the Book: others are not of well-established meaning. But those in whose hearts is perversity follow the part thereof that is not of well-established meaning, seeking discord, and searching for its hidden meanings, but no one knows its true meanings but God and those who are deeply rooted in knowledge. They say "We believe in the Book; the whole of it is from our Lord:" and none will grasp the Message except men of understanding."[66] By deciding to read "God *and* those who are deeply rooted in knowledge," and not ending the sentence after "God," as did the majority of commentators, Averroes raises the possibility that human knowledge can reach a level near to that of God. That is, a complete understanding of the Qur'an and thus of the world itself lies within the grasp of man. Given this view, it is easy to see why Averroes would stress the importance of a belief in secondary causation. In addition, had God not made it clear in the Qur'an that he works through intermediate causes when he declared that he created man from a blood clot?[67] For those who are able to attain the necessary level of knowledge, it is necessary to try to understand the nature of reality. By denying causality, the Ashᶜarī theologians were arraying themselves against an obligation imposed on the knowledgeable by God. Because they insisted that theirs was the only legitimate way of interpretation, they could legitimately be referred to as "oppressors of the Muslims."[68]

Conclusion

Averroes's views on causation and theology were exceptional and found little resonance among other scholars of the Almohad Empire and their successors.

He considered himself a philosopher, and the philosophers of his time, few as they were, chose a path of outward conformity combined with personal inquiry.[69] Theologians of the seventh/thirteenth–ninth/fifteenth centuries in al-Andalus and North Africa paid little attention to Averroes's work and continued to transmit Ashᶜarī occasionalism. Their understanding of what this occasionalism entailed and whether it was compatible with secondary causation, however, varied. As discussed above, many current scholars have argued that al-Ghazālī was able to incorporate an understanding of natural causation within Ashᶜarism, and later jurists such as al-Yūsī (d. 1102/1691), al-Fīlālī (d. after 1252/1836), and Ḥamdān Khoja (d. ca. 1258/1842) were able to make similar arguments, though none of them drew explicitly on al-Ghazālī in this. The ability of Ashᶜarism to encompass nuanced understandings of secondary causation, which nonetheless affirm God as the only true efficient cause, has largely been overlooked in contemporary scholarship. In part, this lapse can be attributed to the paucity of contemporary studies of Islamic theology after the seventh/thirteenth century.[70] In part, however it is also due to an apologetic desire, often on the part of Arab scholars, to reject Ashᶜarī occasionalism as a cause for the perceived intellectual stagnation of the Arab world in the nineteenth and twentieth centuries. Faced with the challenge of colonialism and its argument for Europe's intellectual superiority over the Muslim world because it championed rational empiricism, it was far easier for Arab intellectuals to look back to the figure of Averroes as an Arab rationalist whose thought had sadly been neglected than to tease out the heritage of Ashᶜarī thinkers who had affirmed natural causation.[71]

Preface

1. Classic examples include Crosby, *Columbian Exchange;* McNeill, *Plagues and Peoples;* and Diamond, *Guns, Germs, and Steel.* An interesting exception is Horden and Purcell, *Corrupting Sea,* an admirable geographical and environmental history of the Mediterranean, which barely mentions disease.

2. The basis for the following comments is Reilly, *Medieval Spains,* chaps. 1 and 2.

3. It is possible that there were Arians in Iberia before the arrival of the Visigoths. There was certainly an awareness of the doctrines of Arianism among the Catholic clergy. See Hanson, *Search for Doctrine of God,* 519–26.

4. This is something of a simplification. The literature on the subject of the relationship between reason and revelation is enormous. One of many good places to begin reading is Edward Grant, *God and Reason in the Middle Ages* (Cambridge: Cambridge University Press, 2001).

5. For a review of the many meanings of "al-Andalus," see Stearns, "Representing and Remembering al-Andalus."

6. The now classic study on this topic is Menocal, *Ornament of the World,* which, though well written, is unfortunately the result of the projection of contemporary fantasies onto medieval Iberia. In this regard, Fletcher, *Moorish Spain,* provided a much more accurate survey a decade earlier. Most recently, Maya Soifer has offered an incisive critique of the term *convivencia,* which characterized much of the twentieth-century writing on religious interaction in medieval Iberia. See Soifer, "Beyond Convivencia."

Introduction. Contagion and Causality in the Study of Premodern Muslim and Christian Societies

Epigraphs: Luther, "Whether One May Flee," 127; Quoted in Noordegraaf, "Calvinism and the Plague," 27.

1. See especially Bashford and Hooker, *Contagion;* and Conrad and Wujastyk, *Contagion.*

2. See Cunningham, "Transforming Plague"; and Pelling, "Meaning of Contagion."

3. See the bibliographies in the cited work of Cunningham, Carter, and Worboys, as well as in the more recent article of Brown, "From Foetid Air to Filth."

4. Sontag, *Illness as Metaphor* (1988), 61. See also chapter 2 of this volume.

5. See Carter, *Rise of Causal Concepts.*

6. Ibid., 1.

7. Michael Worboys has noted as well that doctors in the 1860s were usually averse to relying on general principles, privileging instead empirical practices. See

Spreading Germs, 28. It is worth noting, however, that Carter and Worboys have substantially different approaches to the subject; they differ especially on the question of the definition and importance of "theory" in the history of medicine. Compare Carter, *Rise of Causal Concepts,* 6–9, with Worboys's review of Carter's book in the *Bulletin of the History of Medicine.*

8. Carter, *Rise of Causal Concepts,* 126, emphasis in original. Carter's remarks regarding causation are striking, and I will return to them.

9. My characterization of this debate here is abbreviated and simplistic. For greater detail and further references, see Hamlin, "Predisposing Causes," 44–49; Worboys, *Spreading Germs,* 42; and Cooter, "Anticontagionism."

10. See Arrizabalaga, Henderson, and French, *Great Pox,* 244–50; the informative historical overview of developments in the field of medical history in Arrizabalaga, "Problematizing Retrospective Diagnosis"; and the excellent articles of Vivian Nutton in the bibliography.

11. Ibn al-Khaṭīb is discussed at length in chapter 3.

12. See Panzac, *La peste,* 283–86.

13. Perler and Rudolph, *Occasionalimus.*

14. For a brief overview of the context in which Muᶜtazilī thought arose, see Blankinship, "Early Creed."

15. See Perler and Rudolph, *Occasionalismus,* 23.

16. Ibid., 31–34.

17. Ibid., 39–41.

18. Ibid., 44.

19. Ibid., 51–58.

20. For an overview of recent scholarship on Ashᶜarism in the Maghrib in the centuries leading up to the Black Death, see appendix B.

21. The question of al-Ghazālī's stance on the issue of causality has been hotly debated in recent decades. I discuss this issue at greater length in appendix B, arguing that al-Ghazālī accepted secondary causation while emphasizing God's ability to intervene at any moment. I am principally following Perler and Rudolph, *Occasionalismus,* 73–105. For an opposing view, see Dallal, "Ghazali and the Perils of Interpretation," 782–86.

22. The argument offered by G. R. Hawting that Islam emerged into a largely monotheistic environment and that references to polytheism in the Qur'an and Islamic tradition are to be understood as a metaphoric polemic against Christianity and Judaism does not detract from the fact that polytheism was viewed as a grave danger by early generations of Muslim scholars. See Hawting, *Idea of Idolatry.*

23. Perler and Rudolph note that al-Ghazālī's stance on causality had little impact on later Ashᶜaris (*Occasionalismus,* 106), although their survey stops well before al-Yūsī. For further discussion of Ashᶜarism, see chapter 5.

24. This removed occasionalism from the original atomistic framework used by the Muᶜtazila. See Perler and Rudolph, *Occasionalismus,* 134, 249, 258.

25. Ibid., 15.

26. See Cunningham and Grell, *Four Horsemen,* 284–88.

27. Luther, "Whether One May Flee," 121–23. To use terms taken from Islamic law, Luther defined taking care of the sick in a time of plague as a collective, not an individual, duty: if some fulfilled it, others were free to flee. Regarding the source of

the plague, Luther mentions the "filth" of Wittenberg and the actions of some who, inspired by the devil, would try to spread the disease among their fellow men (133).

28. Luther writes: "By the same reasoning a person might forego eating and drinking, clothing and shelter, and boldly proclaim his faith that if God wanted to preserve him from starvation and cold, he could do so without food and clothing" (ibid., 131).

29. See Stearns, "Contagion in Theology and Law." This article is based on material presented here in chapters 3 and 5.

30. Noordegraaf, "Calvinism and the Plague," 28.

31. See Grell, "Conflicting Duties," 139–40.

32. Noordegraaf, "Calvinism and the Plague," 27–28.

33. For a comparison between sixteenth-century Protestant and Catholic writings on the plague, see Klairmont, "Problem of the Plague."

34. An additional reason is to be found in my own academic training, which is in the field of Near Eastern studies.

Chapter 1. Contagion in the Commentaries on Prophetic Tradition

Epigraph: McNeill, *Plagues and Peoples,* 188–89. McNeill relied largely upon Michael Dols's dissertation, "The Black Death in the Middle East" (Ph.D. diss., Princeton University, 1971); and Jacqueline Sublet's article "La peste," on Ibn Ḥajar al-ᶜAsqalānī, for his discussion of the Muslim response to plague. See McNeill, *Plagues and Peoples,* 336.

1. Al-Khaṭṭābī, *Al-Ṭibb wa-l-Aṭibbā' fī-l-Andalus al-Islāmiyya,* 2:188. Compare the text and translation given by Müller in Ibn al-Khaṭīb's "Ibnulkhatîbs Bericht über die Pest," 2:6–8, 18–21. I consider Ibn al-Khaṭīb and his treatise on the plague at greater length in chapter 3. Unless otherwise noted, all translations in this book are my own.

2. Dols, *Black Death,* 93–94; and Ullmann, *Die Medizin im Islam,* 246–47. Ullmann glosses Ibn al-Khaṭīb in a slightly different fashion in his *Islamic Medicine,* 95–96. There he notes that Ibn al-Khaṭīb's belief in contagion was extraordinary only because of the strength of the conviction with which it was professed and that his true contribution lay in distinguishing the plague from other epidemic diseases.

3. See, for example, al-Bazzāz, *Tārīkh al-Awbi'a,* 393, where he writes of the absence of a belief that jinn caused plague in the writing of Ibn al-Khaṭīb's North African contemporary Ibn Haydūr. For another analysis of Ibn al-Khaṭīb as a lone voice of reason, see Congourdeau and Melhaoui, "La perception de la peste," 110. For this last reference I am indebted to Peter Brown.

4. On the process of this canonization, see Brown, *Canonization of al-Bukhārī and Muslim.*

5. I see the collecting of Prophetic traditions and the writing of commentaries on these collections as largely polemical. By polemical I mean here that the collecting and commenting on Prophetic Tradition, as well as the genre of explaining apparent contradictions in the Prophetic Tradition, were primarily directed against those who attacked the validity of that tradition. Thus, I suggest that Vardit Tokatly's classification of al-Khaṭṭābī's *Aᶜlām al-ḥadīth* as a polemical treatise and *therefore* not primarily a commentary may be a false distinction. Tokatly's other observations on the difference between al-Khaṭṭābī's project and that of later commentators are valuable, especially

in describing how the nature of the opponents of the scholars of Tradition differed according to author. Tokatly, "*A^c lām al-Ḥadīth* of al-Khaṭṭābī."

6. I have borrowed the term *hadith folk* from Melchert, "Piety of the Hadith Folk"; he, in turn, took it from Marshall Hodgson's *Venture of Islam.*

7. Those of the hadith folk who did not reject Ash^c arite theology were able to draw upon its methods, well developed in the debates against those whom the Ash^c arites suspected of anthropomorphism. See, for example, Ibn Fūrak's *Bayān Mushkil al-Aḥādīth,* 31/30 of the Arabic/German.

8. See van Ess, *Der Fehlschritt des Gelehrten,* 296–304. See also van Ess, "Ein unbekanntes Fragment des Naẓẓām"; and Strohmaier, "Die Ansteckung."

9. A more complete exploration of early Islamic views on the status of augury would also have to include magic (*siḥr*) and soothsaying (*kihāna*), both of which appear here only tangentially.

10. Van Ess's recent *Der Fehltritt des Gelehrten* is very much an example of the opposite approach.

11. See Edward Lane's entry on ṭ-y-r, in his *Arabic-English Lexicon,* where he writes: "For the Arabs used to augur evil from the croaking of the crow, and from birds going towards the left . . . and *ṭiyara* is an inf. n. [or rather a quasi inf. n.] of *taṭayyara* and signifies auguration of evil. . . . The Arabs used to say, to a man or other thing from which they augured evil . . . *ṭā'ir Allāh lā ṭā'iru-ka* [the quotation is from the *Tāj al-^c Arūs*] . . . meaning *What God doth and decreeth, not what thou dost and causest to be feared.*"

12. While *ṭiyara* in this meaning is at times used interchangeably with *shu'm,* only rarely is *fa'l* replaced with *yumn.* See Ibn al-Athīr, *Jāmi^c al-Uṣūl,* 8:397, where Ibn al-Athīr cites a tradition from al-Tirmidhī: "The Prophet of God said: No evil fortune (*lā shu'm*). And good fortune (*al-yumn*) may be in houses, women, and horses." This is the only tradition I have found that states that good and not evil fortune may be found in houses, horses, and women (the tradition is found in the 58th section of al-Tirmidhī's book on *adab*). For an example of the exchangeability of *ṭiyara* and *shu'm,* see al-Bukhārī, *Ṣaḥīḥ,* 5:2171.

13. I have given here a composite version, which contains all the phenomena whose existence was denied. Individual traditions contain various subsets of the list given above. I have not found a tradition that contains all of these at the same time. See Ibn Ḥanbal, *Musnad,* 3:357, 431; al-Bukhārī, *Ṣaḥīḥ,* 5:2177; Muslim, *Ṣaḥīḥ,* 4:1744; Ibn Māja, *Sunan,* 2:1170–71. For a definition of these phenomena (except the evil omen), see the discussion of the contagion traditions below.

14. See Ibn Ḥanbal, *Musnad,* 3:90; and Ibn Māja, *Sunan,* 2:1170.

15. In the following examples, an alternate wording is often found alongside the one given in the text: *lā ṭiyarata wa-yu'jibunī al-fa'l.* See al-Ṣan^c ānī, *Al-Muṣannaf,* 10:22; Ibn Ḥanbal, *Musnad,* 3:373; 4:237, 262, 308, 346, 355, 500; al-Bukhārī, *Ṣaḥīḥ,* 5:2171, 2178; Muslim, *Ṣaḥīḥ Muslim,* 4:1745–46; Abū Dāwūd, *Sunan,* 3:16. In addition the following variant is of interest because it occurs only here, as far as I can tell: from Suhayl from a man from Abū Hurayra: "That the Prophet of God, peace be upon him, heard a word that pleased him and said: We have taken your good omen from what you said [*min fīka*]." Al-Tirmidhī, *Al-Jāmi^c al-Ṣaḥīḥ,* 4:161.

16. Al-Ṣan^c ānī, *Al-Muṣannaf,* 10:21, where a group of the Prophet's Companions

ask him about going to soothsayers (*kuhhān*) and are told not to do so. Compare Muslim, *Ṣaḥīḥ Muslim,* 4:1748; and Abū Dāwūd, *Sunan,* 3:16, where the generic "Companions" is replaced by the Companion Muᶜāwiya b. al-Ḥakam al-Sulamī. In Muslim, *Ṣaḥīḥ Muslim,* 4:1748, we find that if one has gone to a soothsayer (*ᶜarrāf*), one's prayers will not be accepted for forty nights.

17. Al-Ṣanᶜānī, *Al-Muṣannaf,* 10:22; Abū Dāwūd, *Sunan,* 3:15. There was some confusion as to what *ṭarq* referred to exactly. Abū Dāwūd notes: ᶜAwf said: "*Al-ᶜiyāfa* is divination (*zajr*) from birds and *al-ṭarq* is the line (*al-khaṭṭ*) which is drawn on the ground" (3:15). See also Lane, *Arabic-English Lexicon,* under *ṭ-r-q*, where he equates it with pessomancy, the use of pebbles for purposes of divination.

18. Muslim, *Ṣaḥīḥ Muslim,* 4:1750; and al-Bukhārī, *Ṣaḥīḥ,* 5:2172–73.

19. Al-Ṣanᶜānī, *Al-Muṣannaf,* 10:23; Ibn Māja, *Sunan,* 2:1170–71; Abū Dāwūd, *Sunan,* 3:16; al-Tirmidhī, *Al-Jāmiᶜ al-Ṣaḥīḥ,* 4:161.

20. Ibn Ḥanbal, *Musnad,* 1:380, 2:535; al-Bukhārī, *Ṣaḥīḥ,* 5:2171, 2177; Muslim, *Ṣaḥīḥ Muslim,* 4:1746–47; Abū Dāwūd, *Sunan,* 3:18. See also Ibn al-Athīr, *Jāmiᶜ al-Uṣūl,* 8:397. There are also a small number of traditions in which it is mentioned that an earlier prophet used to be able to foretell the future by drawing lines. Al-Ṣanᶜānī, *Al-Muṣannaf,* 10:22; Muslim, *Ṣaḥīḥ Muslim,* 4:1748–49.

21. Abū Dāwūd, *Sunan,* 3:18.

22. On the importance of names as good omens in early Islam, see Kister, "Call Yourself by Graceful Names," esp. 11–14.

23. Ibn Ḥanbal, *Musnad,* 2:688. It is worth noting that the tradition denounces envy (*ḥasad*) even as it confirms the evil eye. For a similar denial of the power of envy, see al-Ṣanᶜānī, *Al-Muṣannaf,* 10:22, where it is refuted along with the power of thinking poorly of others. The reality of the evil eye is widely attested in the hadith collections (see, for example, Bukhārī's chapter on medicine in *Ṣaḥīḥ*). For later Christian conceptions of the evil eye, see chapter 4.

24. Abū Dāwūd, *Sunan,* 3:18–19.

25. Al-Ṣanᶜānī, *Al-Muṣannaf,* 10:21. Here the Prophet says of seeing omens in the flight of birds: "That is something you find in your souls; it does not hinder you." A similar tradition is found in Muslim, *Ṣaḥīḥ Muslim,* 4:1748–49.

26. Al-Ṣanᶜānī, *Al-Muṣannaf,* 10:22.

27. Ibid., 21. The opinion of Ibn ᶜAbbās is given to the effect that if one stays after seeing an evil omen, one is trusting in God, and that if one recoils, one is not. This has certain general parallels in the traditions on fleeing the plague. Compare Ibn Māja, *Sunan,* 2:1170–71. Abū Dāwūd, *Sunan,* 3:16; al-Tirmidhī, *Al-Jāmiᶜ al-Ṣaḥīḥ,* 4:161, in which ᶜAbd Allāh b. Masᶜūd relates that the Prophet said: "The evil omen is a type of polytheism (*min al-shirk*) and there is no one among us but [that] God abolishes the belief in it through trusting in him."

28. A recent estimate gives the number of traditions in the six canonical books, Mālik's *Muwaṭṭa',* ᶜAbd al-Razzāq's *Muṣannaf,* and Ibn Ḥanbal's *Musnad* as 62,169, well beyond the ability of the average believer to memorize or even be familiar with. See Buhindi, *Akthara Abū Hurayra,* 23.

29. This can be seen in the existence of numerous Web sites where technologically enabled believers can ask questions regarding specific traditions or consult previous responses (see, e.g., www.muslimfr.com, www.maison-islam.com and www.islam

online.net). Among those commentaries that attained exceptional places of respect are al-Nawawī's work on Muslim, Ibn Ḥajar al-ʿAsqalānī's commentary on Bukhārī, and al-Zurqānī's commentary on Mālik's *Muwaṭṭa'*.

30. A possible exception might be commentaries on short selections of traditions, such as al-Nawawī's *Arbaʿīn*.

31. This, admittedly, should not be seen as a process that denied the commentators their own individuality. The choice of opinions may reflect the preference of an older commentary over a more recent one, or the reverse. However, instead of a linear progression of opinion, one should imagine a circling, recursive movement.

32. The later compilers, especially al-Tirmidhī, regularly offer an opinion on the strength of a hadith. See Burton, *Introduction to the Hadith,* 126–30.

33. A telling example of Muʿtazilī attitudes toward Prophetic traditions is found in *Kitāb al-Muʿtamad,* by Abū al-Ḥusayn al-Baṣrī (d. 436/1044), 2:550: "Not everything that was related from him, God's prayers be upon him, is true. This is supported by what was related from him, may God pray for him, when he said: 'People will make false attributions to me (*sa-yakdhibu ʿalayya*).' If this tradition (*khabar*) is true, then false attributions have been made regarding him. If it is false, it has been falsely attributed to him, may God pray for him. The early scholars (*al-salaf*) used to reject many transmissions. It is related from Shuʿba that he said: 'A third of the traditions are lies.' " This passage is especially relevant because it immediately precedes a discussion of various traditions that were falsely attributed to the Prophet, or were misunderstood because the relater came in when the Prophet was speaking and heard only the last half of the tradition. Among the examples given of such traditions are the one stating that the evil omen resides in women, houses, and horses and ʿĀ'isha's assertion that the Prophet was speaking about someone else's beliefs. Abū Hurayra is not mentioned here, but in other sources ʿĀ'isha states that Abū Hurayra came in on the Prophet when he was already speaking and that he had been speaking about the beliefs of either the Jāhiliyya or the Jews. Ibn Ḥajar al-ʿAsqalānī defends this tradition and refutes ʿĀ'isha in his *Fatḥ al-Bārī.* See the section on the historical and Qur'anic background of the debate.

34. See, for example, Conrad's discussion of al-Naẓẓām's views in "Ninth-Century Muslim Scholar's Discussion."

35. Ibn al-Ṣalāḥ, *ʿUlūm al-Ḥadīth,* 284–86. For the same passage, see Ibn al-Ṣalāḥ, *Introduction to the Science of the Ḥadīth,* 205–6. For an excellent introduction to the importance of Ibn al-Ṣalāḥ's work, see Dickinson, "Ibn al-Ṣalāḥ al-Shahrazūrī."

36. Vardit Tokatly has recently argued that al-Khaṭṭābī's work should be considered a polemical treatise against the opponents of the hadith folk instead of a commentary on al-Bukhārī. Tokatly, "*Aʿlām al-Ḥadīth* of al-Khaṭṭābī," 87–88. For the purposes of my argument, however, and considering the extent to which later commentators drew upon al-Khaṭṭābī, I have chosen to consider him as a commentator. Commenting on Prophetic Tradition and refuting the hadith folk's enemies are, in any case, hardly contradictory endeavors.

37. The *Mukammil* of Abū ʿAbd Allāh Muḥammad b. Yūsuf al-Sanūsī al-Mālikī is included in al-Ubbī, *Ikmāl Ikmāl al-Muʿlim.*

38. Ibn Qutayba, *Ta'wīl Mukhtalif al-Ḥadīth,* 97–103. On this passage, see Conrad, "Ninth-Century Muslim Scholar's Discussion." Conrad, however, does not discuss Ibn Qutayba's treatment of augury.

39. For an overview of omens in the larger context of Arab divination, see Fahd, *La divination arabe,* 431–521.

40. Ibn Qutayba, *Ta'wīl Mukhtalif al-Ḥadīth,* 101; Ibn Baṭṭāl, *Sharḥ Ṣaḥīḥ al-Bukhārī,* 9:438; Ibn Ḥajar, *Fatḥ al-Bārī,* 21:340–41. After quoting various poets against the existence of contagion, Ibn Ḥajar notes: "Most of them practiced the augury (*yataṭayyarūna*) and relied on this, and it usually turned out correct for them because Satan embellished it for them (*wa-yaṣiḥḥ ma^ca-hum ghāliban li-tazyīn al-shayṭān dhālik*)." See also Ibn ᶜAbd al-Barr's legal work *Al-Istidhkār,* 8:422–23.

41. Ibn Baṭṭāl, *Sharḥ Ṣaḥīḥ al-Bukhārī,* 9:437–38; Ibn Ḥajar, *Fatḥ al-Bārī,* 11:11. See also al-Qasṭallānī, *Irshād al-Sārī,* 8:412.

42. Here and throughout the book, unless otherwise indicated, I refer to the translation of Abdel Haleem, *Qur'an.*

43. In Qur'anic exegesis the messengers are identified as apostles of Jesus, sent to Antioch. See, for example, al-Qurṭubī, *Al-Jāmiᶜ li-Aḥkām al-Qur'ān,* 15:17–21; and al-Shawkānī, *Fatḥ al-Qadīr,* 4:449–53.

44. There is some difference as to whether the king and some of his subjects convert in the end, or only the king himself. In any event, Gabriel gives a shout and all those who did not convert die as unbelievers, going to hell. Al-Qurṭubī, *Al-Jāmiᶜ li-Aḥkām al-Qur'ān,* 15:19.

45. Ibn Baṭṭāl, *Sharḥ Ṣaḥīḥ al-Bukhārī,* 9:438; Ibn ᶜAbd al-Barr, *Al-Tamhīd,* 9:284; Ibn Abī Jamra, *Bahjat al-Nufūs,* 2:1267–68.

46. This is a tradition not found in the nine collections of traditions examined earlier. See, however, Ibn Baṭṭāl, *Sharḥ Ṣaḥīḥ al-Bukhārī,* 9:437; Ibn ᶜAbd al-Barr, *Al-Tamhīd,* 9:285. Also see *Fatḥ al-Bārī,* 21:341, where Ibn Ḥajar cites *Saḥīḥ,* by Ibn Ḥibbān (d. 354/965), as his source for the tradition.

47. That is, it is not cited after Ibn Abī Jamra (d. 699/1300). Significantly, Ibn Ḥajar does not mention it in his fifteenth-century commentary.

48. See Abū Dāwūd, *Sunan,* 3:18. Ibn al-ᶜArabī notes that the house in question was that of Mukammil b. ᶜAwf, the brother of ᶜAbd al-Raḥmān b. ᶜAwf. *Al-Qabas fī Sharḥ Muwaṭṭa',* 3:1148.

49. Ibn Qutayba, *Ta'wīl Mukhtalif al-Ḥadīth,* 100; Ibn ᶜAbd al-Barr, *Al-Tamhīd,* 9:285. Ibn ᶜAbd al-Barr cites this verse outside the context of the ᶜĀ'isha episode, though he uses it for the same purpose. In addition, he cites Sūrat al-Tawba, 51, to strengthen his argument: "Say, 'Only what God has decreed will happen to us. He is our Master: let the believers put their trust in God.'" Again, it is to Ibn Ḥajar, *Fatḥ al-Bārī,* 11:11–12, that we owe a reference to this tradition's source: the *Musnad* of Abū Dāwūd al-Ṭayālisī (d. 203/818). (I have not been able to find this reference.) On the one occasion when al-Ṭayālisī does include ᶜĀ'isha's comments on women as evil omens, it is her rebuke of Abū Hurayra for taking the Prophet's criticism of Jewish beliefs to refer to Muslims. See his *Musnad Abī Dāwūd al-Ṭayālisī,* 215; al-ᶜAynī, *ᶜUmdat al-Qārī,* 10:196 (quoting from Ibn al-Jawzī [d. 597/1201]; I have not been able to identify which work of his al-ᶜAynī is referring to). This tradition is also quoted in Ibn al-Ḥājj, *Madkhal al-Sharᶜ al-Sharīf,* 4:120; Ibn Rushd, *Al-Bayān wa-l-Taḥṣīl,* 17:275; and Ibn Rushd, *Muqaddimāt,* 2:497.

50. Ibn Qutayba and Ibn ᶜAbd al-Barr were convinced by ᶜĀ'isha's denial, although this did not hinder Ibn Qutayba from supporting the traditions regarding the presence of the evil omen in the house. *Ta'wīl Mukhtalif al-Ḥadīth,* 100. Ibn Qutayba

is not as explicit in his opinion as Ibn ᶜAbd al-Barr, but he does not criticize the legitimacy of ᶜĀ'isha's refutation of Abū Hurayra, and he mentions none of the metaphoric rationales for applying the evil omen to women. Nevertheless, Ibn Baṭṭāl quotes Ibn Qutayba as having refuted the Muᶜtazilī claims that the tradition "no evil omen" contradicts "the evil omen is in three" tradition. *Sharḥ Ṣaḥīḥ al-Bukhārī,* 9:437. Ibn ᶜAbd al-Barr tries to play down the conflict between ᶜĀ'isha and Abū Hurayra, saying that the Arabs used the word *kadhaba* in the meaning of "to err" and not "to lie." He explains the existence of the tradition by its being early, later abrogated by both the Qur'an and Prophetic Tradition. The Prophet's calling the house blameworthy was, according to Ibn ᶜAbd al-Barr, part of his attempt to gradually weaken the Arabs' belief in evil omens. *Al-Tamhīd,* 9:286–91.

51. Ibn al-ᶜArabī is quoted in Ibn Ḥajar, *Fatḥ al-Bārī,* 11:12 (I have not been able to find this reference in *Al-Qabas fī Sharḥ Muwaṭṭa',* where Ibn al-ᶜArabī discusses evil omens in 3:1148–50). Ibn Ḥajar introduces his own opinion here, refuting ᶜĀ'isha's views and then explicitly rejecting Ibn ᶜAbd al-Barr's view that the tradition of the evil omen in three was abrogated. *Fatḥ al-Bārī,* 11:13. On this subject, al-Zurqānī cites the views of Ibn Ḥajar and Ibn al-ᶜArabī. See *Sharḥ al-Zurqānī,* 4:487–88.

52. The Yemeni scholar Muḥammad al-Shawkānī quotes Ibn Ḥajar without mentioning the views on this matter of either Ibn Qutayba or Ibn ᶜAbd al-Barr. See *Itḥāf al-Mahara bi-l-kalām ᶜalā ḥadīth lā ᶜadwā wa lā ṭiyara,* fols. 143–44.

53. For the distressing habit that some people had of seeing evil omens in other people or in certain children, see Ibn Abī Jamra, *Bahjat al-Nufūs,* 2:1269–70. For the continued existence of a belief in both evil and good omens in Morocco, see Ourāb, *Al-Muᶜtaqadāt al-Siḥriyya fī-l-Maghrib,* 202–3. The words *tashā'um* and *tafā'ul* continue to be used in Morocco to describe interpreting something as an evil or a good omen (personal observation, April 2004, Rabat).

54. Conrad, "Ninth-Century Muslim Scholar's Discussion," 167, 177. Conrad notes that it was a characteristic of "emergent Islam" to emphasize God's nature as the sole agent of causation.

55. Compare with note 19. Cited in al-Qasṭallānī, *Irshād al-Sārī,* 8:412; Ibn ᶜAbd al-Barr, *Al-Tamhīd,* 9:285.

56. Mālik's literal understanding of the tradition is attested in al-Nawawī, *Sharḥ Ṣaḥīḥ Muslim,* 14:220; al-Māzarī, *Al-Muᶜlim,* 3:104. Al-Māzarī cites the *Mustakhraja* as his source, and indeed we find this view of Mālik's in *Al-Bayān wa-l-Taḥṣīl,* Ibn Rushd's commentary on the *ᶜUtbiyya. Al-Bayān wa-l-Taḥṣīl,* 17:275. I discuss Ibn Rushd's comments in chapter 5. Al-Māzarī's passage is later cited along with Ibn al-ᶜArabī's interpretation. Ibn Ḥajar, *Fatḥ al-Bārī,* 11:12.

57. Al-Māzarī put it as follows: "Someone other than him [Mālik] said: It is to be understood that its intention is that the decree of God may be in accordance with what the inhabitants of a house hate, and this becomes similar to a cause. And it is permissible to attribute the evil omen to it metaphorically, in an extended sense (*ittisāᶜan*)." Finally, see al-ᶜAynī, *ᶜUmdat al-Qārī,* 10:196.

58. Ibn Ḥajar, *Fatḥ al-Bārī,* 11:12. Ibn Ḥajar is quoting Ibn al-ᶜArabī and then gives his own affirming opinion. See also al-Qasṭallānī, *Irshād al-Sārī,* 8:397.

59. See the discussion in Ibn Manẓūr, *Lisān al-ᶜArab,* 5:60, where the author explains that *dhamīma* in this context has the meaning of the passive participle *madhmūma.*

60. Ibn Qutayba, *Ta'wīl Mukhtalif al-Ḥadīth,* 100; Ibn Baṭṭāl, *Sharḥ Ṣaḥīḥ al-Bukhārī,* 9:438; Ibn Abī Jamra, *Bahjat al-Nufūs,* 2:1269–70; Ibn Ḥajar, *Fatḥ al-Bārī,* 11:12, again quoting Ibn al-ᶜArabī.

61. Al-ᶜAynī, *ᶜUmdat al-Qārī,* 10:196, where the author quotes al-Khaṭṭābī. I have not found this in al-Khaṭṭābī, *Aᶜlām al-Sunan;* cf. *Sharḥ Ṣaḥīḥ Muslim,* 14:221, where al-Nawawī quotes al-Khaṭṭābī and unnamed others.

62. Ibn Abī Jamra describes this possibility in terms of God's attributes, his power and his wisdom. *Bahjat al-Nufūs,* 2:1269. See the views of al-Ubbī and al-Qasṭallānī in the discussion of the commentaries on the contagion traditions.

63. See both the introduction and chapter 5 for a fuller discussion of causation in premodern Islamic theology and law.

64. The term *natural philosophers* designates a group characterized, on the part of their enemies, by their belief in "the properties of temperaments" and the denial of paradise, hell, judgment, and resurrection. Al-Ghazālī described them as a subgroup of the heretics (*zanādiqa*). See Goldziher/Goichon's article on the "Dahriyya" in *Encyclopedia of Islam,* 2nd ed., 12 vols. (Leiden: Brill, 1960–2004), 2:96. It is doubtful that such a group existed outside of the imagination of their opponents as anything more than statements of individual scholars. Carl Ernst has remarked helpfully on the tendency of heresiographers to personify trends or concepts they opposed. *Words of Ecstasy in Sufism,* 120.

65. See al-Māzarī, *Al-Muᶜlim,* 3:106.

66. Ibn Abī Jamra, *Bahjat al-Nufūs,* 2:1270; Ibn Ḥajar, *Fatḥ al-Bārī,* 11:12–13. Ibn Ḥajar first cites a tradition related by ᶜAbd al-Razzāq from Maᶜmar giving these explanations (I have not found this tradition in ᶜAbd al-Razzāq's *Muṣannaf*). See also Ibn Ḥajar, *Fatḥ al-Bārī,* 19:165–66; alᶜAynī, *ᶜUmdat al-Qārī,* 10:196, quoting al-Khaṭṭābī; al-Nawawī, *Sharḥ Ṣaḥīḥ Muslim,* 14:221–22, quoting al-Khaṭṭābī.

67. See note 25. Ibn Abī Jamra, *Bahjat al-Nufūs,* 2:1270; Ibn Ḥajar, *Fatḥ al-Bārī,* 21, 341. Ibn Ḥajar transmits Sulaymān b. Ḥarb's opinion, found in al-Tirmidhī, that the belief that evil omens are in the souls of all Muslims reflects the interpolated words of Ibn Masᶜūd in the Prophetic tradition. Al-Qasṭillānī, *Irshād al-Sārī,* 8:412.

68. Neither of these traditions is found in the nine collections of traditions examined thus far. Ibn Qutayba, *Ta'wīl Mukhtalif al-Ḥadīth,* 101 (the editor gives *Kanz al-ᶜUmmāl* as the source of the first, *Tuḥfat al-Aḥwadhī* of the second). The word for doubt, *ẓann,* clearly meant in a negative fashion here, can also mean "opinion" and is used in this fashion below regarding the good omen. Ibn Baṭṭāl, *Sharḥ Ṣaḥīḥ Bukhārī,* 9:438. On not turning back if one sees an evil omen, see Ibn Abī Jamra, *Bahjat al-Nufūs,* 2:1269.

69. Ibn Ḥajar, *Fatḥ al-Bārī,* 21:341; al-ᶜAynī, *ᶜUmdat al-Qārī,* 10:197; al-Qasṭillānī, *Irshād al-Sārī,* 8:412. An especially interesting example is given in Ibn ᶜAbd al-Barr, *Al-Tamhīd,* 24:200, where the Jewish convert Kaᶜb al-Aḥbār attributes such a prayer to the Torah.

70. Ibn Ḥanbal related one tradition in which the good omen is also explicitly denied. Ibn Ḥanbal, *Musnad,* 4:549.

71. See Ibn Ḥanbal, *Musnad,* 3:90; Ibn Māja, *Sunan,* 2:1170; Ibn Qutayba, *Ta'wīl Mukhtalif al-Ḥadīth,* 102; Ibn ᶜAbd al-Barr, *Al-Tamhīd,* 9:279. Al-Khaṭṭābī sees a clear difference between the good and the evil omen on the basis that the former is spoken, as when a sick person hears someone say, "Oh, Healthy One!" (an example

already given in the tradition), whereas the latter is not. As he notes dryly, birds and beasts do not speak. Al-Khaṭṭābī, *Aᶜlām al-Sunan,* 2:1159. In an unacknowledged quotation from Ibn Qutayba, Ibn Baṭṭāl quotes a tradition related by al-ᶜAṣma'ī from ᶜAbd Allāh b. ᶜAwn (d. 231/845) with the same meaning. *Sharḥ Ṣaḥīḥ al-Bukhārī,* 9:436; Ibn Ḥajar, *Fatḥ al-Bārī,* 21:343.

72. See note 23. The examples given in the commentaries greatly exceed the one mentioned by Abū Dāwūd. Ibn Qutayba records that the Prophet was pleased by the citron tree, the red dove, and the henna blossom and displeased by repulsive names such as "the Sons of Fire" and "the Sons of Sadness." *Ta'wīl Mukhtalif al-Ḥadīth,* 103. This passage is quoted in Ibn Baṭṭāl, *Sharḥ Ṣaḥīḥ al-Bukhārī,* 9:437–38. See also Ibn ᶜAbd al-Barr, *Al-Tamhīd,* 24:71–73; Ibn Ḥajar, *Fatḥ al-Bārī,* 21:344; al-Qurṭubī, *Al-Mufhim,* 6:627.

73. The tradition *la ṭiyarata wa-khayru-hā al-fa'l* can be translated literally as "There is no evil omen and the best of it is the good omen." See Ibn Ḥanbal, *Musnad,* 3:90; Ibn Māja, *Sunan,* 2:1170; and note 15.

74. See al-Nawawī, *Sharḥ Ṣaḥīḥ Muslim,* 14:219–20. Al-ᶜAynī also notes that the word *ṭiyara* had a broader original meaning that also encompassed good omens. *ᶜUmdat al-Qārī,* 10:196–97; *Fatḥ al-Bārī,* 21:342–43, where Ibn Ḥajar quotes al-Kirmānī's views and then appends his own.

75. Ibn Baṭṭāl, *Sharḥ Ṣaḥīḥ al-Bukhārī,* 9:436, quoting al-Khaṭṭābī; al-Nawawī, *Sharḥ Ṣaḥīḥ Muslim,* 14:219–20; Ibn Ḥajar, *Fatḥ al-Bārī,* 21:343.

76. Ibn Qutayba, *Ta'wil Mukhtalif al-Ḥadīth,* 103; Ibn Baṭṭāl, *Sharḥ Ṣaḥīḥ al-Bukhārī,* 9:437; al-ᶜAynī, *ᶜUmdat al-Qārī,* 10:197.

77. Ibn Ḥajar, *Fatḥ al-Bārī,* 11:12; al-ᶜAynī, *ᶜUmdat al-Qārī,* 10:196. A similar line of thought was pursued by Ibn Qutayba. After relating the tradition that one should not enter a plague-struck country, he wrote: "From this [tradition] a woman or a house is known as a bad omen (*tuᶜraf bi-l-shu'm*), for the man receives what is hateful or calamitous (*jā'iḥa*) and he says: She infected me with her evil omen (*aᶜdatnī bi-shu'mi-hā*). This is the contagion of which the Prophet, God bless Him and grant Him salvation, said: 'No contagion.'" *Ta'wīl Mukhtalif al-Ḥadīth,* 99.

78. Ibn Qutayba, *Ta'wīl Mukhtalif al-Ḥadīth,* 99. ᶜIyāḍ Ibn Mūsā recounts that some people saw evil omens in sick camels. Ibn Mūsā, *Ikmāl al-Muᶜlim,* 9:142.

79. The plague and the evil omen are grouped together as early as a tradition that appears in Ibn Ḥanbal's *Musnad,* 1:293.

80. Al-Māzarī, *Al-Muᶜlim,* 3:105. The harm that could come about by fleeing the plague was not spreading the contagion, but leaving the sick untended. See chapter 5. Al-Nawawī relates an abbreviated version of this passage in *Sharḥ Ṣaḥīḥ Muslim,* 14:222.

81. Especially striking is the difference between Ibn ᶜAbd al-Barr and Ibn Ḥajar on the issue of ᶜĀ'isha's refutation of Abū Hurayra. See notes 51–52. Ibn ᶜAbd al-Barr and Ibn Ḥajar also differ on the tradition of the good omen's presence in women, houses, and horses, the former regarding it favorably and the latter describing it as weak. Ibn ᶜAbd al-Barr, *Al-Tamhīd,* 9:279; Ibn Ḥajar, *Fatḥ al-Bārī,* 11:12; see also note 12. Al-Tirmidhī had already described this tradition as weak.

82. Conrad, "ᶜUmar at Sargh"; van Ess, *Der Fehltritt des Gelehrten,* esp. 38–41 and 244–50. Compare "ᶜUmar at Sargh," 498–99, with *Der Fehltritt des Gelehrten,* 38–41.

83. Van Ess, *Der Fehltritt des Gelehrten,* 38–41.

84. See note 13. The many variants of this tradition include some that are bound up with the evil omen more than others. A particularly comprehensive example is found in Ibn Ḥanbal, *Musnad,* 1:380.

85. What I have translated here as tapeworm (*ṣafar*) was known by many of the Companions and followers to be an animal or a worm that lived in the stomach and could be contagious. Ibn Ḥanbal, *Musnad,* 1:577–78. Others saw it as referring to the month of *Ṣafar* and to whether one could carry out certain actions during it. The death bird (*hāma*) is a bird that comes to rest on the grave of a dead man, calling out "Give me to drink!" until the man is avenged. Abū Dāwūd, *Sunan,* 3:17–18. The ghoul (*ghūl*) is a female demon. Ibn Ḥanbal, *Musnad,* 5:186. The malignant star (*naw'*) is not defined in the traditions themselves, but in the commentaries it is described as a star with negative influence.

86. Mālik b. Anas, *Al-Muwaṭṭā',* 476; Ibn Ḥanbal, *Musnad,* 357:431; Ibn Māja, *Sunan,* 2:1171. See also al-Bukhārī, *Ṣaḥīḥ,* 2:740, where Ibn ᶜUmar, after being informed that he had been sold camels that were *huyyām*—afflicted with a sickness of constant thirst—notes that the camels should drink but that he did not need to return them, for the Prophet had said that there is no contagion.

87. Al-Ṣanᶜānī, *Al-Muṣannaf,* 10:25; Ibn Ḥanbal, *Musnad,* 3:449; al-Bukhārī, *Ṣaḥīḥ,* 5:2158–59.

88. It is related that ᶜUmar told a leper by the name of Muᶜayqīb al-Dawsī (d. 39/662) that he would not have approached him closer than an arrow shot if it hadn't been him. Al-Ṣanᶜānī, *Al-Muṣannaf,* 10:25; the comment makes more sense if one knows that ᶜUmar had appointed Muᶜayqīb manager of the treasury. See Ibn Ḥabīb, *Kitāb al-Wāḍīḥa,* 121/122 of the Arabic/Spanish. The Prophet is reported to have said that one should not stare at lepers (Ibn Māja, *Sunan,* 2:1172), and Ibn Māja notes that this tradition was related by trustworthy men; the Prophet is also reported to have sent back a leper from the delegation of Thaqīf before seeing him, saying he had accepted his allegiance. Al-Nasā'ī, *Kitāb al-Sunan al-Kubrā,* 4:375.

Abū Bakr is reported to have eaten with a leper, the Prophet gave a leper who came to him supplies and said "No contagion," and ᶜUmar stepped in front of another man to give a leper a dirham. Al-Ṣanᶜānī, *Al-Muṣannaf,* 10:25. In addition the Prophet is said to have taken the hand of a leper and placed it with his own in a bowl, telling the leper to eat and trust in God. Ibn Māja, *Sunan,* 2:1172; and Abū Dāwūd, *Sunan,* 3:18.

89. Abū Salama (d. 94/712) was a prominent jurist and traditionist. See Ibn Saᶜd, *Al-Ṭabaqāt al-Kubrā,* 5:118–20.

90. The text in the *Ṣaḥīḥ* consulted reads: "I yearned (*ababtu*)." I have taken this to be a misprint and read *abaytu.* This latter reading was adopted by later commentators and is consistent with the other versions in Al-Ṣanᶜānī's *Al-Muṣannaf* and the *Sunan Abī Dāwūd.*

91. Muslim, *Ṣaḥīḥ Muslim,* 4:1743–44; and al-Bukhārī, *Ṣaḥīḥ,* 5:2177. This is the most detailed version of the tradition. Note that in Ibn Ḥanbal, *Musnad,* 3:431, Abū Hurayra does in fact relate as one tradition both the denial of contagion and the admonition not to water sick and healthy animals together.

92. On the complicated status of Abū Hurayra as a Companion of the Prophet and a relater of traditions, see Juynboll, *Authenticity of the Tradition Literature,* 62–100;

Ṣālāḥ al-ᶜAlī, *Dafāᶜ ᶜan Abī Hurayra;* and most recently Muṣṭafā Buhindi, *Akthara Abū Hurayra.*

93. Conrad has noted a widespread belief among the pre-Islamic Arabs in the transmission of disease and even physical defects. The Qur'an spoke against such beliefs in Sūrat al-Nūr, 61: "No blame will be attached to the blind, the lame, the sick." "Ninth-Century Muslim Scholar's Discussion," 166.

94. Al-Ṣanᶜānīᶜ, *Al-Muṣannaf,* 10:24; Ibn Ḥanbal, *Musnad,* 1:578 (camels and mange), 1:703 (sheep and scabies), 3:90; Muslim, *Ṣaḥīḥ Muslim,* 4:1390; al-Bukhārī, *Ṣaḥīḥ,* 5:2177–78.

95. This is a comment that has clear parallels with Sūrat al-Ḥadīd, 22, discussed earlier. For this incident, see Ibn Ḥanbal, *Musnad,* 2:144, 2:252, 3:219; Ibn Māja, *Sunan,* 2:1171, where Ibn Māja notes that the *isnād* (back to Ibn ᶜUmar) is weak; al-Tirmidhī, *Al-Jāmiᶜ al-Ṣaḥīḥ,* 1:450–51. Here the tradition is related by Ibn Masᶜūd, who is praised by al-Tirmidhī due to his authority. The tradition is, appropriately enough, included in the chapter on fate (*qadar*).

96. That *qadar* was not theologically well developed as a concept until the second–third century after the Prophet's death has been suggested by, among others, van Ess in *Der Fehltritt des Gelehrten,* 38–39, 240–41.

97. See the discussion of the eighth/fourteenth-century jurist Ibn Lubb in chapter 5.

98. Mālik, *Al-Muwaṭṭa',* 476. Here helping the sick and sitting with them is seen as praiseworthy rather than an actual imperative. This perspective changed in later commentaries. See also Ibn al-ᶜArabī, *Al-Qabas fī Sharḥ Muwaṭṭa',* 3:1132–33, where similar traditions from al-Tirmidhī and Ibn Māja are quoted.

99. Mālik, a*l-Muwaṭṭa',* 476. None of the other eight collections of traditions preserve this exchange.

100. This episode has been extensively discussed by both Conrad and van Ess. See note 86.

101. Van Ess argues that the Prophetic Tradition was included in the episode at a very late date in its evolution. See *Der Fehltritt des Gelehrten,* 41.

102. Conrad, "ᶜUmar at Sargh," 508.

103. This may indeed have been the way the tradition was understood during the first stages of its evolution. Ibid., 507.

104. Al-Bazzāz discusses the resistance in Morocco on the part of scholars as well as the government to both the idea of contagion and that of a quarantine. *Ta'rīkh al-Awbi'a,* 395–408. Van Ess says the theological arguments have only recently caused public health officials in the Muslim world to step in to prevent the spread of epidemics. *Der Fehltritt des Gelehrten,* 301.

105. Ibn Qutayba, *Ta'wīl Mukhtalif al-Ḥadīth,* 99; Ibn ᶜAbd al-Barr, *Al-Tamhīd,* 6:209–17. One might also choose to argue that when ᶜUmar said "flee from the will of God," he was speaking metaphorically, not of actual flight. See Zurqānī, *Sharḥ al-Zurqānī,* 4:296. This admittedly is not a very convincing argument in this context.

106. See Ibn ᶜAbd al-Barr, *Al-Tamhīd,* 6:211–13.

107. Ibn ᶜAbd al-Barr, *Al-Tamhīd,* 6:213–14; Zurqānī, *Sharḥ al-Zurqānī,* 4:300. See also van Ess, *Der Fehltritt des Gelehrten,* 305.

108. The plague generally was explained as being the remnant of a punishment that God had sent down upon some of the Jews, the group referred to in Sūrat al-Baqara,

243. Al-Ṭabarī and al-Qurṭubī provide abundant details in their Qur'anic exegeses. For a comprehensive overview of information on plagues during pre-Islamic times, see Ibn Ḥajar al-ᶜAsqalānī, *Badhl al-Māᶜūn,* 73–88.

109. The belief in contagious diseases was widespread among the bedouin. ᶜĪsā b. Dīnār relates from Ibn Wahb that the bedouin believe that proximity to the sick is dangerous and quotes a line of poetry to the effect that the places where sick animals had lain down could infect the healthy. Al-Bājī, *Al-Muntaqā,* 9:388–93. On ᶜĪsā b. Dīnār (d. 212/827), one of the most important figures in introducing the Mālikī legal school to al-Andalus, see H. Munis's article in *Encyclopedia of Islam*, 4:87; and Fernández Félix, *Cuestiones legales del Islam temprano,* 22, 33. For other attestations of pre-Islamic beliefs in contagion, see Conrad, "Ninth-Century Muslim Scholar's Discussion," 165.

110. Ibn ᶜAbd al-Barr, *Al-Tamhīd,* 24:191–96. Ibn ᶜAbd al-Barr gives here a Prophetic Tradition that spells out Muḥammad's meaning: "There is no contagion and no evil omen and no owl. Do you not look to the camel in the desert and there appears on its chest or its joints near its stomach a spot of scabies that had not been there before? Who infected the first?" Ibn al-Ṣalāḥ, *ᶜUlūm al-Ḥadīth,* 285; al-Nawawī, *Sharḥ Ṣaḥīḥ Muslim,* 14:217; al-Ubbī, *Ikmāl Ikmāl al-Muᶜlim,* 7:420–21.

111. Al-Bājī, *Al-Muntaqā,* 9:388–93. Al-Bājī is quoting ᶜĪsā b. Dinār, who stresses that God can also create such a disease out of nothing (*ibtidā'an*) and that there is no room for the possibility of contagion; see also al-Ubbī, *Ikmāl Ikmāl al-Muᶜlim,* 7:419.

112. Al-Khaṭṭābī, *Aᶜlām al-Sunan,* 1:583–84; Ibn Baṭṭāl, *Sharḥ Ṣaḥīḥ al-Bukhārī,* 6:230–31; al-Kirmānī, *Al-Kawākib al-Darārī,* 9:217–18, where al-Kirmānī merely quotes al-Khaṭṭābī.

113. Ibn Ḥajar, *Fatḥ al-Bārī,* 9:172–74. Ibn Ḥajar also cites the view of al-Dāwūdī (possibly Aḥmad b. Naṣrallāh [d. 844/1440], a prominent Ḥanbalī jurist in Cairo who wrote on ḥadith; see al-Kaḥḥāla, *Muᶜjam al-Mu'allifīn,* 1:319) that *ᶜadwā* in this context means oppression, a unique view as far as I can tell.

114. Al-Qurtubī, *Al-Mufhim,* 5:621–22; Ibn Ḥajar, *Fatḥ al-Bārī,* 21:377. Ibn Ḥajar alters and abbreviates the passage slightly.

115. See chapter 5, where I discuss the relationship between theology and law in relation to causation and contagion.

116. I have not found any sources that argue this explicitly, but it is implicit in the materials quoted here.

117. See Ibn Mūsā, *Ikmāl al-Muᶜlim,* 9:141–42.

118. Al-Kirmānī, *Al-Kawākib al-Darārī,* 21:45; Ibn Ḥajar, *Fatḥ al-Bārī,* 21:376–77. The quality of Abū Hurayra's memory was relevant because he had reportedly been given by the Prophet the ability to remember all the traditions he heard by spreading out his cloak and then drawing it to his chest while he recited. Ibn Ḥajar cites the views of Ibn al-Tīn (d. 611/1214), author of a previous commentary on al-Bukhārī, who notes that Abū Hurayra may have heard this tradition before the Prophet told him to use his cloak. For a critical view of this episode, see Juynboll, *Authenticity of the Tradition Literature,* 87; and Buhindi, *Akthara Abū Hurayra,* 38. That many besides Abū Hurayra related the Prophet's denial of contagion was noted by Ibn Ḥajar in *Fatḥ al-Bārī,* 21:277.

119. Al-Bājī cites ᶜIsā b. Dīnār's view that the Prophet had abrogated the "do not water" tradition with the "no contagion" tradition—a choice opposite to that of

Abū Hurayra—only to disagree with him, saying that because the order of the traditions was not known, one could not use the argument of abrogation here. *Al-Muntaqā,* 9:388–93. Ibn Ḥajar commented that while Abū Salama thought that the traditions were contradictory, he showed in his chapter on leprosy that they could be reconciled and that there was no need for talk of abrogation. *Fatḥ al-Bārī,* 21:377. Al-Qurṭubī gave the most extensive list of arguments against abrogation among the possible reasons for Abū Hurayra's silence. *Al-Mufhim,* 5:626. See also al-Māzarī, *Al-Muᶜlim,* 3:102–3. Ibn al-ᶜArabī acknowleges the tension between the two traditions (*Al-Qabas fī Sharḥ Muwaṭṭa',* 3:1134), but unequivocally denies the transmission of disease between two animals.

120. Ibn al-Ṣalāḥ, *ᶜUlūm al-Ḥadīth,* 285; Zurqānī, *Sharḥ al-Zurqānī,* 4:425; al-Qasṭillānī, *Irshād al-Sārī,* 8:411–12; al-Ubbī, *Ikmāl Ikmāl al-Muᶜlim,* 7:419. Both al-Ubbī and al-Zurqānī compare being close to a sick person to standing next to a leaning wall.

121. Ibn Qutayba, *Ta'wīl Mukhtalif al-Ḥadīth,* 98; al-Khaṭṭābī explains the moisture that transmits the sickness as a coalesced form of the awful smells given off by the mange, which has a parallel in the discussion of the danger of leprosy and had already been suggested by Ibn Qutayba himself. In addition he notes that some refuse this explanation, seeing it to be at odds with the belief that God created the mange in the camel. *Aᶜlām al-Sunan,* 2:1161–62. Ibn Qutayba's views are also quoted in Ibn Ḥajar, *Fatḥ al-Bārī,* 21:276–81.

122. Ibn Qutayba's rejection of this view is found in *Ta'wīl Mukhtalif al-Ḥadīth,* 98. Supporters of this view can be found in Ibn ᶜAbd al-Barr, *Al-Tamhīd,* 24:197–98; al-Māzarī, *Al-Muᶜlim,* 3:102–3; ᶜIyāḍ, *Ikmāl al-Muᶜlim,* 9:142; al-Qurṭubī, *Al-Mufhim,* 5:620–26. In *Sharḥ Ṣaḥīḥ Muslim,* 14:217, al-Nawawī notes that believing in contagion may lead to apostasy.

123. For a narration of ᶜUmar's turning back at Sargh because he did not want his followers to fall into believing in contagion, see Zurqānī, *Sharḥ al-Zurqānī,* 4:302.

124. Leprosy of course had been present in the Middle East long before the coming of Islam. For a recent evaluation of leprosy in the Bible, see Lieber, "Old Testament 'Leprosy,' Contagion, and Sin." Michael Dols reviewed the historical material on lepers in the Islamic world in "Leper in Islamic Society." Dols addresses the issue of contagion on 895–97.

125. Al-Bājī quotes Yaḥyā b. Yaḥyā al-Maṣmūdī (d. 234/848) on how, even though leprosy is not contagious, the soul is harmed by being close to it. *Al-Muntaqā,* 9:388–93.

126. Ibn Qutayba, *Ta'wīl Mukhtalif al-Ḥadith,* 98. Al-Bājī quotes the views of the Mālikī scholars Yaḥyā b. Yaḥyā, Ibn al-Qāsim (d. 191/806) and Saḥnūn (d. 240/854–55) on the matter. *Al-Muntaqā,* 9:388–93. Whereas leprosy is sufficient reason for a woman to divorce her husband, Ibn al-Qāsim and Saḥnūn differ on whether it is prohibited for a leper to have sex with his slaves, the former forbidding it and the latter permitting it. This passage is also found in al-Khaṭṭābī, *Aᶜlām al-Sunan,* 2:1151–52. Yaḥyā's views on the harmfulness of the smell of lepers are also given in Ibn Baṭṭāl, *Sharḥ Ṣaḥīḥ al-Bukhārī,* 9:449–50. Ibn Qutayba's views are given again in al-Qastallānī, *Irshād al-Sārī,* 8:373–74.

127. Al-Khaṭṭābī, *A'lām al-Sunan,* 2:1151–52. Ibn Baṭṭāl cites Abū Bakr b. al-Ṭayyib al-Baqillānī (d. 403/1013), a Malikī scholar from Baghdad who was known

for his fierce opposition to the Mu'tazila. Al-Baqillānī polemically quotes the famous Mu^c^tazilī polymath, al-Jāḥiz, as relating from his teacher al-Naẓẓām that the two traditions in question stand in conflict to one another. This is nonsense, al-Baqillānī states, because the "no contagion" tradition is specific in its scope, as if to say that there are no transmissible diseases save for leprosy and mange. Ibn Baṭṭāl, *Sharḥ Ṣaḥīḥ al-Bukhārī,* 9:449–50. Al-Ubbī gives a clinical definition of contagion and a list of diseases considered contagious by doctors, cited from a work by al-Ṭībī (possibly Sharaf al-Dīn al-Ḥusayn al-Ṭībī [d. 743/1342]; see Kaḥḥāla, *Mu^c^jam al-Mu'allifīn,* 1:639): the transmission of a sickness (*^c^illa*) from its carrier to another (*al-^c^adwā tajāwuz al-^c^illa ṣāḥibaha ilā ghayrihi*). Doctors see this happening in seven cases: leprosy, mange, smallpox, measles, halitosis, ophthalmia, and epidemic diseases. Al-Ubbī, *Ikmāl Ikmāl al-Mu^c^lim,* 419. Al-Zurqānī gives a slightly altered version of this list at the same time that he notes that most scholars deny the existence of contagion. *Sharḥ al-Zurqānī,* 4:424.

128. Ibn Baṭṭāl cites several examples from al-Ṭabarī (d. 310/923) of how the Prophet and his Companions ate with lepers. In one of these he relates that ^c^Ā'isha denied that the Prophet ever said that one should flee from the leper; he says she herself had a client (*mawlā*) who was leprous and who ate from her plates and slept in her bed. For al-Ṭabarī the matter was clear, as the Prophet had denied the existence of contagious diseases. Ibn Baṭṭāl, *Sharḥ Ṣaḥīḥ al-Bukhārī,* 9:409–12. Ibn Ḥajar cites the same passages of al-Ṭabarī and uses this material to counter those who emphasize that Abū Hurayra retracted the "no contagion" tradition. Ibn Ḥajar, *Fatḥ al-Bārī,* 21:276–81; similarly, al-^c^Aynī, *^c^Umdat al-Qārī,* 10:168–69.

129. The idea that if a person's soul is strong enough to bear it, one should stay with the sick is found in Yaḥyā b. Yaḥyā's comments, quoted in al-Bājī, *Al-Muntaqā,* 9:388–93. This opinion is presented at length in Ibn Abī Jamra, *Bahjat al-Nufūs,* 2:1267–72, where the author argues that the "flee from the leper" tradition was intended as solicitude (*shafaqa*) for common believers. Such a flight is not obligatory, as the Prophet had shown by eating with lepers, but Muḥammad had said "flee" due to his compassion for the common people, since there were smells that would cause harm to body and soul. See Ibn Ḥajar, *Fatḥ al-Bārī,* 21:281.

130. *Fatḥ al-Bārī,* 21:279, where Ibn Ḥajar notes that this is the view held by the majority of the Shāfi^c^ī school and cites al-Bayhaqī (d. 458/1066) to this effect. Al-Qasṭallānī notes that avoiding lepers is a mercy for them as well as for the healthy, because the lepers do not have to be pained by the sight of healthy bodies. *Irshād al-Sārī,* 8:373–74.

131. Al-Bājī again quotes the views of Yaḥyā b. Yaḥyā, who stresses that lepers continue to enjoy all of their property rights and need to be recompensed if their access to a well is hindered. *Al-Muntaqā,* 9:388–93.

132. Al-Bājī continues to quote early Mālikī authorities. Ibid. Compare Ibn Ḥabīb, *Kitāb al-Wāḍīḥa,* 121–22 of the Arabic, 122–23 of the Spanish translation. Ibn Baṭṭāl quotes Yaḥyā b. Yaḥyā to similar effect. *Sharḥ Ṣaḥīḥ al-Bukhārī,* 9:409–12. For his part, al-Māzarī is conspicuous among the commentators on Muslim in that he discusses the subject at all, the "flee from the leper" tradition not being present in Muslim's collection. *Al-Mu^c^lim,* 3:102–3.

133. See, for example, the material analyzed by Mazzoli-Guintard, "Notes sur une minorité d'al-Andalus." I am grateful to Maribel Fierro for this reference.

134. This statement is based on the Prophetic Tradition recorded in the *Muwaṭṭa';* see note 101. Leprosy is not mentioned specifically in the following sources: al-Bājī, *Al-Muntaqā,* 9:388–89; Ibn al-ᶜArabī, *Al-Qabas fī Sharḥ Muwaṭṭā',* 3:1132–33.

135. Ibn Ḥajar al-'Asqalānī's *Badhl al-Māᶜūn* is discussed in greater detail in chapter 5.

136. Ibn Ḥajar, *Fatḥ al-Bārī,* 21:278–81. A similar list is found in al-ᶜAynī, *ᶜUmdat al-Qārī,* 10:168–69.

137. On Abū ᶜUbayd al-Qāsim ibn Sallām al-Harawī, see Conrad, "Ninth-Century Muslim Scholar's Discussion," 170–71.

138. Abū Bakr Muḥammad b. Isḥāq b. Khuzayma was a prominent Nishapuri traditionist from whom both Bukhārī and Muslim transmitted. See Sezgin, *Geschichte des Arabischen Schrifttums* (hereafter *GAS*), 1:601.

139. On the contagiousness of leprosy, see Lieber, "Old Testament 'Leprosy,' Contagion, and Sin," 101. Historians disagree on this issue. Compare Lieber's article with Touati, "Contagion and Leprosy," 179, where he states that leprosy is only mildly contagious.

140. Van Ess, *Der Fehltritt des Gelehrten,* 125–26.

141. Ibn Ḥajar, *Badhl al-Māᶜūn,* 109–22, 155.

142. Ibn Ḥajar did not dispute the Galenic description of the plague's effects upon the body. Indeed, he saw the plague's symptoms as the result of the body's being pierced internally. Yet he completely rejected the miasma theory of transmission. See *Badhl al-Mā'ūn,* 102–5.

143. Conrad, "Ninth-Century Muslim Scholar's Discussion," 173–75. Conrad is citing material from Ibn Qutayba's *ᶜUyūn al-Akhbār.* Compare with Dols, "Leper in Islamic Society," 895, 898–99.

144. Compare with note 80.

145. Al-Ubbī, *Ikmāl Ikmāl al-Muᶜlim,* 7:419.

146. Al-Qasṭallānī, *Irshād al-Sārī,* 8:411–12. For similar views, see notes 125–26.

147. For two examples, see al-Bājī, *Al-Muntaqā,* 9:388–93; and Ibn al-Ṣalāḥ, *ᶜUlūm al-Ḥadīth,* 285.

148. Lest I be misunderstood, it is not so much Ibn al-Khaṭīb who should be corrected for his evaluation of the commentaries on the traditions. Contemporary scholarship often creates what is not there by looking for modern voices in the premodern world. The historiography surrounding Ibn al-Khaṭīb is examined at greater length in chapter 3.

149. This is a sympathetic view. Van Ess offers a slightly different view of the hadith folk's attitude toward the traditions: "Aber dann trotzdem die "Flucht" vor der Lepra zu rechtfertigen, wirkte doch recht gequält; nur Hadithgelehrte konnten auf einen solchen Gedanken kommen. Wer dagegen die Prophetentradition grundsätzlich ablehnte oder ihr misstraute—und das taten zu Anfang noch recht viele—konnte an dieser Stelle eigentlich nur einen Widerspruch sehen." Van Ess, *Der Fehltritt des Gelehrten,* 297.

150. Conrad and Wujastyk, *Contagion,* xvii.

151. This would seem to be one of the more practical measures to which Conrad is referring in "Ninth-Century Muslim Scholar's Discussion," 176.

152. See al-Bazzāz, *Tārīkh al-Awbi'a,* 403–8; and chapter 6.

Chapter 2. Contagion as Metaphor in Iberian Christian Scholarship

Epigraph: Sontag, *Illness as Metaphor* (1988); and *AIDS and Its Metaphors.* For an example of Sontag's continued influence in discussions of contagion in the humanities, see Davis, "Contagion as Metaphor." Davis's essay is an introduction to a special volume of *American Literary History* on "Contagion and Culture."

1. Sontag acknowledges that withholding metaphoric significance from disease might not be possible: "Of course one cannot think without metaphors. But that does not mean there aren't some metaphors we might well abstain from or try to retire. As, of course, all thinking is interpretation. But that does not mean it isn't sometimes correct to be 'against' interpretation." *AIDS and Its Metaphors,* 5.

2. The premodern period figures predominantly in her critique of how AIDS was discussed in the eighties. Ibid., 35, 46.

3. Ibid., 43. Compare with her similar views from ten years previously: "The fantasy that a happy state of mind would fend off disease probably flourished for all infectious diseases, before the nature of infection was understood. Theories that diseases are caused by mental states and can be cured by will power are always an index of how much is not understood about the physical terrain of a disease." Sontag, *Illness as Metaphor* (1988), 55.

4. Ibid., 61.

5. Ibid., 58. François-Olivier Touati has incisively criticized the characterization of the leper and his contagious nature in the prevailing literature. See the subsequent discussion of Touati, "Contagion and Leprosy."

6. See Sontag, *AIDS and Its Metaphors,* 93.

7. For example: "Modern—that is, effective—medicine is characterized by far more complex notions of what is to be observed inside the body." Ibid., 35.

8. For a discussion of these passages in Christian exegetical writings of antiquity and the early medieval period, see appendix A.

9. Jarcho, *Concept of Contagion.* Greek discussions of disease transmission are described by Nutton, "Did the Greeks Have a Word for It?"

10. Jarcho, *Concept of Contagion,* 28.

11. In thinking about metaphor, I have found the following essays useful: Travis, "Chaucer's Heliotropes"; Mansell, "Metaphor as Matter"; Cohen, "Metaphor and the Cultivation of Intimacy"; and Booth, "Metaphor as Rhetoric."

12. See Lienhard, "Christian Reception of the Pentateuch."

13. Firey, "*The Letter of the Law,*" 205, 210.

14. For Claudius's and Hrabanus's reliance on Isidore, see ibid., 218–19n48.

15. See Bischoff, "Der Werke Isidors von Sevilla," 187.

16. Ibid., 172. Bischoff notes that this had much to do with the late flowering of Roman-Patristic culture in Spain after Reccared's sixth-century conversion from Arianism to Catholicism.

17. Ibid., 178.

18. Ibid., 187.

19. Little is known of Isidore's life. I have drawn here on Sharpe, "Isidore of Seville." Isidore's qualities as an historian have been discussed by Basset, "Use of History."

20. While Isidore may not have made certain connections explicit, that does not imply ignorance of them on his part. For example, his failure to comment upon 1 Corinthians 5 in his writings does not mean he was not aware of previous discussions of the passage's meaning. This is suggested by his references to the pure and unleavened (*azymi*) nature of those who are baptized; he was also likely recalling earlier exegesis when he said that Sarah's preparing three loaves (Gen. 18:6) prefigured the woman Jesus speaks of in Luke 13:21. *Patrologia Latina* (hereafter *PL*), 84.244C. For further discussion of contagion in biblical exegesis, see appendix A.

21. I have used Sharpe's translation of *De medicina* in his "Isidore of Seville," 55–64, in association with the Latin given in San Isidoro de Sevilla, *Etimologías,* 1:488–97.

22. Sharpe, "Isidore of Seville," 57.

23. It is worth recalling that no distinction was made between "contagious" and "infectious." Once public authorities began to take responsibility for organizing an official response to epidemic disease, including enforcing the costly strategy of quarantine, the exact manner of the transmission of the plague had to be more carefully defined. For an excellent discussion of the practical problems faced by doctors and rulers when trying to determine the nature of "contagious" disease, see Carmichael, "Contagion Theory and Contagion Practice."

24. Isidore defined viscera in his discussion of man and his parts in book 9 of the *Etymologiae.* Sharpe, "Isidore of Seville," 46.

25. Isidore does not discuss this process explicitly. Yet, see Sharpe, "Isidore of Seville," 55–56.

26. The history of Galen's suggestive but vague reference to "seeds of disease" has been ably discussed by Nutton in two articles: "Seeds of Disease"; and "Reception of Fracastoro's Theory."

27. Sharpe, "Isidore of Seville," 66. The Latin can be found at *PL,* 83.1011A.

28. Vivian Nutton has noted that this passage was identified by Renaissance commentators on Isidore as referring to *De rerum natura,* by Lucretius (d. 55 BCE). "The Seeds of Disease," 20, where he gives a slightly different translation from that of Sharpe. Lucretius's contemporary Varro (d. 27 BCE) had written that "swamps are the source of invisible tiny animals which enter the human body and cause disease." Jarcho, *Concept of Contagion,* 11.

29. For a fuller discussion of this point, see chapter 4.

30. Isidore seems to depart from Leviticus in that he also applied the term "leprosy" when all of a person's skin changed color. Leviticus 13:13 states that if a leper is entirely covered with leprosy, and his entire skin becomes white, he is to be declared pure again. See the discussion in appendix A and Baruch Schwartz's marginal commentary on Leviticus 13–14 in *The Jewish Study Bible,* ed. Adele Berlin and Marc Zvi Brettler (Oxford: Oxford University Press, 2004), 234–41.

31. The development of what became known as anagogic interpretation of the Bible began systematically with Origen (d. ca 254). For the difficulties the Old Testament caused for early Christian exegetes, see Lienhard, "Christian Reception of the Pentateuch." Lienhard sees Isidore's efforts at exegesis as a distinct decline from those of earlier Christian writers (379).

32. See *PL,* 83.109A–B.

33. Lienard, "Christian Reception of the Pentateuch," 382–83.

34. Isidore, *Letters of St. Isidore,* 26–27.

35. *PL,* 83.327C–D.
36. *PL,* 83.327D–328D.
37. *PL,* 83.328A.
38. *PL,* 83.328C.
39. *PL,* 83.290C–291A. There were still occasions when Isidore discussed leprosy as something that was merely ritually impure, with no association with sin. See his comparison of a leper with a woman who has just given birth and is considered impure for a week thereafter. *PL,* 83.327B–C.
40. Lienhard comments perceptively on interpretations of the plague up to the time of Isidore. "Christian Reception of the Pentateuch," 381.
41. The words *pestilentia* and *plaga* were not synonymous for Isidore, though they may have become so in recent discussions and translations of his work. The former was instead a subcategory of the latter, a specific type of blow or affliction.
42. Compare with his discussion of pestilence in *De natura rerum,* where human sin is the cause of the appearance of the blow (*plaga*) of pestilence. *PL,* 83.963.
43. Isidore, *Las historias,* 256–57, 296–97, and 300–301. On Jerome's linking of Arianism with pestilence, see appendix A.
44. In his *Regula,* Isidore counseled his reader to avoid the contagion of cupidity like a deadly plague (*Philargyriae contagium ut lethiferam pestem abhorreat*), but there is no explicit statement that greed is transmitted from one person to another. *PL,* 103.558A.
45. I have consulted the edition and translation of Joaquín González Echegaray, Alberto Del Campo, and Leslie G. Freeman, Beato of Liebana, *Obras completas.*
46. See the volume of *Historia de España* authored by Claudio Sánchez-Albornoz, *El Reino Astur-Leonés,* 616–17. Sánchez-Albornoz suggests the possibility, acknowledging the lack of evidence either way, that Beato himself may have been the son of one of the Christians who fled north after 711 (615).
47. Ibid., 616. See also Díaz y Díaz, "Isidoro en la Edad Media Hispana," 166–67.
48. The adoptionism controversy, which with Elipando's friend Felix de Urgel became a subject of debate beyond the Pyrenees in Carolingian France, has been carefully studied by Cavadini, *Last Christology of the West.* A useful brief overview can be found in McWilliam, "Context of Spanish Adoptionism."
49. In Alberto Del Campo's introduction to the *Apologético,* he notes this fact and his inability to explain it. Beato, *Obras completas,* 693. See also the recent article of Wolf, "Muḥammad as Antichrist," 3–4.
50. Mikel de Epalza has argued that in Iberia Islam was not yet considered to be a theological threat, and that potential Islamic influence on Christianity would have most likely appeared as Judaizing. See his "Félix de Urgel," 42.
51. Beato, *Obras completas,* 442. Compare with a similar characterization of plagues as words at 548–50.
52. Some recent scholarship confirms his worries. See Del Campo's remarks in Beato, *Obras completas,* 680–93; and de Epalza's "Félix de Urgel." For the opposing view that there was no Muslim influence on Elipando, see Cavadini's argument in *Last Christology of the West,* 16, 27, 149. The two sides of the argument address different possibilities. De Epalza is concerned with the *unconscious* influence of Islam on the Mozarabs, whereas Cavadini sees no reason for the Christians to have expected any benefit if they changed their beliefs. Instead, he sees the context of the Christian com-

munity in Iberia as sufficient explanation for the appearance of adoptionism. Ibid., 24–44. Compare with Dominique Urvoy's "Les conséquances christologiques de la confrontation islamo-chrétienne en Espagne au VIII siècle," in *Das Frankfurter Konzil von 794* (Mainz: Selbstverl. der Ges. für Mittelrheinische Kirchengeschichte, 1997), 981–92, reprinted in *The Formation of al-Andalus, Part 2*, ed. Maribel Fierro and Julio Samsó (Brookfield, VT: Ashgate, 1998), 37–48.

53. Beato, *Obras completas,* 544.

54. Cavadini, *Last Christology of the West,* 105–6. For the writings of Beato, see 45–70.

55. For a detailed look at contagion in commentaries on 1 Corinthians 5:6–8, see appendix A.

56. Beato, *Obras completas,* 752.

57. Ibid.

58. Ibid., 866. Compare with 916.

59. Ibid., 938; and the second book of the *Apologetico* in general.

60. Beato, *Obras completas,* 944. There is some confusion here due to Beato's use of *testes* (witnesses) and *testiculi* (testicles). The editors suggest that at times Beato means the latter when using the former. The beast of which God is speaking, Behemoth, is, along with Leviathan, commonly taken to represent Satan. Consider how Elipando refers to Behemoth subsequently.

61. *PL,* 83.221A.

62. Beato, *Obras completas,* 952.

63. See Elipando, *Obras,* 157–58 (Spanish)/227 (Latin).

64. Ibid., 163/231.

65. Touati dates the first appearance of views on the contagiousness of leprosy to ca. 1220–30. See Touati, "Contagion and Leprosy"; and *Maladie et societé au Moyen Age,* 102–51 and 709–67.

66. See especially Touati, "Contagion and Leprosy," 187.

67. Ibn Sīnā, *Al-Qānūn fī-l-Ṭibb,* 8:2616.

68. Ibid. Compare with the Latin of the sixteenth-century Venetian printing of *Liber canonis,* given in Touati, "Contagion and Leprosy," 194.

69. On the growing Christian awareness that Islam had arrived in Iberia to stay, see the excellent article of Safran, "Identity and Differentiation"; and Tolan, *Saracens,* 79–104.

70. See Tolan, *Saracens,* 135–69.

71. For two examples of such reevaluations, see Burns, "Alfonso X of Castile"; and Callaghan, "Image and Reality."

72. The biography is given in Alfonso El Sabio, *Primera crónica general de España,* 1:260–74. As early as 743 in the writings of John of Damascus, Muhammad is said to have been instructed by an Arian monk, and in the work of Peter the Venerable from the 1140s, he is grouped together with Arius and the Antichrist. See Tolan, *Saracens,* 52, 158.

73. Hanlon, "Islam and Stereotypical Discourse."

74. I am not arguing that such a reading was the intended one of the compilers (intention always being difficult to prove) but that the structure of the narrative suggests that the *Estoria* could be approached in this way.

75. Wolf, *Christian Martyrs in Muslim Spain.*

76. I am indebted to Isabel Alfonso for this reference. The *Partidas* were not implemented as law until the second half of the fourteenth century and then not completely.

77. Alfonso El Sabio, *Las siete partidas,* partida 6, chap. 2, fol. 16. The word *gafedad* may have its origin in the Arabic *q-f-*[c], which can refer to the shriveled hand of a leper. See the entry for *gafedad* in Corominas and Pascual, *Diccionario crítico etimológico.*

78. The belief that sex with a menstruating woman can cause leprosy was widespread in the later Middle Ages. See Jacquart and Thomasset, *Sexuality and Medicine,* 186 ff. The authors describe the difficulty of knowing exactly which symptoms or conditions were referred to as leprosy in the Middle Ages.

79. See Alfonso El Sabio, *Las siete partidas*, partida 6, chap. 2, fol. 16. The parallel can be seen to continue, for the daughters of a traitor are able to inherit up to one-fourth of their mother's goods because they, unlike their brothers, are not likely to help their fathers. Similarly, women were believed to be able to pass on leprosy without suffering from it themselves. See Byron Grigsby, "The Doctour Maketh This Descriptioun," 101, 132.

80. Even so, those who plot but do not carry out treason may be forgiven, for, so claims the text, a man cannot be responsible for the initial feelings that stir in his heart. One may read this with some skepticism. Alfonso himself had not yet been confronted with the treachery of his son Sancho, who overthrew him some twenty years after the composition of the *Partidas.*

81. On the genre and structure of the *General estoria,* see Rico, *Alfonso el Sabio.*

82. Alfonso El Sabio, *General estoria,* 534. All Bible quotations are from the King James Version unless otherwise indicated.

83. The Bible states regarding the plague of frogs that after they died, the land stank (Exod. 8:14), without mentioning any effects this had. For Alfonso, however, the death of the frogs brought about a change in the air, a corruption that was the cause of death of many men. *General estoria,* 336. The text cites here Josephus Flavius, the first-century Jewish historian, but Josephus, in the second book of his *Antiquities,* though he says that the frogs corrupted the water and fouled people's dishes, does not mention a corruption of the air or that people died from the stink of the frogs. Flavius Josephus, *Antigüedades Judías,* 1:122.

84. Ibid., 1:172.

85. Alfonso El Sabio, *General estoria,* 534.

86. I have been unable to identify either of these authorities. Stefano Mula has pointed out to me that in Josephus's *Against Apion,* translated by John Barclay (Leiden: Brill, 2007), book 1, chap. 31, the Egyptian priest Manetho (third century BCE) is identified as the source of this story.

87. Alfonso El Sabio, *General estoria,* 534.

88. Ibid., 535.

89. Characterizing leprosy as contagious in the middle of the thirteenth century is a comparatively early development. Touati sees the influence of Ibn Sīnā becoming widespread only in the late thirteenth, and especially in the fourteenth, century. See esp. Touati, "Contagion and Leprosy," 187. Considering that the Alphonsine corpus was produced in Toledo, the same city where Gerard of Cremona had translated the Canon, this early reference to leprosy as contagious is perhaps not that surprising.

90. For Ferrer's sermons, I have consulted (1) the six volumes of his collected sermons (*Sermons* [Barcelona: Barcino, 1932–88]); volumes 1–2 were edited by Josep Sanchis Sivera in 1932 and 1934, and volumes 3–6 were edited by Gret Schib in 1975, 1977, 1984, and 1988; (2) *Sermons de quaresma;* (3) Cátedra, *Sermón, sociedad y literatura;* (4) Perarnau, "Sermons de Sant Vicent Ferrer."

91. See Ferrer's *Tratado del cisma moderno,* in De Garganta and Forcada, *Biografía y escritos de San Vicente Ferrer.* The king of Aragon, Pere the Ceremonious—after Ferrer's unsuccessful attempts to sway him from his neutral stance—forbade Ferrer to preach on the subject from 1380 onward. *Sermons de quaresma,* 1:9.

92. *Sermons de quaresma,* 9. The charge leveled against Ferrer was that he believed in the efficacy of Judas's penitence for his betrayal of Christ and that he was subsequently forgiven by God. Ferrer was fortunate to have the Avignon pope as a friend. Eymerich, the author of *Directorium inquisitorum,* the main manual used by inquisitors in Spain at that time, was a powerful opponent. He was also a biblical exegete, though his exegetical work has only recently begun to be published. See Reinhardt, "Nicolás Eymerich."

93. *Sermons de quaresma,* 33.

94. Ferrer's influence on Queen Catalina is dated to the period of his preaching in Castile in 1411. On Ferrer's belief that the Antichrist was born in 1403 and that the world would end in 1437, see the fascinating article of Guadalajara Medina, "La edad del Antichristo." Ferrer's attitude toward the Jews has been discussed repeatedly. For a recent example, see Nirenberg, "Enmity and Assimilation."

95. See Baer, *History of the Jews,* 2:166–69; Nirenberg, "Enmity and Assimilation," 144. For the text of the chronicle that attributed this decision to Ferrer's influence, see Cátedra, "La Predicación Castellana," 243–45, 309. Also see Cátedra, *Sermón, sociedad y literatura,* 241–51.

96. See *Un sermonario Castellano medieval,* 1:46–47. Here Sánchez contrasts Ferrer's sermons with those he edited in this volume, which are model sermons, fixed in writing before they were given.

97. Deyermond, "Sermon and Its Uses," 128, 132.

98. Ibid., 128–29. I have consulted the edition of Sánchez Sánchez (*Un sermonario Castellano medieval*) as well as Cátedra's *Los sermones en romance;* and Cátedra's *Los sermones atribuidos a Pedro Marín.* Cátedra has suggested in the latter volume that the sermons collected there be assigned to Ferrer (44–45).

99. Almazan, "L'exemplum chez Vincent Ferrer," 290.

100. The most dramatic case of this was documented and commented upon by Floriano, "San Vicente Ferrer." See especially the documents in appendixes 27 and 28 on 579–80. It should be noted, however, that while the Jews were forced to move to a *judería,* Floriano describes their economic influence in the town council as continuing unchanged (567).

101. The literature here is extensive. For an introduction to Augustine's discussion of Christ as doctor, see the article of Martin, "Paul the Patient," esp. his note on 222, where Martin has collected references to Augustine and medicine.

102. On man's repeated tendency to sin, see Augustine's analysis of Paul in Martin, "Paul the Patient," 228. Believing in the possibility of a sinless life, Pelagian authors saw things differently, and Augustine took pains to address their error. See 241–

42. For the Pelagian viewpoint, in which Augustine denied medicine its own rightful sphere of influence, see Lössl, "Julian of Aeclanum on Pain," 238.

103. Martin, "Paul the Patient," 225.

104. On the Eucharist in the Middle Ages, see Ruben, *Corpus Christi.*

105. Martin, "Paul the Patient," 225, emphasis in original.

106. Ferrer, with characteristic vividness, describes preachers as the dogs of Christ, who heal with their tongues (Luke 16:21; misidentified by the editor as Ps. 67:24): "Canes vanienbant [*sic*], et lingebant ulcera eius," a reference to a beggar whose sores were licked by dogs. In Luke, the action of the dogs does not necessarily encourage a positive interpretation. See *Sermons de quaresma,* 1:159. Here the importance of the medicinal properties of speech is emphasized, as opposed to the infection of heresy that can be caused by listening to heretics.

107. *Sermons de quaresma,* 1:71. The anonymous author of the sermons edited by Sánchez claims the same. *Un sermonario Castellano medieval,* 1:272–73.

108. See Sánchez, *Un sermonario Castellano medieval,* 1:252.

109. The sacraments in general are referred to as medicines. See *Un sermonario Castellano medieval,* 1:253.

110. Ferrer, *Sermons,* 4:241–43, referencing Luke 8:11: "Semen est verbum Dei."

111. This is a curious equation. Original sin would have seemed a more natural meaning for the fever.

112. See Ferrer, *Sermons,* 1:184. On how Jews and Muslims, not enjoying the light of baptism, will remain beneath the earth in the caverns of the law of, respectively, Moses and Muhammad, see 1:126.

113. Cátedra, *Sermón, sociedad y literatura,* 384.

114. Admittedly, Ferrer does not suggest that baptism heals the actual sickness of leprosy.

115. On the nature of the exemplum, a short narrative piece often including dialogue, which bears interesting parallels with the *khabar* of Arab historians, see Almazan, "L'exemplum chez Vincent Ferrer," 288; and Cátedra, *Sermón, sociedad y literatura,* 195 ff. Ferrer often singled out Jews or Muslims in his sermons, and Cátedra has argued for the presence, however unwilling, of both communities at his sermons. *Sermón, sociedad y literatura,* 244–45.

116. Ferrer, *Sermons,* 1:104–5.

117. Perarnau, "Sermons de Sant Vicent Ferrer," 257–59. See Nirenberg's thesis in "Enmity and Assimilation" on how a distrust of new Christians was not yet prominent at the time of Ferrer. On another occasion Ferrer explained Jesus's circumcision as a proof against later heretics who would deny his human nature. He notes as well that Mary saw in the circumcision of her son a sign of the Jews' later sentencing and killing him. See *Sermons,* 6:251.

118. In a sermon delivered on the text "Hoc facite in meam commemorationem," 1 Corinthians 11, referring to the taking of the Host, Ferrer gives the Host five separate meanings, the first of which is medicinal. See *Sermons de quaresma,* 2:163–65. Compare with 1:76.

119. See especially ibid., 2:163–64, where, in a sermon on 1 Corinthians 11, Ferrer defines the Host as a new fruit that functions as a medicine against that other fruit through which man committed his first sin.

120. Ferrer, *Sermons,* 3:211. Ferrer justifies this by quoting Ezekiel 36:25: "Then will I sprinkle clean water upon you, and ye shall be clean: from all your filthiness, and from all your idols, will I cleanse you." The doctrine of *fomes peccati* (literally "the tinder of sin"), adopted formally by the Council of Trent in 1546, was that the sacrament of baptism does not purify the believer of all sin but leaves a small amount. See also appendix A, note 18.

121. See *Sermons de quaresma,* 1:9.

122. Ibid., 1:72–76.

123. Medicine was not wholly metaphoric for Ferrer. He differentiated between a physical and a spiritual medicine, the former existing through the decree of God, the latter spiritual in nature. Less clear is Ferrer's distinction between a "medecina de ciència," which is used to cure those who sin out of ignorance, and the spiritual medicine of loving God needed by those who sin out of weakness. *Sermons de quaresma,* 2:150. When this first medicine proves ineffective, one should turn to the cross of Jesus to seek further healing (1:124). It is also possible that, if the patient's disposition and state do not allow it, doctors will not be able to cure a physical illness. This is different from the case of spiritual illness, where a cure seems to be guaranteed as long as the patient repents of his sins. Ferrer recounts the case of a king who suffered mightily from hemorrhoids and whom the doctors were afraid to treat because the treatment might itself be the cause of his death. This is not the fault of medicine, he notes. On the same page he states that "the sweet syrup of contrition with hot tears" preserves one from spiritual death (2:164).

124. Cátedra, *Los sermones en romance,* 173–74. This legend has most recently been discussed by Peregrine Horden, who argues that Gregory and other Church officials may have played an active role in combating epidemic disease. See Horden, "Disease, Dragons, and Saints."

125. Like many commentators before him, Ferrer reads the plagues of Egypt allegorically. The frogs of the second plague (Exod. 8) are to be understood as heretics. He explains that heretics, like frogs, begin in water (that of baptism), and once they have left the water, they walk the world, croaking meaninglessly. *Sermons,* 1:202–3.

126. See Cátedra, *Los sermones en romance,* 181. A similar sentiment is expressed in another preacher's citation of the book of Job. See *Un sermonario Castellano medieval,* 1:313.

127. See *Un sermonario Castellano medieval,* 1:314. Compare with *Sermons,* 3:212.

128. Ibid., 1:315–16.

129. See also ibid., 2:520.

130. Ibid., 1:307–8.

131. In contrast to Ferrer's sermons, this and the other sermons edited by Sánchez Sánchez are models, not based upon the notes of those who listened. The seeming awkwardness of this passage cannot, then, be ascribed to poor note-taking.

132. Compare with Ferrer, *Sermons,* 3:212, where the contrition of the heart is equated with Jesus's touching of the leper.

133. See ibid., 6:250.

134. See ibid., 3:214.

135. Ibid., 3:216–17.

136. Nirenberg, "Enmity and Assimilation," 143–45.

137. Ferrer, *Sermons,* 4:61. The episode in its entirety is given in 4:58–61. Compare with *Sermons de quaresma,* 2:69. In Ferrer's mind, much of the world was once Christian but had fallen away through the sins of the Christians, particularly simony.

138. See Ferrer, *Sermons,* 5:16. This image of pride as a tumor was a favorite of Augustine's. See Martin, "Paul the Patient."

139. Much of traditional Christian historiography is structured according to the framework of seven ages, the last beginning with the Second Coming. This was a narrative of progress. See Patrides, *Grand Design of God.* Ferrer's choice of Daniel is perhaps in part explained by his belief that he was living in the last days and that the world would end in 1436.

140. Cátedra, *Sermón, sociedad y literatura,* 638–39.

141. *Sermons de quaresma,* 2:68. At times Ferrer addresses the Muslims directly, explaining the doctrine of the Trinity to them or mocking Muhammad by citing the Qur'an as proof that he once worshipped idols. See 2:75, 88.

142. Ibid., 1:156.

143. For Ferrer's ingenious explanation that Christ gave Jerusalem to the Muslims because he did not want Christians sinning on holy land, see ibid., 2:64.

144. Ferrer, *Sermons,* 3:112–13; compare with 6:250. In other sermons Ferrer also called for the segregation of Jews and Muslims based on their being impure due to their sins. See Perarnau, "Sermons de Sant Vicent Ferrer," 231–32, 248; and compare with Nirenberg, *Communities of Violence,* 169.

145. Compare with the portrayal of Jews and crypto-Jews in the late-fifteenth- to early-sixteenth-century *Memorias del reinado de los reyes Católicos* of Andrés Bernáldez (d. 1516). See Gerli, "Social Crisis and Conversion," esp. 149–53, where Jews are described as, among other things, "fomes peccati" and accused of spreading the plague in Andalusia.

146. An example of such a debate is found in Ferrer, *Sermons,* 2:206–7.

147. See ibid., 3:23–24.

Chapter 3. Contagion Contested

Epigraphs: Gigandet, "Trois *maqālāt* sur la prevention des épidémies," 261; Himmich, *Polymath,* 73–74. While it is certainly possible that Ibn Khaldūn had read the plague treatise of Ibn al-Khaṭīb (whose views are inaccurately presented here)—whom he had met in Fez in 1360–61 and in Granada shortly thereafter—we have no conclusive proof that he had read it.

1. On the arrival and initial impact of the Black Death in al-Andalus, see Lirola Delgado, Garijo Galán, and Lirola Delgado, "Efectos de la epidemia de peste negra"; and Calero Secall, "La peste en Málaga." A more general overview of the spread of the Black Death throughout Iberia is given by Ubieto Arteta, "Cronología des desarrolló."

2. Lirola Delgado, Garijo Galán, and Lirola Delgado, "Efectos de la epidemia de peste negra," 179.

3. Calero Secall, "La peste en Málaga," 66.

4. The literature on the subject is substantial, and the following references are by no means comprehensive: Arié, "Un opuscule Grenadin"; Ullmann, *Die Medizin im Islam,* 241–50; Conrad, "Arabic Plague Chronologies and Treatises"; Millán, "Tres opúsculos inéditos"; Lirola Delgado, Garijo Galán, and Lirola Delgado, "Efectos de

la epidemia de peste negra"; Gigandet, "Trois *maqālāt* au sujet des épidémies"; "Trois *maqālāt* sur la prévention des épidémies." For further references, see the next note.

5. For an excellent survey of the history of the medicine practiced in Islam, see Pormann and Savage-Smith, *Medieval Islamic Medicine.* The following study is still useful: Dols, *Medieval Islamic Medicine.* The first part of Dols's book is much more than an introduction to the treatise of Ibn Riḍwān; it gives a perceptive overview of the state of the scholarship.

6. For a comprehensive discussion of the translation movement, see Gutas, *Greek Thought, Arabic Culture.* While administrative records were translated from Greek to Arabic during the Umayyad period, scientific and medical texts (with a small number of possible exceptions) were first translated under the Abbasids (23–24). On the importance of the second Abbasid caliph al-Manṣūr as the originator of the translation movement (including medical texts), see 28–34 and 53–56. See also an earlier article by Dols, "Syriac into Arabic."

7. In some cases, such as that of Ibn Sahl b. Rabbān al-Ṭabarī, who was from a Nestorian family, these doctors converted to Islam.

8. The most comprehensive and perceptive discussion of the nature and development of Prophetic medicine is that of Perho, *Prophet's Medicine.* Other comments on Prophetic medicine can be found in Bürgel, "Medieval Arabic Medicine"; and Karmi, "Al-Tibb al-Nabawi."

9. See Savage-Smith, "Medicine," 929. See Ibn Khaldūn, *Muqaddima,* bk. 6, chap. 25, for a review of Muslim medical achievements. For a more sectarian justification of the need for Muslims to study medicine, see Ibn al-Ḥājj, *Madkhal al-Shar*ᶜ *al-Sharīf,* 4:107–24.

10. In his classic work on the Black Death, Michael Dols comments on the difference between contagion and infection as follows:

> In my discussion of the Muslim prohibition of the idea of infection, I have interpreted "infection" (*ᶜadwā*) in the Arabic texts in a broad sense to mean both contagion and infection. In modern medical terminology . . . this is unacceptable. "Contagion" means the transmission of the disease by an agent while "infection" implies the lack of such an agent and the communication of the bacilli directly. With regard to plague, the distinction is an important one; bubonic plague is contagious, whereas pneumonic plague is infectious. While this distinction is helpful in understanding the historical phenomenon of the Black Death, no such distinction was made in the medieval treatises on plague. Moreover, the statement that there is no infection should be understood to mean that the disease came directly from God. In this sense, infection should not be interpreted as distinct from contagion. *Black Death,* 74.

See also the remarks of Ullmann, *Islamic Medicine,* 86–96.

11. Ibn Sahl b. Rabbān al-Ṭabarī, *Firdaws al-Ḥikma fī l-Ṭibb.* On this work see Ullman, *Die Medizin im Islam,* 119–22.

12. Al-Ṭabarī, *Firdaws al-Ḥikma fī l-Ṭibb*, 225. Plagues and the possibility of warding them off by burning sweet-smelling wood, following the example of Hippocrates, are mentioned on 233.

13. Qustā Ibn Lūqā, *Abhandlung über die Ansteckung.* On Ibn Lūqā's life, see Ger-

rit Bos, *Qusṭā Ibn Lūqā's Medical Regime for the Pilgrims to Mecca: The Risāla fī tadbīr safar al-ḥajj* (Leiden: Brill, 1992), 1 ff.

14. Ibn Lūqā, *Abhandlung über die Ansteckung,* 12–13.

15. Ibid., 18–21.

16. Ibid., 24–25.

17. For support, Ibn Lūqā refers here to the homily of Gregory Nazianzen (d. 389) on giving alms to the poor, in which the bishop laments that lepers are driven away even from rivers. Ibid., 26–27.

18. Ibn Lūqā remarks on the lack of detail in Galen's comments on contagion: "These are the sicknesses that Galen mentioned as contagious, though he mentioned no reason for this nor devoted speech specifically to it." Ibid., 28–29. Ibn Lūqā's editor, Harmut Fändrich, notes that this is most likely a reference to Galen's *De febrium differentiis,* which was translated into Arabic by Ḥunayn b. Isḥāq (d. 260/873), the greatest and most prolific representative of the third/ninth-century translation movement. For an overview of his works, see Sezgin, *GAS,* 3:247–56.

19. Travaglia, *Magic, Causality, and Intentionality,* 20 ff.

20. Ibn Lūqā, *Abhandlung über die Ansteckung,* 28–29.

21. Meyerhof, "Book of Treasure," 60–61. For arguments that Ibn Qurra was not the author of this work, see Ullmann, *Die Medizin im Islam,* 136, 244; and Sezgin, *GAS,* 3:260–61.

22. Al-Rāzī, *Al-Ḥāwī fī l-Ṭibb,* 8:3823–24.

23. The identity of al-Ḥarrāni is unclear, although it is reported that he left the Middle East for al-Andalus during the reign of Muḥammad b. ᶜAbd al-Raḥmān (rl. 238–273/857–886). See Sezgin, *GAS,* 3:258.

24. Al-Rāzī, *Al-Ḥāwī fī l-Ṭibb,* 8:3823–24.

25. For later views of contagion in association with leprosy, see Ibn Sīnā, *Al-Qānūn fī-l-Ṭibb,* 8:2616; and Ibn al-Nafīs (d. 687/1288), *Al-Mūjaz fī l-Ṭibb,* 303.

26. Al-Ṭabarī, *Firdaws al-Ḥikma fī l-Ṭibb,* 233; Ibn Sīnā, *Al-Qānūn fī l-Ṭibb,* 8:2616.

27. Perho, *Prophet's Medicine,* 11.

28. Here I follow Perho's description closely. Ibid., 44–46.

29. Ibid., 44.

30. For generally disparaging estimations of Prophetic medicine, see Ullmann, *Islamic Medicine,* 4–5; Savage-Smith, "Medicine," 927–30; and Gallagher, *Medicine and Power in Tunisia,* 8–10.

31. For two examples of such citations of Ibn Khaldūn, see the previous note. The passage in question can be found in *Muqaddima,* bk. 6, chap. 25, where Ibn Khaldūn cites the Prophet as saying, "You are more knowledgeable concerning your worldly affairs," and notes that following medical traditions related by the Prophet constituted an act of faith, not of Galenic medicine (*al-ṭibb al-mizājī*) (490–91). The same tradition was cited by Ibn Qayyim and was later invoked by Ḥamdān Khoja in the nineteenth century. See Perho, *Prophet's Medicine,* 98; and Ḥamdān Khoja, *Itḥāf al-munṣifīn,* 66.

32. Perho, *Prophet's Medicine,* 31, 70–71.

33. For Ibn Taymiyya's aversion to speculative theology (*kalām*), see Henri Laoust's article on him in the *Encyclopedia of Islam,* 2nd ed., 12 vols. (Leiden: Brill,

1960–2004); and for his relationship with al-Dhahabī, see Little, "Did Ibn Taymiyya Have a Screw Loose?"

34. The earliest example of the genre of Prophetic medicine was written by ᶜAbd al-Malik ibn Ḥabīb al-Sulamī al-Qurṭubī (d. 238/853). Perho, *Prophet's Medicine,* 53. This has now been translated. See Ibn Ḥabīb, *Mujtaṣar fī l-Ṭibb.*

35. Perho, *Prophet's Medicine,* 56–57.

36. Ibid., 63.

37. The section on Prophetic medicine has now been translated into English: Ibn Qayyim al-Jawziyya, *Medicine of the Prophet.*

38. Ibid., 27–32 and 110–16.

39. Ibid., 28–30. Where I have modified Johnstone's translation, I have added the Arabic in parentheses. See also Ibn Qayyim al-Jawziyya, *Al-Ṭibb al-Nabawī,* 29–34.

40. Perho, *Prophet's Medicine,* 127–28.

41. Ibn Qayyim al-Jawziyya, *Medicine of the Prophet,* 31–32.

42. This transmission is described as follows: "Avoiding of proximity to the sick who have fallen ill of plague, for by [*sic*] such proximity infection is inevitable. In the *Sunan* of Abū Dāwūd (*marfūᶜ*) it says: from *ᶜirq* comes destruction. Ibn Qutayba explains *ᶜirq* as: coming close to the pestilence and the sick." Ibid., 31–32.

43. Ibid., 111 ff.

44. Ibid., 114. Ibn Qayyim also notes that the contagion denied by the Prophet was that described in the tradition regarding the woman who had experienced misfortune in a house and wished to move elsewhere. Ibid. Perho discusses this tradition in *Prophet's Medicine,* 92–93.

45. Perho, *Prophet's Medicine,* 99. See Ibn Qayyim al-Jawziyya, *Miftāḥ Dār al-Saᶜāda,* 3:372–79.

46. Further evidence for Ibn Qayyim's support of a qualified theory of secondary causation is found in his *Madārij al-Sālikīn,* 3:494–501.

47. Perho, *Prophet's Medicine,* 99–100.

48. Based on manuscript evidence, Perho has argued convincingly that *Al-Ṭibb al-Nabawī* could not have been written by Jalāl al-Din al-Suyūṭī, as it has traditionally been widely believed, and that al-Dhahabī is the most likely author. See Perho, *Prophet's Medicine,* 36–40 (Perho is able to date this work to the late seventh/thirteenth or early eighth/fourteenth century, but her argument for Dhahabī's authorship, though strong, is not conclusive; further evidence may confirm or refute her identification). *Al-Ṭibb al-Nabawī* has been translated by Elgood, "Tibb-ul-Nabbi." Elgood believed the author of the treatise to be al-Suyūṭī. For an edition of this work, see al-Dhahabī, *Al-Ṭibb al-Nabawī.*

49. Elgood, "Tibb-ul-Nabbi," 150; al-Dhahabī, *Al-Ṭibb al-Nabawī,* 130.

50. Elgood, "Tibb-ul-Nabbi," 137; al-Dhahabī, *Al-Ṭibb al-Nabawī,* 116–17.

51. Elgood, "Tibb-ul-Nabbi," 149–51; al-Dhahabī, *Al-Ṭibb al-Nabawī,* 130–32. A hadith is cited here from the collection of Abū Dāwūd, which reads, in Elgood's translation: "From contact comes destruction" (*inna min al-qaraf al-talaf*); Ibn Qutayba also commented that what the Prophet meant by this was proximity to plague and pestilence. A tradition very similar to this one can be found in the 29th chapter of Abū Dāwūd's collection, entitled *Kitāb al-kihāna wa-l-taṭayyur,* related on the authority of Farwa ibn Musayk (d. 30/650) of Yemen. This tradition, and Ibn Qutayba's

comment explaining the meaning of *qaraf,* is also found in al-Ḥamdān al-Khūja, *Itḥāf al-munṣifīn,* 88–89. Elgood's translation of the hadith is tendentious considering that *qaraf* is generally defined as proximity and not contact (see the supplement to Lane's *Arabic-English Lexicon*).

52. See Perho, *Prophet's Medicine,* 146.

53. Ibn Ḥajar does acknowledge the skill of Ibn Sīnā', but he claims that no doctor of true ability is practicing in his own day. See the section "Ibn Ḥajar al-ᶜAsqalānī's Intervention."

54. Ibn Qayyim divides the practice of medicine into three types, in ascending order of validity: that practiced by soothsayers (*al-ṭarqiyya* [my understanding of this word is tentative, but see Lane's entry under "ṭāriq" in his *Arabic-English Lexicon*]), that of the doctors, and Prophetic medicine. Although he privileged Prophetic medicine above Greco-Islamic medicine, he and his contemporaries writing in the genre emphasized the importance of seeking out a well-trained doctor, who, in turn, would of course benefit from the study of Prophetic medicine. Perho, *Prophet's Medicine,* 115–17; Ibn Qayyim, *Medicine of the Prophet,* 101–9 (chap. 26).

55. See Dols, *Black Death,* 93–94; Ullmann, *Die Medizin im Islam,* 246–47; Ullmann, *Islamic Medicine,* 92–96; Rofail Farag, "Muslims' Medical Achievements," 303; Vásquez de Benito, "La materia médica de Ibn al-Jaṭīb," 140–41; Arjona Castro, "Las epidemias de peste bubónica," 58; Calero Secall, "La peste en Málaga," 58; al-Bazzāz, *Ta'rīkh al-Awbi'a,* 393; Congourdeau and Melhaoui, "La perception de la peste," 110.

56. This narrative has now been challenged in numerous recent studies. See, for example, Powers, *Law, Society, and Culture;* Hallaq, *Law and Legal Theory.*

57. Not everyone has misread the treatises in this way. See Ullmann, *Die Medizin im Islam* and *Islamic Medicine,* for a more nuanced view.

58. For biographical information on Ibn al-Khaṭīb, see Lirola Delgado's excellent entry, "Ibn al-Khaṭīb," in *Biblioteca de al-Andalus;* Molina López, *Ibn al-Jatib;* and ᶜInān, *Lisān al-Dīn ibn al-Khaṭīb.*

59. Portions of the following discussion appear in Stearns, "Contagion in Theology and Law."

60. Some scholars have suggested that Ibn al-Khaṭīb's criticism of religious authorities in his plague treatise played a role in his trial. See Dols, *Black Death,* 98; and Aberth, *Black Death,* 114. This seems unlikely. On the trial of Ibn al-Khaṭīb, see the excellent article of Calero Secall, "El proceso de Ibn al-Jaṭīb." She deals with the accusations against Ibn al-Khaṭīb on 432–45. Many if not most of the allegations against him were doubtless politically motivated; but in the charges that have been preserved, no reference to his views on causality, contagion, or disease is to be found. Most objectionable, instead, seem to have been several of Ibn al-Khaṭīb's comments in his writings on Sufism.

61. Al-Khaṭṭābī, *Al-Ṭibb wa-l-Aṭibbā' fī-l-Andalus al-Islāmiyya,* 2:188. This passage is difficult at times. Compare the text and translation given by M. J. Müller in Ibn al-Khaṭīb, "Ibnulkhatîbs Bericht über die Pest," 2:6–8/2:18–21; the partial English translation (based on Müller's edition) given in Aberth, *Black Death,* 114–16; and the partial translation found in Ullmann, *Islamic Medicine,* 86–96. Ildefonso Garijo Galán, Jorge Lirola Delgado, and Pilar Lirola Delgado are currently preparing a schol-

arly edition of all three Andalusian plague treatises, and once it appears, that edition will greatly facilitate further research into the Muslim response to the plague in al-Andalus.

62. Hallaq, *History of Islamic Legal Theories,* 132. Compare with Masud, *Shatibi's Philosophy of Islamic Law,* 142.

63. Masud, *Shatibi's Philosophy of Islamic Law,* 119–20, 151. Compare with Hallaq, *History of Islamic Legal Theories,* 166–67, 182–83. For discussions of *maṣlaḥa* in the modern period, see Hallaq, *History of Islamic Legal Theories,* 207–55; and Opwis, "*Maṣlaḥa* in Contemporary Islamic Legal Theory." Ibrahim's recent dissertation on *maqāṣid al-sharīʿa* is also useful: "The Spirit of Islamic Law and Modern Religious Reform."

64. Masud, *Shatibi's Philosophy of Islamic Law,* 142.

65. Ibid., 161. See also Hallaq, *History of Islamic Legal Theories,* 166–67, 205–6.

66. A similar fear is expressed by al-Ghazālī in his *Iḥyā' ʿUlūm al-Dīn.* See *Al-Ghazali,* 143.

67. It is difficult to know to what degree Ibn al-Khaṭīb's interpretation of Q2:195 ("Spend in God's cause: do not contribute to your destruction with your own hands, but do good, for God loves those who do good.") was shared by his contemporaries. Many commentators seem to have understood the verse to refer to the (spiritual) danger of *not* taking part in the *jihād* against the enemies of God. While Ṭabarī mentions the prohibition of suicide as one of the many interpretations given to the verse, Ibn Kathīr and al-Qurṭubī interpret it as primarily emphasizing the importance of carrying out and supporting *jihād.* See Kuramustafa, "Suicide"; Ibn Kathīr, *Tafsīr al-Qur'ān al-ʿAẓīm,* 1:200–201; and al-Qurṭubī, *Tafsir al-Qurtubi,* 1:499–501.

68. On the medical training of Ibn al-Khaṭīb, see Castrillo Márquez, "Yaḥya b. Hudhayl." On his medical works, see Molina López, *Ibn al-Jatib*, 195–96; and Vásquez de Benito, "La materia médica de Ibn al-Jatīb."

69. A full edition of this treatise is in preparation by Garijo Galán, Lirola Delgado, and Lirola Delgado, as mentioned in note 61, and I am grateful to Jorge Lirola Delgado for sending me a copy of their edition of the final section (chaps. 7–10) of Ibn Khātima's treatise, previously unpublished and untranslated, in which the author examines the Prophetic traditions relevant to the plague and contagion. For the other sections of the treatise, I have depended on the Arabic text partially edited in al-Khaṭṭābī, *Al-Ṭibb wa-l-Aṭibbā' fī-l-Andalus al-Islāmiyya,* 2:161–87; and Ibn Khātima "Die Schrift ueber die Pest." For biographical information on Ibn al-Khātima, see Lirola Delgado and Garijo Galán's entry "Ibn al-Khaṭīb" in *Biblioteca de al-Andalus.*

70. Dols, *Black Death,* 92–94, 110. Compare with Ullmann, *Islamic Medicine,* 95. Ullmann, by emphasizing that Ibn al-Khaṭīb's true contribution was his description of plague and not his defense of its contagious nature, groups Ibn Khātima and Ibn al-Khaṭīb together, instead of seeing them as at odds with each other. Other evaluations of Ibn Khātima's treatise include Antuña, "Abenjátima de Almería"; Fermart, "Contribución al estudio de la medicina árabe española"; Molina López, "La obra histórica de Ibn Jātima de Almería"; Lirola Delgado, Garijo Galán, and Lirola Delgado, "Efectos de la epidemia de peste negra."

71. Al-Khaṭṭābī, *Al-Ṭibb wa-l-Aṭibbā' fī-l-Andalus al-Islāmiyya,* 2:179–80. I benefited from consulting Ibn Khātima, "Die Schrift ueber die Pest," 49–51.

72. Since this section of Ibn Khātima's treatise has not yet been edited or trans-

lated, I have referred here to the forthcoming edition of Garijo Galán, Lirola Delgado, and Lirola Delgado. When I cite a passage, I refer to the folio number of the manuscripts used in this edition (they have based their edition on manuscripts of the *Taḥṣīl* in Berlin [B], Escorial [E], Istanbul [S], and a partial manuscript in Rabat [R]).

73. Ibn Khātima, "Taḥṣīl," E 99v, B 66v.

74. Ibid., E 98v, B 64v. The Mu'tazilī attacks of al-Jāḥiẓ and al-Naẓẓām on Prophetic tradition and their belief that things are able to influence each other and that people create their own acts are summarily dismissed on E 102r, B 70r.

75. Ibid., E 94r, B 58v. Ibn Khātima's reference to places of danger (*mahālik*) is reminiscent of Ibn al-Khaṭib's allusion to Q2:195.

76. Ibn Khātima, "Taḥṣīl," E 100v, B 68r.

77. Ibid., E 101r, B 68r.

78. Ibid., E 98r, B 66r. This tradition is still today often recited in Egypt in order to counter arguments thought to be fatalistic. While I have found references to the tradition's being in Tirmidhī, I have not found it there. See, however, Ibn al-Jawzi (d. 597/1201), *Talbīs Iblīs,* 270, where the tradition is related from Anas b. Mālik (d. 93/711) as part of a conversation between an unnamed man and the Prophet.

79. One of the many facets of Ibn al-Khatīb's thought that has received too little attention—certainly in this context—is his interest in Sufism and the amount of energy he devoted to writing on the subject. See, for example, de Santiago Simón, "Un opúsculo inédito de Ibn al-Jaṭīb sobre sufismo." In this treatise, entitled *Kitāb Istinzāl al-Luṭf al-Mawjūd fī Asrār al-Wujūd,* Ibn al-Khaṭīb emphasizes that patience and reliance upon God is the only true cure (1246). Taken outside the greater context of Ibn al-Khaṭīb's work, such a statement may be read as fatalistic—quite different from the standard depiction of Ibn al-Khaṭīb as a rational predecessor to modern empiricism.

80. Abū ᶜAbd Allāh Muḥammad b. ᶜAlī b. ᶜAbd Allāh al-Lakhmī al-Shaqūrī was born in 727/1327 into a family of doctors. For more on him and his plague treatise, see Gigandet, "Trois *Maqālāt* sur la prévention des épidémies"; and Arié, "Un opuscule grenadin sur la peste."

81. See Gigandet, "Trois *Maqālāt* sur la prévention des épidémies," 257. An edition of al-Shaqūrī's treatise is currently being prepared by Garijo Galán, Lirola Delgado, and Lirola Delgado.

82. Admittedly, in Gigandet's translation we read, "Nous commençons, avant d'exposer nos propos, par une introduction, en affirmant que la véritable cause [de l'épidémie] est l'infection qui se répand dans l'air respirable; les médecins ordonnent donc de purifier cet air, et c'est une tâche des plus dificiles." "Trois *Maqālāt* sur la prévention des épidémies," 256. I have been able to acquire a copy of the al-Bannūnī manuscript used by Gigandet, however, and on page 26 (as on Escorial 1785, 106r), what she translated as "infection" is *fasād* in the original; a literal translation would be "corruption." Similarly, Arié's claim that Shaqūrī went beyond his Christian contemporaries by believing that contamination could be transmitted by contact seems forced. See Gigandet, "Trois *Maqālāt* sur la prévention des épidémies," 258. For Arié's position, see "Un opuscule Grenadin," 195, 199.

83. See Dols, "Ibn al-Wardī's *Risālah al-naba' ᶜan al-waba'*"; "Al-Manbijī's 'Report of the Plague.' "

84. See Dols, *Black Death,* 101, and compare 326–28. Note that Dols fails to credit Ibn Abī Ḥajala with believing in a type of contagion.

85. The consideration of plague treatises written in the Mashriq from the fifteenth to nineteenth centuries lies beyond the scope of this study, but I expect that future research will show a similar trend there.

86. This treatise has previously been discussed by Sublet, "La peste"; and at length by Dols, *Black Death,* 110–21. Since the publication of Dols's book, the treatise has been edited with a useful introduction: Ibn Ḥājar al-ᶜAsqalānī, *Badhl al-Māᶜūn.* The title of the treatise is somewhat unclear, as it would appear to refer to Q107:4–7, "Woe to those who pray but are heedless of their prayer; those who are all show and forbid common kindnesses (*yamnaᶜūna al-māᶜūn*)."

87. These are examined in chapter 6. The influence of Ibn Ḥajar on later writers on the plague is emphasized by his editor, Aḥmad ᶜAṣṣām. Ibn Ḥājar al-ᶜAsqalānī, *Badhl al-Māᶜūn,* 6.

88. Ibid., 9.

89. Ibn al-Wardī died of the plague in Aleppo in 749/1349. This work has been studied by Dols, in "Ibn al-Wardī's *Risālah al-naba' ᶜan al-waba'.*" For Ibn al-Wardī's stance on contagion, see 454.

90. Ibn Ḥajar, *Badhl al-Māᶜūn,* 109–22. Ibn Ḥajar distinguishes between the plague and other epidemics on 102–8, arguing, in part, that it is precisely because the plague has no cure that it is different from other epidemic diseases (106).

91. Ibid., 105.

92. Ibid., 105–6.

93. Ibid., 105. Ibn Ḥajar was well informed on the views of doctors working within the Islamo-Greek tradition. See 306 for another instance of his criticism of miasma theory, and see 341 for his praise of Ibn Sīnā and his disparagement of the doctors of his own time.

94. Ibid., 106.

95. Ibn Ḥajar tells us that Shihāb al-Dīn b. ᶜAdnān was the private secretary (*kātib al-sirr*) of the Mamluk sultan and that he died of the plague in 833/1429. See Ibn Ḥajar, *Inbā' al-Ghumr fī Abnā' al-ᶜUmr,* 3:441–42.

96. Ibn Ḥajar, *Badhl al-Māᶜūn,* 155.

97. Ibid., 145–50.

98. See esp. ibid., 192–202.

99. Ibn Ḥajar denies the phenomenon of contagion explicitly at ibid., 294–301.

100. Ibid., 295–96.

101. Not found in the *Fatḥ al-Bārī* is Ibn Ḥajar's lengthy discussion of the report that late in his life the caliph ᶜUmar repented of turning back from the plague at Sargh. After sifting through previous opinions on the strength of this report and its interpretation, Ibn Ḥajar states that this tradition is valid, that ᶜUmar most probably repented because he had returned instead of waiting until the plague ended and then continuing. *Badhl al-Māᶜūn,* 286–87.

102. *Badhl al-Māᶜūn,* 341. Tāj al-Dīn al-Subkī, who died of the plague in Damascus, authored a work on the plague—*Juz' fī l-Ṭāᶜūn*—that is no longer extant and to which Ibn Ḥajar refers repeatedly in his *Badhl al-Māᶜūn.* See 32.

103. Ibid., 342.

104. Ibid., 342–44.

105. Ibid., 341.

106. See, for example, Savage-Smith, "Medicine," 930. Dols identified the genre

with what he called "orthodox Islam," and he characterizes Ibn Ḥajar's treatise as representative of the genre as a whole. See his *Black Death,* 110.

Chapter 4. Situating Scholastic Contagion between Miasma and the Evil Eye

Epigraphs: Foucault, *Order of Things,* 23–24; Cunningham, "Transforming Plague," 241.

1. On the dangers of applying modern notions of disease to medieval narratives, I have been chiefly influenced by Arrizabalaga, Henderson, and French, *Great Pox;* and by Cunningham, "Transforming Plague." See also Van Arsdall, "Reading Medieval Medical Texts."

2. See Cunningham, "Transforming Plague," 209.

3. I have been guided in my thinking on this issue by a handful of excellent exceptions, including the already cited studies of Arrizabalaga, Henderson, and French and Cunningham as well as Temkin, "Historical Analysis of the Concept of Infection"; Grmek, "Le concept d'infection"; Nutton, "Did the Greeks Have a Word for It?"; and "Reception of Fracastoro's Theory."

4. See the references in the preceding notes, but especially Arrizabalaga, Henderson, and French, *Great Pox,* 121–26, 234 ff.

5. See, among others, Arrizabalaga, "Facing the Black Death," 287; and Carmichael, "Contagion Theory and Contagion Practice," 215.

6. See Cunningham, "Transforming Plague," 217.

7. For an excellent discussion of the historiography surrounding early-nineteenth-century debates between contagionists and miasmists in England, see Hamlin, "Predisposing Causes." For the influence of the Church on late medieval and early modern conceptions of contagious disease, see Palmer, "Church, Leprosy, and Plague."

8. For Sudhoff's invaluable efforts, see Sudhoff, "Pestschriften." Sudhoff provides an overview and an index of the treatises he published in the last installment of the series in *Archiv für Geschichte der Medizin* 17 (1925): 241–91. For a recent and exhaustive study of the spread and demographic effects of the Black Death, see Benedictow, *Black Death.* An overview of the spread of the Black Death in Christian Iberia is given in Phillips, "*Peste Negra.*" For an overview of recent publications on the Black Death, see Stearns, "New Directions in the Study of Religious Responses to the Black Death."

9. See Campbell, *Black Death and Men of Learning;* Palazzotto, "Black Death and Medicine." See also Singer, "Some Plague Tractates." Along with the articles already cited, see also Chase, "Fevers, Poisons, and Apostemes"; and Wray, "Boccaccio and the Doctors."

10. Notable and relevant exceptions include Amasuno Sárraga, *La peste en la Corona de Castilla;* and York, "Experience and Theory in Medical Practice." Another is Cohn, *Cultures of Plague,* a copy of which I received only in the final stages of this project.

11. For an overview of the treatises written in response to the first wave of the Black Death, see Campbell, *Black Death and Men of Learning,* 9–33; and Palazzotto, "Black Death and Medicine," 31–52.

12. Cunningham, "Transforming Plague," 221.

13. See especially Chase, "Fevers, Poisons, and Apostemes," 162–63, where she

argues that the emphasis many authors placed on the poisonous nature of the air that infected the victims of the plague was due to their dissatisfaction with the Galenic humoral paradigm. But the cases of Alfonso and Jacme were more specific, and both of them have been linked to the theory that the Jews had somehow been the cause of the Black Death. See especially Amasuno Sárraga, *La peste en la Corona de Castilla,* 41–48; and also Campbell, *Black Death and Men of Learning,* 53; as well as Arrizabalaga, "Facing the Black Death," 257–61. For their own words, see Alfonso of Cordoba, "Epistola et regimen Alphontii Cordubensis de pestilentia," 224. An English translation is found in Aberth, *Black Death,* 45–47. For Jacme d'Agramont, see Jacme d'Agramont, *Regiment de preservació de pestilència,* 27 (the editors' commentary), 56. An English translation can be found with Jacme d'Agramont, "Regiment de preservació a epidimia," 65.

14. On the implementation of the first actual quarantine (i.e., the isolation of the healthy, not the sick, until a period of time had passed) in Dubrovnik (Ragusa), see Grmek, "Le concept d'infection," 38–53. Chase, in "Fevers, Poisons, and Apostemes," 155, stressed the prominence given to contagion in the plague treatises written at Montpellier immediately following the Black Death.

15. See Wray, "Boccaccio and the Doctors," 314–19, where she disagrees with the opinions advanced by Cohn, *Black Death Transformed,* passim, but for an example see 233. See now, however, Cohn's argument in *Cultures of Plague* that writing on the plague in Italy changed drastically in the late sixteenth century.

16. An interesting example of a study that takes up precisely the larger questions I am avoiding here is York, "Experience and Theory in Medical Practice."

17. See Palazzotto, "Black Death and Medicine," 150; and Jacme d'Agramont, *Regiment de preservació de pestilència,* 31 (introduction). Other examples of scholars who believed that disease was caused or its passage facilitated by focusing on negative thoughts are easy to find. Two examples from the Iberian Peninsula include Licenciado Fores's plague treatise of 1481, in Velasco de Taranta, Fores, Álvarez, and Álvarez Chanca, *Tratados de la peste,* 106; and Lluis d'Alcanyiz's plague treatise, published in 1490. See Lluis d'Alcanyiz, "Lluis d'Alcanyiz," 44–45. Examples from the treatises edited by Sudhoff are numerous and include the plague treatises of an anonymous German doctor of Munich in the fifteenth century in Sudhoff, "Pestschriften aus den ersten 150 Jahren," 4 (1911): 389–424, at 423; an anonymous fourteenth-century author in 6 (1913): 313–79, at 330; Johannes Aygels von Korneuburg, written between 1412 and 1428, at 371; and Sigmund Albich (d. 1427) in 7 (1913): 57–114, at 92–93.

18. Jacme d'Agramont, "Regiment de preservació a epidimia o pestilència," 84. For the original, see Jacme d'Agramont, *Regiment de preservació de pestilència,* 64.

19. For the suggestion that breeders may have been following Jacob's example into the nineteenth century, see *The Interpreter's Bible* (New York: Abington Press, 1952), 1:709–10.

20. For Gui de Chauliac, see Aberth, *Black Death,* 63–64. The relevant passage from the treatise of the anonymous practitioner of Montpellier is translated by Campbell, *Black Death and Men of Learning,* 61–62. See also the views of the Siennese chronicler Agnolo de Tura (fl. 1348–51) in his *Cronaca senese,* in Aberth, *Black Death,* 81.

21. Campbell, *Black Death and Men of Learning,* 61–62. Another translation of this passage is found in Horrox, *Black Death,* 182–84.

22. A. I. Sabra has written at length on Ibn al-Haytham. See, among others, Sabra, "Ibn al-Haytham's Revolutionary Project in Optics." The earlier work of David Lindberg is also of use here. See his two articles, "Alkindi's Critique of Euclid's Theory of Vision"; and "Alhazen's Theory of Vision."

23. See Lindberg, "Alhazen's Theory of Vision," 339–41.

24. On Enrique de Villena's life and works, see Torres-Alcalá, *Don Enrique de Villena.* For an overview in English of his life and works, including a useful bibliography, see Miguel-Prendes, "Enrique de Villena."

25. Enrique de Villena obtained the annulment by having his wife claim that he was impotent. See Pedro Cátedra's comments in Enrique de Villena, *Obras completas,* 1:xiv–v.

26. On this event see Gascón Vera, "La quema de los libros."

27. See Gilbert-Santamaría, "Historicizing Vergil," where the author argues that Villena, while articulating a critique of many of the conventions of the Middle Ages, was also very much a product of them.

28. Enrique de Villena, *Obras completas,* 1:115–30, 327–41. On Alonso de Chirino, see Maria Teresa Herrera's introduction in his *Menor daño de la medicina.*

29. See Alonso de Chirino, *Menor daño de la medicina,* xvi. On the later history of the Chirino family, who may well have been conversos, see Ruiz, *Spanish Society,* 75–9. For his part, Pedro Cátedra has no doubt that Alonso Chirino was a converso. See Enrique de Villena, *Obras completas,* 1:xxii.

30. Enrique de Villena, *Obras completas,* 1:117.

31. His authority for leprosy's affect on oak trees is the tenth-century Muslim physician al-Zahrāwī (Zaharahui), on whom see Sezgin, *GAS,* 3:323–25. On equating the oxidization of metal to leprosy, Villena refers to Jābir ibn Ḥayyān (Ageber) (d. ca. 199/815) and *De turba philosophorum.* For the latter text and the debate on its origin, see Rudolph, "Christliche Theologie."

32. Enrique de Villena, *Obras completas,* 1:123.

33. Ibid., 1:124. For a general overview on Galenic medicine as practiced in fourteenth- and fifteenth-century Spain, see García Ballester, "Nuevos valores y neuvas estrategías en medicina."

34. Enrique de Villena, *Obras completas,* 1:124–27.

35. Ibid., 1:129. On the danger of reading medical references in medieval literature as only metaphor, see Gasse, "Practice of Medicine in *Piers Plowman.*"

36. Enrique de Villena, *Obras completas,* vol. 1. For other contemporary metaphoric uses of contagion in Castile and Aragon, see chapter 2, and for al-Shāṭibī's admonition not to sit with heretics, see chapter 5.

37. Enrique de Villena, *Obras completas,* 1:130. Considering Alonso's opening references to the Talmud and the possibility that he was a converso, Villena's comments here may have carried a not-too-veiled warning. For evidence that Villena was sympathetic to both Jews and conversos, see Gascón Vera, "La quema de los libros," 319 ff. The literature on accusations of Judaizing in the early fifteenth century is growing. See Nirenberg, "Enmity and Assimilation."

38. Alonso of Chirino, *Menor daño de la medicina,* 34. On precautions against pestilential disease, see also 39 ff. Like Villena, Alonso emphasized the importance of maintaining a proper Catholic faith in times of disease (46).

39. See Chase, "Fevers, Poisons, and Apostemes," 156–59, for the importance of

poison in the etiologies of the plague proposed by the authors of plague treatises from Montpellier.

40. See Salmón and Cabré, "Fascinating Women," 56.

41. Enrique de Villena, *Obras completas,* 1:xxii–xxiii.

42. Ibid., 1:329. Villena refers to the *Cosmography*—presumably of Ptolemy—which places these women in Ciçia. I have not been able to identify this passage.

43. On the history of the basilisk in classical and medieval times, see Alexander, "Evolution of the Basilisk."

44. Enrique de Villena, *Obras completas,* 1:330.

45. Salmón and Cabré, "Fascinating Women," 58.

46. Ibid.; Campbell, *Black Death and Men of Learning,* 62.

47. On the enigmatic figure of the fourteenth-century doctor Philippe Éléphant, see Beaujouan, "Philippe Éléphant."

48. Villena's knowledge was based not only on his scholarship but also on personal communications: "E otras muchas diversidades d'esta nature e condiçión, segúnt cuenta Cancaf el Indiano e *Mushaf al-camar* el corto, segúnt oí dezir a un sabiador morisco que dezían Xarifi Viejo de Gaudalhajara." Enrique de Villena, *Obras completas,* 1:335. General positive references to the authority of the teachings of the Kabbala are found, among other places, on 1:333, 335, and esp. 338. Yet note that Villena also insists that the methods of the Jews to prevent the evil eye that he describes are used only by Jews, not Christians (1:333).

49. Enrique de Villena, *Obras completas,* 1:340–41.

50. Ibid., 1:xxii–xxiii. See also see Carmen Parrilla's introduction in El Tostado, *Las çinco figuratas paradoxas,* 39–41. Parrilla agrees with Cátedra that many of the questions discussed in the *Paradoxas* would have been of interest to courtly circles at the time (39).

51. For an overview of the content of El Tostado's *Las çinco figuratas paradoxas* and its context, see Carmen Parrilla's introduction, 1–63.

52. See ibid., 7, where Parrilla suggests that in the early fifteenth century, scientific questions were discussed in a cultural environment that had its foundations in the thirteenth-century Castile of Alfonso the Wise.

53. See ibid., 38. The Jews, of course, had repented and asked Moses to pray for them before God told Moses to make a serpent of brass and place it on a pole. The discussion of the evil eye is found in 432–62.

54. Ibid., 432. For examples from the sixteenth and later centuries on the powers of menstruating women, see Salmón and Cabré, "Fascinating Women," 60 ff.

55. See El Tostado, *Las çinco figuratas paradoxas,* 433.

56. The following is a summary of views expressed ibid., 433–47.

57. For the true nature of sight, see ibid., 445: "Pues necessaries que la vision se faga non enbiando de los ojos algunos spíritos, según los platónicos entendieron, mas fázesse resçibiendo alguna cosa dentro. Ca todas las cosas multiplican sus species o figures, las quales vienen fasta los ojos de los animals veyentes, et ansí se causa vision." The poisonous nature of the basilisk and the infected eyes of wolves and menstruating women are discussed on 446–47. As noted above, the misogynistic construction of the menstruating woman as both infected and contagious has been explored by Salmón and Cabré, "Fascinating Women."

58. El Tostado, *Las çinco figuratas paradoxas,* 448.

59. Ibid., 448–50.

60. Although El Tostado does not mention Aquinas's discussion of the subject of the evil eye in his *Summa Theologiae* (part 1, chap. 117), he may well have had it in mind. Aquinas wrote:

> Avicenna attributes the phenomenon of bewitchment (*fascinationis*) to the fact that matter innately obeys non-material beings rather than opposing natural agents. So when the soul's imaginative power is strong, matter is changed by it. This, he says, is the cause of the "evil eye" (*oculis fascinantis*). But it has been shown above that matter does not obey non-material beings at will, but rather the Creator alone. Thus it is preferable to say that the *spirits* joined with the body are changed by the imagination's power. This change occurs mainly in the eyes, which the more subtle *spirits* reach. Now the eyes infect the air to a certain definite distance, just as new and untarnished mirrors become tarnished from the glance of a menstruating woman, as Aristotle says. Thus, when certain souls are strongly stirred by wickedness, as happens especially with old women, their looks become spiteful and poisonous, particularly to children with tender and impressionable bodies. It is also possible that by God's permission, or by virtue of some hidden arrangement, the spitefulness of the demons (with whom the witches have some sort of compact) also plays a part in this. Aquinas, *Summa Theologiae,* 15:141.

My attention was drawn to this passage by Salmón and Cabré, "Fascinating Women," 58. The influence of the passage in Iberia can in part be seen by its being cited in later treaties dealing with the subject of the evil eye, such as the sixteenth-century *De superstitionibus* of Martín de Andosilla. See Goñi Gaztambide, "El tratado 'De Superstitionibus,'" 287–88.

61. El Tostado, *Las çinco figuratas paradoxas,* 452–54.

62. Ibid., 457–59.

63. The section of El Tostado's *Las çinco figuratas paradoxas* is not mentioned in Salmón and Cabré, "Fascinating Women."

64. On Enrique de Villena, see Sol Miguel-Prendes, "Enrique de Villena." On the importance of Iberian scholars in the Renaissance and the Scientific Revolution, see, among others, Cañizares-Esguerra, "Iberian Science in the Renaissance." For an example of acceptance of visual contagion in Italy in the fifteenth century, see the statement of Giovanni Calora (doctor of Lorenzo of Medici) in Singer, "Some Plague Tractates," 198: "No wonder that contagion passes from one to another since the mere sight of a basilisk will kill."

Chapter 5. Contagion between Islamic Law and Theology

Epigraph: Nagel, *History of Islamic Theology,* 90–91.

1. On the history of the establishment of the Mālikī school in al-Andalus, including a very useful overview of the state of the field, see Fernández Félix, *Cuestiones legales del Islam temprano,* 337–48.

2. On Ibn Abī Zayd, see now Rahman, "Thought of Ibn Abī Zayd al-Qayrawānī."

3. For both a historical overview of Ashᶜarism's arrival in the Maghrib and the debates around causality taking place in this school of theology, see appendix B.

4. The multiple meanings of *sabab* are reflected in the translations in this chapter, in which I have chosen "occasion" or "cause" depending on context. Contemporary European and American philosophers continue to wrestle with how to understand causation. For one example, see Mellor, *Facts of Causation.*

5. See "The *Muqaddimāt* of al-Sanusī" for the example of the ninth/fifteenth-century theologian and scholar of medicine al-Sanūsī (d. 895/1490).

6. For Ibn Rushd al-Jadd's views on Ashʿarism, see appendix B.

7. On this work and its place in the history of law in al-Andalus, see Fernández Félix, *Cuestiones legales del Islam temprano.*

8. For biographical information on al-ʿUtbī, see ibid., 17–24.

9. Ibid., 66, 76–77. On the various generations of Mālikī scholars whose opinions are preserved in the *ʿUtbiyya,* see 117–20.

10. Ibid., 97.

11. Ibid., 283–85.

12. Ibid., 335. For the trial and persecution of the traditionist Baqī b. Makhlad, see ibid. On the introduction of hadith into al-Andalus, see also Fierro, "Introduction of *ḥadīt.*"

13. Fernández Félix, *Cuestiones legales del Islam temprano,* 347. Fernández Félix sees the consolidation process coming to a close in the first decades of the fourth/tenth century with the writing of *Mukhtaṣars,* legal manuals or summaries (392). For a later dating of the rise of the *Mukhtaṣar,* see Fadel, "Social Logic of *Taqlīd.*"

14. See Fernández Félix, *Cuestiones legales del Islam temprano,* 348. As late as the first quarter of the fourth/tenth century, the ‘Umayyad caliph ‘Abd al-Raḥmān III appointed a prayer leader who was described as having no knowledge of ḥadīth. See ibid., 200.

15. Ibid., 292.

16. Ibid., 270–71.

17. Ibn Rushd al-Jadd, *Al-Bayān wa-l-Taḥṣīl,* 17:396–99.

18. See Conrad's discussion in "ʿUmar at Sargh," 492. Compare with the alternate version given in the *gharā'ib al-ḥadīth* literature, in which ʿUmar turns back because many of his companions are *qarḥānūn*—i.e., they had never been exposed to smallpox and were thus especially susceptible to epidemic disease. See 495–96. I have not encountered this second version in any of the hadith commentaries or plague treatises.

19. To my knowledge, Ibn Rushd is the only scholar ever to propose such a reading. By doing so he offered an innovative use of the legal principle *sadd al-dharā'iʿ* (avoiding means that lead to prohibited ends), which hadith commentators and later scholars writing on the issue of contagion (such as Ibn Ḥajar al-ʿAsqalānī and al-Shawkānī) employed to argue against approaching lepers and plague victims on the grounds that believers can be led into the temptation of thinking that something other than God has causative power.

20. Ibn Rushd al-Jadd, *Al-Bayān wa-l-Taḥṣīl,* 17:396–97.

21. See chapter 2.

22. ʿUmar's argument is discussed in "An Exceptional Voice." Ibn Rushd's opinion was reproduced with greater fidelity in Ibn Juzayy (741/1340), *Al-Qawānīn al-Fiqhiyya,* 452–53.

23. On lepers, compare Ibn Rushd, *Al-Bayān wa-l-Taḥṣīl,* 8:360–61, 9:390–93, 18:261–62; with Ibn Rushd, *Masā'il Abī al-Walīd Ibn Rushd,* 2:932–34. For Ibn

Rushd's use of the material from the *ʿUtbiyya* on which he was commenting at the time in his fatwas, see Fernández Félix, *Cuestiones legales del Islam temprano,* 253–54.

24. Ibn Rushd, *Al-Bayān wa-l-Taḥṣīl,* 8:360–61. On Muḥammad b. Dīnār, see Ibn Mūsā, *Tartīb al-Madārik,* 1:291–92. By acknowledging the authority of doctors regarding leprosy, Muḥammad b. Dīnār took a stance similar to that of Tāj al-Dīn al-Subki (d. 771/1370) in his *Risālah fi'ṭ-ṭāʿūn,* which, while no longer extant, is quoted in Ibn Ḥajar's treatise on the plague. See Dols, *Black Death,* 327–28; and the discussion in chapter 3.

25. Ibn Rushd, *Masā'il Abī al-Walīd Ibn Rushd,* 2:932–34. The issue of the degree to which lepers should be allowed to mix with other Muslims has been discussed, with regard to al-Andalus, by Mazzoli-Guintard in her "Notes sur une minorité urbaine d'al-Andalus."

26. Ibn Rushd, *Al-Bayān wa-l-Taḥṣīl,* 9:390–93.

27. For al-Sakūnī, I have drawn on al-Sakūnī, *ʿUyūn al-Munāẓarāt;* and Latham, "Content of the *Laḥn al-ʿAwāmm.*" For biographical information on the al-Sakūnī family, see al-Sakūnī, *ʿUyūn al-Munāẓarāt,* 10–26 (of the French text). I am grateful to Maribel Fierro for referring me to the works of al-Sakūnī and the article of Latham, "Content of the *Laḥn al-ʿAwāmm.*"

28. Al-Sakūnī, 'Uyūn al-Munāẓarāt, 18–22.

29. Since Latham's article, this work has been edited and published by Saʿd Ghrab in *Ḥawliyyāt,* no. 12 (1975), 109–255. I have not been able to consult this edition.

30. Latham, "Content of the *Laḥn al-ʿAwāmm,*" 304.

31. Ibid., 302.

32. Ibid., 306.

33. Al-Sakūnī, *ʿUyūn al-Munāẓarāt,* 16–17 (this and all subsequent references are to the Arabic text).

34. Ibid., 18.

35. Ibid., 19.

36. Ibid., 151–52.

37. On the life of Ibn Lubb, see Zomeño, "Ibn Lubb." Ibn al-Khaṭīb wrote respectfully of Ibn Lubb in *Al-Iḥāṭa,* 4:253–55. I have compared the views of Ibn al-Khaṭīb and Ibn Lubb in Stearns, "Contagion in Theology and Law."

38. The *Miʿyār* has been the subject of much, though hardly exhaustive, study in recent years. The most recent and comprehensive study is Powers, *Law, Society, and Culture.* The earlier study by Lagardère, *Histoire et société en occident musulman,* is also useful.

39. With regard to the *maqāṣid al-sharīʿa,* I have found Yasir Ibrahim's recent study of use, "Spirit of Islamic Law and Modern Religious Reform." Al-Ghazālī defined the *maqāṣid* as the preservation of religion, life, private property, mind, and offspring, whereas the eighth/fourteenth-century Māliki jurist al-Shāṭibī gave the principle its first extensive discussion in his *Muwāfaqāt* (7–10). Al-Shāṭibī's views on contagion are discussed in "Causality in the Writings of the Contemporaries of Ibn Lubb."

40. See al-Wansharīsī, al-*Miʿyār,* 11:355, for one example. On *sadd al-dharīʿa* in general, see Kamali, *Principles of Islamic Jurisprudence,* 310–20. An overview of the status of *sadd al-dharīʿa* in the Māliki school can be found in al-Jīdī, *Al-Tashrīʿ al-Islāmī,* 118–19. See also Fierro, "El principio mālikī." Al-Shāṭibī discusses it in his *Muwāfaqāt,* 2:556–58.

41. Al-Wansharīsī, al-*Mi^{c}yār,* 11:352–60.

42. I was first directed to these fatwas by a reference in a Moroccan master's thesis to which Rashid Hour had referred me. See al-Qijīrī, "Al-Āfāt wa-l-Kawārith al-Ṭabī^{c}iyya bi-l-Maghrib bayna al-Qarnayn 11 wa 15," 7. Van Ess cites the fatwas in passing in *Der Fehltritt des Gelehrten,* 300.

43. Al-Wansharīsī, al-*Mifiyār,* 11:353.

44. Wensinck, *Concordance et indices,* 1:108. This tradition is found in Muslim (Iman, 71, 72), al-Bukhārī (Imān, 7), al-Tirmidhī (Qiyāma, 59), al-Nasā'ī (Imān, 19, 22), Ibn Māja (Muqaddima, 9), and Abū Dāwūd (Rifq, 29).

45. Wensinck, *Concordance et indices,* under *kh-dh-l.* The tradition is found only in Ibn Hanbal's *Musnad,* 2:68, 277, 311, 360; 3:491; 4:66, 69; 5:24, 25, 71, 379, 381.

46. I have not been able to locate this tradition in the six canonical collections. It can be found in al-Ghazālī, *Iḥyā' ^{c}Ūlūm al-Dīn,* in the chapter entitled *Ḥuqūq al-Muslim.* Describing the religious community as a body has, naturally, far-reaching metaphoric implications, as seen in chapter 2 of the present volume.

47. See chapter 1.

48. I have not been able to locate this passage.

49. Al-Wansharīsī, al-*Mifiyār,* 11:357.

50. Ibn Lubb is possibly referencing the concept of *al-maqāṣid al-shar^{c}iyya,* developed at length by his student al-Shāṭibī (whose treatment of contagion is considered in "Causality in the Writings of the Contemporaries of Ibn Lubb").

51. This treatise is addressed in chapter 3. On the weakness of the tradition equating death by plague with martyrdom, see van Ess, *Der Fehltritt des Gelehrten,* 43.

52. For Jābiya, see Yaqūṭ, *Mu^{c}jam al-Buldān,* 2:106–7. Ibn Lubb cites the famed traditionist al-Zuhrī (d. 124/742) as his source for the subsequent episode.

53. ^{c}Amwās (Emmaus) was a small village in Palestine. See under ^{c}Amwās in *Encyclopedia of Islam,* 2nd ed., 12 vols. (Leiden: Brill, 1960–2004), 1:460. On Mu^{c}ādh, see van Ess, *Der Fehltritt des Gelehrten,* 127–56. In an aside, van Ess describes the destruction of Emmaus by the Israeli Defense Forces in 1967 (404).

54. Since ^{c}Amr later conquered Egypt, he can be understood to have reached greater prominence in this world. For the ^{c}Amr-Mu^{c}ādh confrontation, see van Ess, *Der Fehltritt des Gelehrten,* 25–40. In van Ess's opinion, much of this episode originated in the generation following Mu^{c}ādh's death (162).

55. Al-Shāṭibī, *al-Muwāfaqāt,* 1:313–17.

56. Ibid.

57. See the following Qur'anic ayas: *al-Ṣāfāt,* 96; *al-Zumar*, 62; *al-Takwīr*, 29; *al-Shams*, 7–8.

58. Al-Shāṭibī seems to have gotten his *ṣaḥāba* confused. Traditionally it was Abū ^{c}Ubayda who argued against flight from the plague, saying, "Do we flee from the will of God?" See chapter 1. As discussed previously in the context of Ibn Lubb's fatwas, ^{c}Amr b. al-^{c}Āṣ argued that one should flee the plague, not approach it.

59. Compare al-Shāṭibī, *Al-I^{c}tiṣām,* 400–402 (chap. 10, sections 22, 23), with Ibn Waḍḍāḥ al-Qurṭubī, *Kitāb al-Bida^{c},* 190–97; Spanish translation, 313–19.

60. Literally, "stickier than the mange." Compare with the proverbial expression, given in Lane's *Arabic-English Lexicon* under *j-r-b*: "More transitive, or catching (*a^{c}dā*), than the mange, or scab, among the Arabs." The quotation is from al-Shāṭibī, *al-I^{c}tiṣām,* 400.

61. There may have been occasional exceptions. Ibn Waḍḍāḥ cites the following example: "From Muḥammad b. Wāsiᶜ, he said: I saw Ṣafwān b. Muḥriz and near him an old man. They were arguing. I saw him get up and shake his clothes and say: Truly, you are mangy." *Kitāb al-Bidaᶜ,* 196; Spanish translation, 318–19. Compare with the injunction of Ibn al-Jawzī (d. 597/1200) not to sit with storytellers, in his *Kitāb al-Quṣṣāṣ wa-l-Mudhakkirīn,* 101/180 (Arabic/English).

62. Al-Shāṭibī, *al-Iᶜtiṣām,* 402.

63. A few words should be said here about the son of one of al-Shāṭibī's students, Abū Yahyā Muḥammad b. ᶜĀṣim al-Gharnāṭī (d. 857/1452), who addressed the issue of contagion in passing in his *Garden of Satisfaction in Submitting to the Decree and Ordinance of God* (*Jannat al-Riḍā fīl-Taslīm li-mā Qaddara Allāh wa Qaḍā*) On Abū Yaḥyā Ibn ᶜĀṣim, see Morales Delgado, "Abū Yaḥyā Ibn ᶜĀṣim." Abū Yaḥya, though not al-Shāṭibī's direct student, did claim to have seen him in a dream (*fī ᶜālim al-nawm*) and to have conversed with him. See Ibn ᶜĀṣim al-Gharnāṭī, *Jannat al-Riḍā fīl-Taslīm li-mā Qaddara Allāh wa Qaḍā,* 1:141–42. The title of the book suggests, correctly, that its author was interested in proclaiming the virtues of submitting to the will of God. Of relevance here is that Ibn ᶜĀṣim offers an analysis of what happens to the soul of the believer who is confronted with imminent danger or death (2:31–39). The answer to any fear one might experience at such a time is found in prayer to God and in testifying that God is the Creator of all. The universality of this remedy can be measured by the different examples given by Ibn ᶜĀṣim: strong winds, thunder, evil omens, injustice, oppression, sickness, tyranny, and disease, especially leprosy. The causes of these events are beyond the comprehension of man. Ibn ᶜĀṣim's argument with regard to leprosy is largely implicit, but it is reminiscent of the argument that lepers should be avoided because being close to them may cause the believer anguish, not because they are dangerous in and of themselves (see chapter 1, the section "Leprosy, the Other Contagion"). In this, leprosy is identical to evil omens: in both cases one comes to harm if one thinks one will come to harm.

64. Ibn Khaldūn, *Introduction to History,* 353. Admittedly, Ibn Khaldūn goes on to argue that speculative argumentation can be useful to the orthodox believer.

65. Ibid., 349–50.

66. I have referred to two editions of this work: the edition and translation of J. D. Luciani, al-Sanūsī, *Les prolégomènes théologiques de Senoussi;* and the more recent Arabic edition, al-Sanūsī, *Sharḥ al-Muqaddimāt.* The Arabic texts established by Luciani and Ahnāna (the editor of the Arabic edition) are slightly different; the title given in each citation indicates which version of the text I used. For an evaluation of al-Sanūsī as a strict Ashᶜarī, see Gimaret, *Théories de l'acte humain,* 234.

67. Al-Sanūsī, *Les prolégomènes théologiques de Senoussi,* 6–9. I have based my translation on that of Luciani, but where he translates *ᶜādī* and *naẓarī* as "expérimental" and "discursive," I use "habitual" and "inductive."

68. Ibid., 32–33.

69. Al-Sanūsī, *Sharḥ al-Muqaddimāt,* 23–24.

70. See appendix B.

71. Al-Sanūsī, *Les prolégomènes théologiques de Senoussi,* 68–69.

72. Ibid., 44–45.

73. For other passages where a belief in causality is portrayed as leading to unbelief or heterodoxy, see ibid., 110–13, 120–23.

74. See esp. al-Sanūsī, *Khayr al-Bariyya min Ghāmiḍ asrār al-Ṣinā*ᶜ*a al-Ṭibbiyya.*

75. Ibid., 47. The editors of this work note that the tradition on which the book is based does not go back to the Prophet but is linked to the Arab doctor al-Ḥārith b. Kalada al-Thaqafī (d. 50/669). In their view, only the last section of the tradition—the origin of every sickness is poor digestion—can be attributed to the Prophet (27).

76. Ibid., 49.

77. Ibid., 87–89.

78. Wolfson, *Philosophy of the Kalam,* 559–66, 577.

79. Al-Sanūsī, *Les prolégomènes théologiques de Senoussi,* 72–73.

80. Ibid., 92–95. For the stupidity of the Qadariyya, see 60–61. The analogy of the blind man used here by al-Sanūsī is similar to but distinct from an argument employed by al-Ghazālī against philosophers. See Kogan, *Averroes and the Metaphysics of Causation,* 90.

81. For al-Qurṭūbī's discussion, see chapter 1.

82. On this point al-Sanūsī cites as an authority one Ibn Dahhāq (I have not been able to identify this scholar). See al-Sanūsī, *Les prolégomènes théologiques de Senoussi,* 108–9.

83. Ibid., 96–97.

84. Al-Maqqarī, *Azhār al-Riyāḍ,* 2:125–32. The *maqāma* was analyzed and translated by de la Granja, "La maqama de la peste." De la Granja was unable to identify the author of the poem, whom we know only by his first name, ᶜUmar, and that he was from Málaga. See the brief entry in Makhlūf, *Shajrat al-Nūr al-Zakiyya,* 248.

85. For the tradition "Flee from the leper as you flee from the lion," see chapter 1.

86. Al-Maqqarī, *Azhār al-Riyāḍ,* 2:129.

87. For an overview of what the historical sources do tell us regarding the presence and influence of epidemic disease in the two centuries following the Black Death, see al-Bazzāz, "Al-Ṭāᶜūn al-Aswad bi-l-Maghrib fī-l-qarn 14 milādī"; and Renaud, "Les 'pestes' des XVe et XVIe siècles." The effects of epidemic disease in North Africa in the centuries before the Black Death are addressed in Bulaqṭīb, *Jawā'iḥ wa Awbi'at Maghrib ᶜAhd al-Muwaḥḥidīn.*

88. Al-Mawwāq and al-Raṣṣāᶜ, *Al-Ajwiba al-Tūnisiyya.* I am exceedingly grateful to Jocelyn Hendrickson for providing me with a copy of this work.

89. Al-Mawwāq is reported to have studied with Abū Bakr Ibn ᶜĀṣim (d. 829/1426), who was a student of al-Shāṭibī (d. 790/1388), a student of Ibn Lubb. The editor of *Al-Ajwiba,* Muḥammad Ḥasan, writes: "Al-Mawwāq is to be counted of the school of traditional jurisprudence represented by Ibn Lubb, relying on knowledge (*al-dirāya*), displaying an interest in *ijtihād* more than in conservation and imitation. This is in contrast to the school of the supporters of the sunna, which is represented by Abū Isḥāq al-Shāṭibī." Ibid., 26–27. For his part, al-Raṣṣāᶜ studied with many of Ibn ᶜArafa's students, most notably al-Burzulī (d. 841/1438) (33). On Ibn ᶜArafa, see Ghrab, *Ibn ᶜArafa et le Malikisme.* Ibn ᶜArafa's view of the plague is briefly discussed in chapter 6 of the present volume.

90. The nuanced nature of this text strongly suggests that it is worthy of translation in its entirety, a task I am not able to address at this time.

91. Al-Mawwāq and al-Raṣṣāᶜ, *Al-Ajwiba al-Tūnisiyya,* 89–93.

92. Abū Jaᶜfar Aḥmad al-Mālaqī Ibn Ṣafwān was a well known jurist from Má-

laga. I have been unable to ascertain what work is being referred to here. See Ibn al-Khaṭīb, *Al-Iḥāṭa,* 1:221–32; and al-Tinbuktī, *Nayl al-Ibtiḥāj,* 100.

93. Qāsim b. ^{c}Īsā b. Nājī was a prominent jurist in Qayrawan, famous for his commentaries on the *Mudawwana* and on Ibn Abī Zayd's *Risāla.* See al-Tinbuktī, *Nayl al-Ibtiḥāj,* 364. I am not sure to which of his works reference is being made here.

94. This is the famous Egyptian scholar and author of *Ṭabaqāt al-Shafi^{c}iyya.* See al-Kaḥḥāla, *Mu^{c}jam al-Mu'allifīn,* 2:343. I have not been able to ascertain the source referred to here.

95. Al-Ḥusayn b. Mas^{c}ūd Ibn al-Farā' al-Baghawī was a prominent Shāfi^{c}ī scholar from Khurasan who is known for his works on hadith and Shāfi^{c}ī fiqh. See al-Kaḥḥāla, *Mu^{c}jam al-Mu'allifīn,* 1:644. Which of his works is referred to here is unclear to me.

96. Al-Raṣṣā^{c} makes a remarkably explicit admission that the (Shāfi^{c}ī) scholars of the East are superior to the scholars of the West in matters of hadith, seeing this as being especially the case with Ibn Ḥajar, whose authority on the matter of the plague had previously been acknowledged by Ibn Marzūq al-Ḥafīd (d. 842/1439) (the editor confuses him with his grandfather, who could not have known the work of Ibn Ḥajar), Abū Qāsim al-^{c}Abdūsī (d. 837/1433), and Aḥmad al-Shammā^{c} (d. 873/1459). See Al-Mawwāq and al-Raṣṣā^{c}, *Al-Ajwiba al-Tūnisiyya,* 109. On contemporary Mālikī polemics against Shāfi^{c}īs, see Dutton, *Original Islam;* and my review of Dutton's book, "Considering the Maliki madhhab in Nasrid Granada." For an earlier Mālikī awareness of Shāfi^{c}ī thought in al-Andalus and the need to address the criteria employed by Shāfi^{c}ī jurists, see Fierro, "Proto-Malikis, Malikis, and Reformed Malikis."

97. Al-Mawwāq and al-Raṣṣā^{c}, *Al-Ajwiba al-Tūnisiyya,* 115.

98. Ibid., 111–15.

99. Ibid., 115–19.

100. Al-Raṣṣā^{c} spends some time on the debate around whether it is permissible to pray for the plague to end, ultimately citing both Ibn Ḥajar and Ibn Khātima in favor of doing so. See ibid., 120–23. It is worth drawing attention to a remarkable statement attributed by al-Raṣṣā^{c} to Ibn ^{c}Arafa, who, after praying for the cessation of plague, uttered the following foreign words he claims were names of God: "*Inūmī dūmī mar baṭarī kanā sanadām mamnu^{an} binaṭās*" (119). This would appear to be a very garbled rendition of the opening of the Lord's Prayer in Latin.

101. Ibid., 125.

102. On al-Saqalli, see al-Kaḥḥāla, *Mu^{c}jam al-Mu'allifīn,* 1:170.

103. Al-Mawwāq and al-Raṣṣā^{c}, *Al-Ajwiba al-Tūnisiyya,* 130, 133, 144–47.

104. Ibid., 140–45.

105. Ibid., 145–46. Compare with 155–58 and 172–74.

106. Ibid., 153–43.

107. Ibid., 158–61. Note that al-Raṣṣā^{c} places so much importance on one's intention to endure the plague that he suggests that if one does not flee the plague and later becomes sick and then recovers or dies due to a reason other than the plague, one may receive the reward of martyrdom.

108. Ibid., 138.

109. Ibid., 149.

110. On the life of al-Yūsī, see Honerkamp, "Al-Ḥasan ibn Mas^{c}ūd al-Yūsī"; Berque, *Al-Yousi;* al-Madgharī, *Al-Faqīh Abū ^{c}Alī al-Yūsī.*

111. Al-Yūsī, *Al-Muḥāḍarāt,* 96.
112. Ibid., 98.
113. See chapter 6 for more on Ashᶜarism in the plague treatises of the Maghrib in the eighteenth and nineteenth centuries.
114. See, for example, Olshewsky, "Classical Roots of Hume's Skepticism," esp. 282.
115. Ibn Rushd presents a notable exception to those scholars who thought that the smell of leprosy could cause harm.

Chapter 6. Contagion Revisited

Epigraphs: Leibniz, *Theodicy,* 153. I was guided to this passage by Ormsby, *Theodicy in Islamic Thought,* 25. Ḥamdān Khoja, *Itḥāf al-Munṣifīn wa-l-Udabā' fī al-Iḥtirāz ᶜan al-Wabā',* 43.

1. See especially Sabra, "Greek Science in Medieval Islam"; "Science and Philosophy in Medieval Islamic Theology." The many methodological issues raised in the following article by George Saliba are also of great relevance to the argument presented here: "History of Arabic Astronomy."
2. For nuanced and discerning comments on Sufism in early modern Moroccan history, see Munson, *Religion and Power in Morocco,* 81–87.
3. For a readable, if at times sensational, account of this discovery, see Marriott, *Plague.*
4. See, for example, Zuckerman, "Plague and Contagionism"; and Ackerknecht, "Anticontagionism."
5. This list of works, while arguably representative, is hardly a comprehensive collection of all the texts written on plague or contagion in the Muslim West during these centuries.
6. Al-Khizāna al-Mālikiyya, Rabat, Morocco, no. Az 12,369, fols. 79–95. It is worth noting that although the author cites the plague treatise of Aḥmad b. Mubārak, he predeceased him by almost thirty years. Considering that Aḥmad b. Mubārak was born in 1090/1679, it is nonetheless quite feasible that Ibn al-Ḥājj knew him. On Muḥammad b. Aḥmad al-Ḥājj, see Makhlūf, *Shajarat al-Nūr al-Zakiyya,* 332. On Aḥmad b. Mubārak, see al-Kaḥḥāla, *Muᶜjam al-Mu'allifīn,* 1:235.
7. Al-Khizāna al-ᶜĀmma, Rabat, Morocco, no. 2716 (D 1348), fols. 125–28. This treatise was included in al-Wazzānī, *al-Miᶜyār al-Jadīd,* 2:234–41.
8. Mustapha, Histoire de la medicine, 211–16.
9. Al-Khizāna al-ᶜĀmma, Rabat, Morocco, no. d1854, fols. 44–48.
10. Ibid., no. d2589, 1–22.
11. Ibid., no. d2251, 1–48. Along with Aḥmad b. Mubārak's treatise, this has been partially included in al-Wazzānī, *al-Miᶜyār al-Jadīd,* 2:241–57 (the first 17 pages are omitted).
12. Al-Khizāna al-ᶜĀmma, Rabat, Morocco, no. d2251, 49–79.
13. Ibid., no. d640 (791), 46–110.
14. Al-Khizāna al-Mālikiyya, Rabat, Morocco, no. 2054, fols. 1–131.
15. Ibn Rushd's views, and often his opinion that it is permissible to both enter and leave a plague-struck land, are cited in Ibn Aḥmad al-Ḥājj, *Mas'ala fī Ḥukm al-ᶜAdwā,* 81v, 85v, 91r; Ibn Mubārak, *Jawāb ᶜamman Ḥalla bi-Bilādihim Ṭāᶜūn,*

239 (briefly); Ibn ᶜAjība, *Sulūk al-Durar,* 13; al-Rahūnī, *Jawāb fī Aḥkām al-Ṭāᶜūn,* 243, 249; al-Fīlālī, *Risāla,* 5v, 6r, 9r (by way of Ibn Juzayy); Ibn ᶜAlī Junūn, *Kalām al-A'imma,* 104 (briefly).

16. Ibn Lubb's fatwa is favorably cited in Ibn Aḥmad al-Ḥājj, *Mas'ala fī Ḥukm al-ᶜAdwā,* 90r–90v, 91r; al-Rahūnī, *Jawāb fī Aḥkām al-Ṭāᶜūn,* 254, 256.

17. The extent of Ibn Ḥajar's authority in this group of Mālikī scholars, even though he belonged to the Shāfiᶜī law school, can be measured by the fact that none of those who cited him disagreed with him. We find favorable references to his opinions, including often his refutation of al-Subkī, and especially the sixth way in which the traditions on this issue could be reconciled (in *Fatḥ al-Bārī,* discussed in chapter 1), in Ibn Aḥmad al-Ḥājj, *Mas'ala fī Ḥukm al-ᶜAdwā,* 84v–85r, 86r–87v, 92v; Ibn Mubārak, *Jawāb ᶜamman Ḥalla bi-Bilādihim Ṭāᶜūn,* 235–40; al-Rahūnī, *Jawāb fī Aḥkām al-Ṭāᶜūn,* 242 (where al-Rahūnī notes, defensively, that opinions like that of Ibn Ḥajar are also found in famous Mālikī works), 244, 252; al-Banānī, *Risāla fī al-Ṭaᶜn wa-l-Ṭawāᶜīn,* 45r–47r; Ibn ᶜAbī Junūn, *Kalām al-A'imma,* 50–54; al-Gharīsī, *Aqwāl al-Maṭāᶜīn,* 93r–93v, 108v, 114r.

18. This list is far from comprehensive. In addition to earlier authors of plague treatises, these authors drew upon the substantial literature on contagion found in the hadith commentaries examined in chapter 2. For Qalshānī, see al-Tinbuktī, *Nayl al-Ibtihāj,* 116–17. I am not aware of an extant copy of this work. Ibn Abī Zayd mentions the plague briefly in the second-to-last chapter of his *Al-Risāla,* 120–21, quoting the Prophet's injunction to neither leave nor enter a plague-struck country. Aḥmad Zarrūq's life has recently been examined at length by Kugle, *Rebel between Spirit and Law.* I have not been able to identify which of Zarrūq's many works these authors drew upon. For Muḥammad b. Muḥammad al-Ḥaṭṭāb, see *Nayl al-Ibtihāj,* 592–94, where al-Tinbuktī gives the title of his work on the plague as *ᶜUmdat al-Rāwiyīn fī Aḥkām al-Ṭawāᶜīn.* To my knowledge, the only extant copy of this work is in the National Library of Medicine, no. MS A 80. Despite repeated attempts, I have not been able to procure a copy.

19. Explicitly Ashᶜarī-informed arguments can be found in Ibn Aḥmad al-Ḥājj, *Mas'ala fī Ḥukm al-ᶜAdwā,* 87v–88r; al-Sūsī, *Rāḥat al-Insān fī Ṭibb al-Abdān,* 212; Ibn ᶜAjība, *Sulūk al-Durar,* 11; al-Rahūnī, *Jawāb fī Aḥkām al-Ṭāᶜūn,* 2 (in manuscript, not included by al-Wazzānī), 250–51; al-Fīlālī, *Risāla,* 12r, 13v; Ibn ᶜAlī Junūn, *Kalām al-A'imma,* 62–63.

20. See, for example, Leibniz, *Theodicy,* 153.

21. See Reinert, *Die Lehre vom* tawakkul, 13, 25.

22. Ibid., 145–46, 162.

23. Ibid.,165. The sources for these anecdotes are, respectively, al-Ṭabarī (d. 310/923), *Ta'rīkh;* and Abū Nuᶜaym Aḥmad b. ᶜAbd Allāh (d. 430/1038), *Ḥilyat al-Awliya.* For a detailed discussion of the different traditions around Abū ᶜUbaydah b. al-Jarrāḥ's attitude toward the plague, see van Ess, *Fehltritt des Gelehrten,* 30–32.

24. See Reinert, *Die Lehre vom* tawakkul, 207–11.

25. Ibid., 217–26. For an analysis of the relationship between asceticism and mysticism in early Sufism, see now Kuramustafa, *Sufism.*

26. Reinert, *Die Lehre vom* tawakkul, 227, 230, 235.

27. Ibid., 268.

28. See al-Ghazālī, *Al-Ghazali,* 125–26.

29. Ibid., 134.
30. Ibid., 134–35.
31. Ibid., 135.
32. For later criticisms of extreme interpretations of *tawakkul,* see the comments of the Ḥanbalī scholars Ibn al-Jawzi (d. 597/1201), *Talbīs Iblīs,* 269–76; and Ibn Qayyim al-Jawziyya, *Madārij al-Sālikīn,* 3:494–501. The latter's work is especially interesting, for it is itself a work on Sufism and a commentary on the earlier *Manāzil al-Sā'irīn* by the Ḥanbalī Sūfī ᶜAbdallāh al-Anṣārī al-Harawī (d. 481/1089).
33. Ibn Mubārak, *Jawāb ᶜamman Ḥalla bi-Bilādihim Ṭāᶜūn,* 231. On this treatise, see also al-Bazzāz, *Ta'rīkh al-Awbi'a,* 397–98.
34. Al-Wazzānī, *Al-Miᶜyār al-Jadīd,* 2:241. Al-Wazzānī's choice of these two treatises, his privileging of al-Rahūnī over Aḥmad b. Mubārak, and his placement of them in his chapter on the pilgrimage (*ḥajj*) all deserve further investigation.
35. On al-Rahūnī, see Makhlūf, *Shajarat al-Nūr al-Zakiyya,* 378. At the beginning of his treatise, al-Rahūnī states that he wrote it in response to a series of questions from ᶜAbdallāh, the son of his teacher Muḥammad Ḥasan al-Janawī (d. 1220/1805). Makhlūf, *Shajarat al-Nūr al-Zakiyya,* 375.
36. Al-Rahūnī, *Jawāb fī Aḥkām al-Ṭāᶜūn,* 252.
37. See chapter 1 and Ibn Ḥajar, *Fatḥ al-Bārī,* 21, 278–81.
38. Al-Rahūnī, *Jawāb fī Aḥkām al-Ṭāᶜūn,* 252. This sounds very much like a call for the isolation of the sick.
39. This is possibly Abū ᶜAbbās Aḥmad b. Muḥammad al-Mubārak al-Qusanṭīnī (d. after 1265/1849), although I have not been able to find any work of his that would be a likely source. See al-Kaḥḥāla, *Muᶜjam al-Mu'allifīn,* 1:290.
40. See chapter 3 and al-Ghazālī, *Al-Ghazali,* 143.
41. Al-Rahūnī, *Jawāb fī Aḥkām al-Ṭāᶜūn,* 253.
42. Ibid., 254.
43. Ibid., 255.
44. The episode is related by his student al-Ubbī, whose views on contagion are discussed in chapter 1. It is also mentioned by Ghrab in *Ibn ᶜArafa et le Malikisme,* 2:518.
45. Al-Rahūnī, *Jawāb fī Aḥkām al-Ṭāᶜūn,* 256–57.
46. It is difficult to find extensive material on al-Fīlālī. See Ziriklī, *Al-Aᶜlām,* 7:8; Makhlūf, *Shajarat al-Nūr al-Zakiyya,* 386; and al-Bazzāz, *Ta'rīkh al-Awbi'a,* 400–401.
47. Al-Fīlālī, *Risāla,* 6r.
48. Ibid., 7v–10r. Citing a fatwa of Ibn Hilāl (d. 903/1498), al-Fīlālī emphasizes that even if the *mujtahid*'s opinion is weak, it can still be followed (9r). On Ibrāhīm b. Hilāl, see Makhlūf, *Shajarat al-Nūr al-Zakiyya,* 268. Similarly, al-Filālī emphasizes the famous tradition that difference of agreement among the scholars is a mercy from God. See 10v.
49. Al-Fīlālī, *Risāla,* 10v.
50. Ibid., 11r.
51. Ibid., 12r–12v.
52. For example, ibid., 13v–14r. In this he is followed by Muḥammad b. al-Madanī b. ᶜAlī Junūn, a prominent mufti and Sufi, who, in turn, favorably cited al-Yūsī's views on causality. See Ibn 'Alī Junūn, *Kalām al-A'imma,* 56, 62–63, 67–68, 70, 89.
53. Al-Fīlālī, *Risāla,* 15v–16r.

54. Ibid. 16v. For a discussion of Q2:195, see chapter 3.

55. On al-Banānī, see al-Bazzāz, *Ta'rīkh al-Awbi'a,* 396; Makhlūf, *Shajarat al-Nūr al-Zakiyya,* 357; al-Kattānī, *Salwat al-Anfās,* Dār al-Thaqāfa, 1:174–76; Lévi-Provençal, *Les historiens des chorfas,* 146–47. For Ibn ᶜAjība, see al-Bazzāz, *Ta'rīkh al-Awbi'a,* 398–99; Makhlūf, *Shajarat al-Nūr al-Zakiyya,* 400, where it is stated that he reconciled "the law and truth" (*al-sharīᶜa wa-l-ḥaqīqa*); Lévi-Provençal, *Les historiens des chorfas,* 336. I do not mean to imply that the concept of *tawakkul* was embraced only by Sufis, or that all Sufis denied secondary causation (see the counter-examples of Ibn al-Khaṭīb and Muḥammad Junūn above).

56. Al-Banānī, *Risāla fī-l-Ṭaᶜn wa-l-Ṭawāᶜīn,* 45v–46r. It was generally understood that the jinn that attacked Muslims were not Muslims themselves, but rather Jews and Christians.

57. See al-Bazzāz, *Ta'rīkh al-Awbi'a,* 398.

58. Ibn ᶜAjība, *Sulūk al-Durar,* 12.

59. Ibid., 13.

60. Ibid. 12–13. Ibn ᶜAjība cites the view that the Prophet's advice to flee lepers was meant for those weak in faith. Ibn ᶜAjība's treatise is of additional interest because he alone among his colleagues seems to have seen in the plague a sign of the end of days. Citing al-Būnī (d. 622/1225), *Shams al-Maᶜārif,* he claims that if Christians were to enter Egypt and an epidemic were to strike Morocco, then when the Christians left Egypt—as the French did in 1801—it would herald the coming of the Mahdi and Jesus. See 15.

61. See al-Bazzāz, *Ta'rīkh al-Awbi'a,* 398; Lévi-Provençal, *Les historiens des chorfas,* 336. On Muᶜādh b. Jabal, see van Ess, *Fehltritt des Gelehrten,* 20–25, 127–34.

62. Indispensable here are Gallagher, Medicine and Power in Tunisia; Panzac, La peste; Kuhnke, Lives at Risk; and al-Bazzāz, *Ta'rīkh al-Awbi'a.*

63. Gallagher, Medicine and Power in Tunisia, 31–33, 52–53.

64. Ibid., 37–45. Muḥammad 'Alī imposed a quarantine in Egypt as early as 1812. See Kuhnke, *Lives at Risk,* 94.

65. On instances of plague in Morocco in the eighteenth and nineteenth centuries, see the excellent articles of Renaud: "La peste de 1799"; "La peste de 1818"; "Un nouveau document marocain": "Les pestes du milieu du XVIIIe siècle"; "Les 'pestes' des XVe et XVIe siècles." Of special relevance to issues of power and sovereignty is "La peste de 1818," 15–21 and 34–35.

66. See Gallagher, *Medicine and power in Tunisia,* 83, 98, 101; Kuhnke, *Lives at Risk,* 105–6. Kuhnke observes differences between the various colonial powers' attitudes on the issue of the quarantine; Britain, where the anticontagion lobby was strong, argued against restrictive implementation of the quarantine. Ibid., 106.

67. In Tunis, *ᶜulamā'* were called upon to advise the government on the issue of quarantine and contagion until at least 1850. See Gallagher, *Medicine and Power in Tunisia,* 52–53.

68. Daniel Panzac argues that attitudes toward the plague began changing in the Ottoman Empire between 1812 and 1835. Panzac, *La peste,* 336–38. Belief in the jinn's agency in spreading epidemic disease continued in Egypt until the 1940s, and citing the same tradition on fleeing the leper, Egyptians broke a quarantine as late as 1947. See Gallagher, *Egypt's Other Wars,* 118–20.

69. See Panzac, *La peste,* 583–85.

70. See Kuhnke, *Lives at Risk,* 81–82, 202.

71. On Ḥamdān Khoja, see Muḥammad b. ᶜAbd al-Karīm's introduction to Ḥamdan Khoja, *Itḥāf al-Munṣifīn,* 11–33. For more on Ḥamdān Khoja's life and especially his political activities, see Abdelkader Djeghloul's introduction to Hamdan Khodja, *Le miroir,* 11–32; Yver, "Si Hamdan ben Othman Khodja"; Temimi, "Sidi Hamdan Bin Othman Khudja"; and "L'activité de Hamdan Khudja." On his legal studies, see Yver, "Si Hamdan ben Othman Khodja," 97. For the possibility that Ḥamdān Khoja's *Miroir* never had an Arabic original and was written in French, see 110.

72. The one treatment of this treatise that I have found is the succinct but valuable article of al-Ṣaghīr, "Mulāḥaẓāt ḥawl rudūd fiᶜl baᶜḍ mufakkirī al-maghrib al-ᶜarabī tujāh mushkilat al-wabā' wa-l-ḥijr al-ṣiḥḥī fī-l-qarnayn 18 wa 19." Al-Ṣaghīr's article, which compares the treatises of Ibn ᶜAjība and Ḥamdān Khoja, suffers from being informed by a general bias against Sufism.

73. References to both the *Iḥyā'* and *Munqidh min al-Ḍalāl* can be found, for example, in ibid., 67, 75.

74. On the structure of the quarantine system, see Ḥamdān Khoja, *Itḥāf al-Munṣifīn,* 137–44; and Kuhnke, *Lives at Risk,* 93 ff. Ḥamdān Khoja is not mentioned by Panzac in any of his works on the establishment of a quarantine system in the Ottoman Empire in the 1830s and 1840s.

75. For this biographical information, I have drawn on Muḥammad b. ᶜAbd al-Karīm's introduction in Ḥamdān Khoja, *Itḥāf al-Munṣifīn,* 11–21.

76. Ibid., 43–47.

77. Ibid., 57–58.

78. Ibid., 58–59.

79. Ibid., 60–63.

80. Ibid., 65–70.

81. Ibid., 70.

82. Ibid., 71–72.

83. Ibid., 72–77.

84. Ibid., 78.

85. Ibid., 79–80.

86. Ibid., 105. I have not been able to determine whether this work is extant.

87. Ibid., 96. This work does not seem to be in print, nor have I been able to locate a manuscript.

88. Ibid., 110. For earlier examples of this argument, see chapter 1, note 132.

89. On al-Zayyānī, see Lévi-Provençal, *Les historiens des chorfas,* 142–200; for al-Zayyānī's opinion of the quarantine, see al-Zayyānī, *Al-Turjamāna al-Kubra,* 363–65 (cited in al-Bazzāz, *Ta'rīkh al-Awbi'a,* 404). Compare with the more descriptive, but still skeptical, comments of the earlier Moroccan ambassador to Spain, al-Miknāsī (d. 1212/1798), *Al-Iksīr fī Fikāk al-Asīr,* 9–10.

90. Ḥamdān Khoja, *Itḥāf al-Munṣifīn,* 115–17.

91. Ibid., 119–21.

92. The example had already been given by al-Ghazālī. See Goodman's discussion of the *Tahāfut:* "Did al-Ghazālī Deny Causality?" 92.

93. Ḥamdān Khoja, *Itḥāf al-Munṣifīn,* 124–25.

94. Ibid., 125–26.

95. Ibid., 126–27.

96. Ibid., 131.

97. Ibid., 132. Compare with al-Banānī, *Risāla fī-l-Ṭaᶜn wa-l-Ṭawāᶜīn,* 45r, where we find the older view that the jinn's internal piercing of humans causes plague buboes to emerge.

98. Ḥamdān Khoja, *Itḥāf al-Munṣifīn,* 137–43.

99. Ibid., 145–48.

100. Ibid., 151.

101. Ibid. 152–54.

102. See al-Kaḥḥāla, *Muᶜjam al-Mu'allifīn,* 1:332.

103. Ḥamdan Khoja, *Itḥāf al-Munṣifīn,* 159–62.

104. Ibid., 24. In his edition of the text, Muḥmmad b. ᶜAbd al-Karīm was able to find only one extant copy of the text, written by the author himself and now preserved in the National Library in Paris. Ibid., 37.

105. See Panzac, "Tanzimat et santé publique."

106. Ibid., 84–85. See also Panzac, *Quarantaines et lazarets,* 102–13.

107. See Low, "Empire of the Hajj."

108. See Moulin, "Construction of Disease Transmission"; and Kuhnke, *Lives at Risk,* 70, 75.

109. Kuhnke, *Lives at Risk,* 52–53.

110. See al-Bazzāz, *Tārīkh al-Awbi'a,* 403–8.

111. See Amster, "Many Deaths of Dr. Emile Mauchamp"; C. R. Pennell, *Morocco since 1830: A History* (New York: New York University Press, 2000), 49–53. For a more general look at how medicine functioned within the broader program of European colonialism, see Paul, "Medicine and Imperialism in Morocco."

112. Amster, "Many Deaths of Dr. Emile Mauchamp," 413.

113. Ibid., 409, passim. On the Mauchamp affair, see also Katz, *Murder in Marrakesh.*

114. See Dols, *Black Death,* 121–42. As Dols notes, this tradition was certainly present in the genre of plague treatises as well. See, for example, Ibn Ḥaydūr and Ibn Manẓūr in Gigandet, "Trois *Maqālāt* sur la prevention des épidémies," 267 and 276, respectively.

Conclusion. Reframing Muslim and Christian Views on Contagion

1. Al-Mawwāq, M. and M. al-Raṣṣāᶜ, *Al-Ajwiba al-Tūnisiyya,* 58.

2. Dols, "Comparative Communal Responses."

3. Ibid., 272. In this article, Dols neither defines contagion nor discusses at any length what he means by it.

4. Ibid., 272–75.

5. Ibid., 287.

6. Ibid., 275n25, 285.

7. Ibid., 279.

8. Ibid.

9. Ibid., 286.

10. "It will become evident that the European Christian and the Muslim reactions were quite dissimilar, and the comparison of these differences tells us much about what is essential to the identity of each culture." Ibid., 272. But see also Dols's view

that "the Black Death did not create these forms of reaction or the ideology that lay behind them; it was a stimulus, despite its irregularity of attack, which exposed the nerve system of late medieval Christian society" (275). Finally, for Dols, "Christian," "Western," and "Europe" have a disturbing tendency to become interchangeable, a stance that is especially problematic when seen from the perspective of al-Andalus. See notably Dols's opposition of "Western man" and "the Islamic tradition" (287).

11. Ibid., 287. Admittedly, the sharp edges of Dols's contrast between the Muslim and Christian intellectual traditions do soften when he notes that Muslim scholars differed in their interpretations of Prophetic Tradition on the theme of whether it is permissible to flee, as well as in his observation that some Muslims also saw the plague as a punishment (277).

12. Much of the following is taken from Stearns, "New Directions in the Study of Religious Responses to the Black Death."

13. On evolving Protestant attitudes toward the plague, see the references given in the introduction.

14. See Leibniz, *Theodicy,* 153.

15. For Jewish views, see R. Barkai, "Jewish Treatises on the Black Death (1350–1500): A Preliminary Study," in *Medicine from the Black Death to the French Disease,* edited by R. French, J. Arrizabalaga, A. Cunningham, and L. García-Ballester (Burlington, VT: Ashgate, 1998), 21.

16. See for example Aberth, *Black Death,* 97, 114; and J. P. Byrne, *Daily Life during the Black Death* (Westport, CT: Greenwood Press, 2006), 263–74. See also S. Einbinder, *No Place of Rest: Jewish Literature, Expulsion, and the Memory of Medieval France* (Philadelphia: University of Pennsylvania Press, 2009), 128–30, 215–16.

17. See Perho, *Prophet's Medicine,* 91–100; Conrad, "Ninth-Century Muslim Scholar's Discussion"; and J. Stearns, "Infectious Ideas: Contagion in Medieval Islamic and Christian Thought" (Ph.D. diss., Princeton University, 2007).

18. On Ibn al-Khaṭīb's trial, see Calero Secall, "El Proceso de Ibn al-Jaṭīb," where the charges against him are discussed on 432–45. The fatwa collection referred to here is Al-Mawwāq and al-Raṣṣā^c, *Al-Ajwiba al-Tūnisiyya.*

19. For two edited collections of primary sources regarding the plague, see Horrox, *Black Death;* and Aberth, *Black Death.* Horrox's book offers a wide array of materials on Christian processions, sermons, and prayers (111–157), whereas Aberth's contains excerpts of Muslim sources and a single Jewish source.

20. For Jewish views that the plague was a punishment of God, see Barkai, "Jewish Treatises on the Black Death," 16–18, 21.

21. Compare the various views given in Horrox, *Black Death,* 114, 116, 120, 130, 131, 134; and Aberth, *Black Death,* 99. For the plague as a general punishment from God for Jews, see Barkai, "Jewish Treatises on the Black Death," 18, 21. See, however, Einbinder, *No Place of Rest,* 125–27, where Jacob b. Solomon's fourteenth-century *Evel Rabbati,* citing many of the same biblical passages that Christian authors cited, implies that the plague is a punishment for disobedience.

22. Compare Horrox, *Black Death,* 134–35 and 146.

23. See van Ess, *Der Fehltritt des Gelehrten,* 125–26.

24. Hanska, *Strategies of Sanity and Survival,* chap. 3. Compare with Horrox, *Black Death,* 111–120.

25. Hanska, *Strategies of Sanity and Survival,* 45–47.

26. Dols, *Black Death,* 245–54.
27. Ibn Ḥajar, *Badhl al-Mā'ūn,* 317–18.
28. Dols, *Black Death,* 247.
29. For a fascinating study of the interconnected worlds of Christian, Jewish, and Muslim doctors in Spain, see L. García-Ballester, "A Marginal Learned Medical World: Jewish, Muslim, and Christian Medical Practitioners, and the Use of Arabic Medical Sources in Late Medieval Spain," in *Practical Medicine from Salerno to the Black Death,* edited by L. García-Ballester, R. French, J. Arrizabalaga and A. Cunningham (Cambridge: Cambridge University Press, 1994), 353–94. See here also R. Barkai, "Between East and West: A Jewish Doctor from Spain," in *Intercultural Contacts in the Medieval Mediterranean,* edited by B. Arbel and D. Jacoby (Portland, OR: F. Cass, 1996), 49–63.
30. Barkai, "Jewish Treatises on the Black Death," 21. For a later Jewish plague treatise, which similarly identifies God as the origin of the plague, see Barkai, "Between East and West," 60. For more recent works on Jewish plague treatises, see the works of Gerrit Bos in the bibliography.
31. Einbinder, *No Place of Rest,* esp. 129–30. Here the study of rabbinical responsa is of additional value in proving that many rabbis called for fleeing the plague. Still unsurpassed in this regard is H. J. Zimmels, *Magicians, Theologians, and Doctors: Studies in Folk-Medicine and Folk-Lore as Reflected in the Rabbinical Responsa (12th-19th Centuries)* (London: Edward Goldston, 1952), 99–105.
32. For a rich description of the origins of the plague, see Ibn Ḥajar, *Badhl al-Mā'ūn,* 81–86. Clement VI's mass is found in Horrox, *Black Death,* 122. That the passage from 2 Samuel was cited in the mass is bewildering, for the sin for which David chooses the punishment of plague is that of carrying out a census.
33. Al-Mawwāq and al-Raṣṣāᶜ, *Al-Ajwiba al-Tūnisiyya.*
34. Ibid., 43. The claim that quarantines were being implemented in North Africa in the fourteenth century is anachronistic, because initial attempts to apply quarantines to prevent the spread of the plague occurred first in the eighteenth and nineteenth centuries. See al-Bazzāz, *Ta'rīkh al-Awbi'a,* 403–6.
35. See Congourdeau and Melhaoui, "La perception de la peste."
36. Hanska, *Strategies of Sanity and Survival.*
37. Dols, Comparative Communal Responses," 287.
38. See, for example, Wray, "Boccaccio and the Doctors."
39. David Nirenberg argues that the interreligious relations that characterized Christian-Jewish interactions during the thirteenth and early fourteenth centuries ended in 1348. Nirenberg, *Communities of Violence,* 245–48. To my knowledge, a detailed exploration of Jewish-Christian relations in Christian Iberia in the second half of the fourteenth century has not yet been undertaken.

Appendix A

1. See Lieber, "Old Testament "Leprosy," Contagion, and Sin," 99–136. Lieber believes that *ṣara'at* actually referred to chronic psoriasis or bejel. While Lieber is the only author I have found who identifies a distinct disease for Levitical leprosy, her reading should be compared with earlier studies to which she does not refer: Lewis, "Lesson from Leviticus"; and Brody, *Disease of the Soul,* 110–19.

2. Brody, *Disease of the Soul,* 117.

3. "The case of Miriam shows that evil speech or a lying tongue causes leprosy. Gehazi's disease shows that leprosy comes from profanation of the Divine Name or from feet that are swift in running to evil. Uzziah's instance connects leprosy with the sin of wicked thoughts . . . and with . . . usurping an undeserved dignity and overweening pride. That haughty eyes are punished with leprosy is proved through the haughty daughters of Zion (Isaiah 3:16–17), whom the Lord will smite with a scab. . . . One of the exegetes presents the experience of Goliath as evidence that blaspheming the Divine Name produces leprosy" (ibid., 116).

4. Ibid., 113.

5. Ibid., 125. For the works of two other exegetes of Leviticus, neither of whom discussed contagion, see the articles of Beryl Smalley, "An Early Twelfth-Century Commentator on the Literal Sense of Leviticus"; and "Ralph of Flaix on Leviticus," in *Studies in Medieval Thought and Learning.*

6. Compare with Galatians 5:9, "A little leaven leaveneth the whole lump."

7. The identity of Ambrosiaster remains a mystery, although it its agreed that the text is from the fourth century. This work was thought to have been authored by Saint Ambrose (d. 397) until the sixteenth century, when Erasmus challenged the attribution. I have referred to the text in the *Patrologia Latina,* 17.209A–210A. Saint Cyprian (d. 258) had written briefly on 1 Corinthians 5:7 in his *Liber de Habitu Virginum,* but, not having mentioned the previous verse, he had not focused so explicitly on the transmission of sin. See *PL,* 4.455B–457A.

8. *PL,* 4.209A–B.

9. A reference to Exodus 13:3–7, where Moses tells the Jews that to commemorate their rescue from Egypt they are eat no leavened bread during the Passover feast. It would remind them that they did not have time to leaven the bread they took with them as they fled from Egypt (Exod. 12:39). The eating of unleavened bread has remained a part of the Jewish celebration of Passover until today.

10. This passage of Ambrosiaster is quoted at length and without acknowledgment by the ninth-century German archbishop Rabanus Maurus (d. 856) in his commentary on Corinthians. *PL,* 112.51D–52A.

11. *PL,* 26.402D–403B.

12. As in the confrontation between the Prophet and the bedouin, the observation that scabies was contagious is attributed to popular wisdom.

13. For the complicated literary history of cancer, see Demaitre, "Medieval Notions of Cancer."

14. The text of the Vulgate: "Profana autem inaniloquia devita multum enim proficient ad impietatem: et sermo eorum ut cancer serpit, ex quibus est Hymenaeus et Philetus, qui a veritate exciderunt, dicentes resurrectionem iam factam et subvertunt quorundam fidem." (But shun profane and vain babblings: for they will increase unto more godlessness. And their word will eat as doth a canker: of whom is Hymenaeus and Philetus; Who concerning the truth have erred, saying that the resurrection is past already; and overthrow the faith of some.) The Vulgate's use of *serpit* is interesting because both the King James Version and Luther translated the activity of *cancer* as one of eating. The New American Standard Version and many other modern editions translate the disease as "gangrene," which spreads, consumes, or eats.

15. *PL,* 4.492A. The use of the verb *transilire* parallels the Arabic *ᶜadā,* in that both refer an act of crossing over, of exceeding a boundary.

16. An earlier example of creeping sin can be found in Seneca (d. 39), *On Tranquility of Mind,* where he describes how vices creep and leap from one person to the next and cause harm by contact (*serpunt etiam vitia et in proximum quemque transiliunt et contactu nocent*). See Jarcho, *Concept of Contagion,* 17.

17. Nutton, "Reception of Fracastoro's Theory," 200.

18. Ibid., 203; and Nutton, "Seeds of Disease," 34. Nutton notes that the doctrine of *fomes peccati* was formally adopted at the Council of Trent in 1546, a council attended by Fracastoro in his capacity as doctor. While the phrase is found as far back as Augustine, in *PL,* 43.1356, the first use of it in a technical fashion to refer to the sin left after baptism is in the commentary on the letters of Paul of Walafrid Strabo (d. 849). *PL,* 114.481B–C. It was generally understood to refer to the concupiscence spoken of in Romans 7:7–8 as well as the lust mentioned in Romans 6:12.

19. *PL,* 117.537A.

20. *PL,* 116.624C, 667C; 118.918B.

21. *PL,* 117.536D.

22. *PL,* 170:208A.

23. On Rupert's life, see Wesseling, "Rupert von Deutz." Rupert wrote at length on *azymi* in his commentary on Exodus and in his *Libro de Divinis Officiis. PL,* 167.618A–619A; 170.48C–51D.

24. *PL,* 181.859C.

25. *PL,* 181.860B. For a similar opinion, see the commentary on Paul of Peter Lombard (d. ca. 1160–64). *PL,* 191.1573B–D.

26. *PL,* 196.258B–259C. The reference to infection reads: "Fermentum illud merito dicitur verus unde animus est infectus, et in infectione corruptus" (259C).

27. *PL,* 196.260B.

Appendix B

1. The argument that Ashᶜarism was on the wane from the fifth/eleventh century onward is advanced by Nagel in *History of Islamic Theology,* 181, 184, 195. Similar sentiments are found in his "Ibn al-ᶜArabī und das Asch'aritentum," 213, 238. More than forty years ago, George Makdisi argued that Ashᶜarism failed to become widely accepted or to be successfully taken up by the law schools. See his "Ashᶜarī and the Ashᶜarites (Part 1)," 44, 47–48; and esp. "Ashᶜarī and the Ashᶜarites (Part 2)," 36. Makdisi's articles were criticized by Wilfred Madelung in his "Spread of Māturīdism and the Turks," 110.

2. Scholars who argue for the prevalence and importance of Ashᶜarism in North Africa and al-Andalus before and during the Almoravid and Almohad periods include Idris, "Essai"; Serrano Ruano, "Los Almorávides y la teología Ashᶜarí"; "Por qué llamaron los almohades antropomorfistas a los almorávides?"; Dandash, "Mawqif al-Murābiṭīn min ᶜIlm al-Kalām wa-l-Falsafa"; Lagardère, "Une théologie dogmatique"; al-Hintati, "Taṭawwur Mawqif ᶜUlamā' al-mālikiyya"; al-Maghrāwī, "Taṭawwur al-Madhhab al-Ashᶜarī"; and al-Manṣūrī, "Al-Ashᶜariyya fī Bilād al-Maghrib." In addition, Dominque Urvoy's recent biography *Averroès* gives a useful overview of

the intellectual climate in the Maghrib in the tenth–twelfth centuries. See Urvoy, *Pensers d'al-Andalus,* 165–74.

3. Lagardère, "Une théologie dogmatique," 71–78; al-Hintati, "Taṭawwur Mawqif ᶜulamā' al-Mālikiyya," 298–300; al-Manṣūrī, "Al-Ashᶜariyya fī Bilād al-Maghrib," 76; a later date is proposed in al-Maghrāwī, "Taṭawwur al-Madhhab al-Ashᶜarī," 137.

4. See Idris, "Essai," 127–28; and al-Manṣūrī, "Al-Ashᶜariyya fī Bilād al-Maghrib," 76. Other schools of theology may have been present in North Africa considerably earlier than this. Some scholars think Muḥammad b. Saḥnūn (d. 256/870) introduced the study of theology to Qayrawān in the third/ninth century. Al-Manṣūrī, "Al-Ashᶜariyya fī Bilād al-Maghrib, 86.

5. Lagardère, "Une théologie dogmatique," 74–78; and Idris, "Essai," 139. Compare with al-Maghrāwī, who dates the entry of Ashᶜarism into al-Andalus to the teaching of 'Abd al-Ḥaqq b. 'Aṭiyya (d. 541/1147). "Taṭawwur al-Madhhab al-Ashᶜarī," 137.

6. One of Abū ᶜImrān's Moroccan students, Wajjāj b. Zalū al-Lamṭī, from the deep Sūs, studied with Abū ᶜImrān in Qayrawān and then returned to his country and opened a center of study under the name Dār al-murābiṭīn. ᶜAbd Allāh b. Yāsīn, the founder of the Almoravid movement, was a student of Wajjāj's, and when Yaḥyā b. Ibrāhīm, head of the Lamtūna, stopped in Qayrawān on the way back from the pilgrimage and asked Abū ᶜImrān al-Fāsī to choose one of his students to go with him to convert his countrymen to Islam, Abū ᶜImrān chose Wajjāj, who chose Ibn Yāsīn, possibly with Abū ᶜImrān's consent. See Lagardère, "Une théologie dogmatique," 80.

7. I draw here on Serrano Ruano, "Los Almorávides y la teología Asᶜarí," 461–65.

8. Ibn Rushd's *Fatāwā* were assembled by his student Ibn al-Wazzān (d. 543/1148). See Oßwald, "Spanien unter den Almoraviden."

9. The Almoravids confused this title with the "Qāḍī al-Quḍāt" used by the Abbasids, whom they wished to emulate. See Urvoy, *Averroès,* 21–22.

10. Al-Maghrāwī, "Taṭawwur al-Madhhab al-ashᶜarī," 146–48.

11. Serrano Ruano argues convincingly against Lagardère's claim that the fatwa placed Ashᶜarism in question. See "Los Almorávides y la teología Asᶜarí," 483. In this she is supported by al-Maghrāwī, "Taṭawwur al-Madhhab al-Ashᶜarī," 147; and Urvoy, *Averroès,* 27–28.

12. Serrano Ruano, "Los Almorávides y la teología Asᶜarí," 474.

13. For an example of Ibn Rushd's ability to provide a subtle discussion of the foundations of law, see Hallaq, "Murder in Cordoba." Compare with Urvoy, *Averroès,* 29.

14. Serrano Ruano, "Por qué llamaron los almohades antropormistas a los almorávides?" 819.

15. Ibid., 819–20. In addition, Abū Bakr b. al-ᶜArabī exercised the position of Grand Qāḍī of Seville from 1134 until its fall to the Almohads in 1148. See Urvoy, *Averroès,* 21, 47.

16. Serrano Ruano, "Los Almorávides y la teología As'arí," 481, 492; Urvoy, *Pensers d'al-Andalus,* 165.

17. Urvoy, *Averroès,* 31. Neither Urvoy nor Frank Griffel give this legend much credence. See Griffel, "Ibn Tumart's Rational Proof," 2:754.

18. See Urvoy, *Averroès,* 30, 47–49; but now also the much more detailed discussion in Garden, 'Al-Ghazālī's Contested Revival," 156–79.

19. Serrano Ruano, "Why Did the Scholars?"

20. Ibid, 151.

21. Asín Palacios, "Un Faqîh Siciliano." I am grateful to Delfina Serrano for this reference.

22. Asín Palacios's source for both Māzarī's criticisms and al-Subkī's defense of al-Ghazālī was al-Subkī (d. 771/1370), *Ṭabaqāt al-Shāfiᶜiya,* 4:122–32 (within the biography of al-Ghazālī, 101–82). For biographical information on al-Māzarī, see Charles Pellat's article in the *Encyclopedia of Islam,* 2nd ed., 12 vols. (Leiden: Brill, 1960–2004), 6:942–43.

23. Asín Palacios, "Un Faqîh Siciliano," 226–28.

24. Ibid., 231–37.

25. al-Subkī, *Ṭabaqāt al-Shāfiᶜiya,* 4:129. I have benefited from consulting Aṣín Palacios's translation of the same passage, "Un Faqîh Siciliano," 244.

26. I have drawn here on al-Ṣaghīr, "Al-Buᶜd al-Siyāsī." I am grateful to Delfina Serrano for this reference.

27. Al-Ṣaghīr, "Al-Buᶜd al-Siyāsī," 182, 189. On the messianic movements in the 1140s in al-Andalus that Ibn al-ᶜArabī may have connected with the Bāṭinīs of the Mashriq, see Urvoy, *Averroès,* 32–33.

28. He set out his criticisms of al-Ghazālī in his *Al-'Awāṣim min al-Qawāṣim.* Frank Griffel offers a different reading of this book, seeing it as a simplified version of al-Ghazālī's *Tahāfut al-Falāsifa.* See Griffel, "Relationship between Averroes and al-Ghazālī," 55. I am grateful to Professor Griffel for sending me a copy of this article.

29. Al-Ṣaghīr, "Al-Buᶜd al-Siyāsī," 187.

30. For a recent analysis of the relationship of al-Ghazālī, Ibn Tūmart, and Ashᶜarism, see Griffel, "Ibn Tumart's Rational Proof," 757–65. For a substantially different view of the relationship between al-Ghazālī and Ibn Tūmart, see Urvoy, *Averroès,* 49, 52. One of the many points on which the two views of Ibn Tūmart differ is the degree to which he was influenced by Muᶜtazilism. Urvoy sees him as more influenced by Muᶜtazilism than by Ashᶜarism (52), whereas Griffel depicts Ibn Tūmart as shaped by the Ashᶜarism and philosophy taught at the Niẓāmiyya in Baghdad. On Ashᶜarism in North Africa in the eighth/fourteenth century, especially in the work of Ibn ᶜArafa, see Ghrab, *Ibn ᶜArafa et le Malikisme;* and, by the same author, "Manzilat al-ᶜAql ᶜInd Ibn ᶜArafa."

31. The literature on this subject is substantial and the following is hardly comprehensive: Frank, "Structure of Created Causality"; Courtenay, "Critique on Natural Causality"; Wolfson, *Philosophy of the Kalam;* Goodman, "Did al-Ghazālī Deny Causality?"; Gimaret, *Théories de l'acte humain,* esp. 168–70; Alon, "Al-Ghazālī on Causality"; Perler and Rudolph, *Occasionalismus;* Halevi, "Theologian's Doubts"; McGinnis, "Occasionalism, Natural Causation, and Science in al-Ghazālī"; and Duart, "Al-Ghazālī's Conception of the Agent." I have also found the following two articles useful: Bernard, "La critique de la notion de nature"; and Morrison, "Portrayal of Nature."

32. Frank, "Structure of Created Causality," 25. Al-Ashᶜarī was in part reacting to his former Muᶜtazilī teacher al-Jubbā'ī's teaching that it is either God or man who can be held to be the author of an act, not both at once.

33. For a more detailed and nuanced account of the stance of Ashᶜarism on this question, see Gimaret, *Théories de l'acte humain,* 233–34. Note that Gimaret, unlike Frank, finds that Ashᶜarism as a whole, as opposed to Māturīdism, tended to deny man any part in his actions.

34. Frank, "Structure of Created Causality," 30. This is admittedly a rather fine line for al-Ash[c]arī to walk. Frank's comments are apposite: "A great part of the misunderstanding of al-As[c]arî's position on this whole question and the tendency of some scholars to see in it a merely verbal (and not entirely honest) affirmation of human causality while at the same time upholding a conservative notion of the universal creativity of God, would seem in great part to find its source in a failure to grasp distinctly and clearly the meaning of the terms of the problem as the author construed it and parallel failure to restrict the problem to the limits within it was conceived and formulated" (31).

35. Ibid., 26. Frank notes that al-Ash[c]arī does not deny secondary causality in nature; he simply does not discuss it (25).

36. Wolfson, *Philosophy of the Kalam,* 544–46.

37. See the exceptional views of al-Yūsī in chapter 5.

38. Ormsby, *Theodicy in Islamic Thought,* 212–13. Compare, however, with Ormsby's more recent remarks in *Ghazali,* 77–86.

39. Besides the above-cited studies of Alon, Courtenay, and Halevi, see Griffel, "Ibn Tumart's Rational Proof," 778. The chief holdout in seeing al-Ghazālī as an Ash[c]arī occasionalist is Michael Marmura: Marmura, "Al-Ghazālī's Second Causal Theory"; and "Al-Ghazālī on Bodily Resurrection and Causality." See also Kukkonen, "Plenitude, Possibility, and the Limits of Reason," 543.

40. Courtenay, "Critique on Natural Causality," 86.

41. Goodman, "Did al-Ghazālī Deny Causality?" 108–9.

42. Ibid., 115–19.

43. Alon, "Al-Ghazālī on Causality," 401–3.

44. Wolfson, *Philosophy of the Kalam,* 550. Al-Ghazālī's tendency to reintroduce "causes" under different names was later noted by Averroes.

45. Perler and Rudolph, *Occasionalismus,* 102–4.

46. Halevi, "Theologian's Doubts," 28.

47. Ibid., 38–39.

48. Griffel, "Ibn Tumart's Rational Proof," 778. For al-Ghazālī's remarks on how medicines can be considered to be effective to the same extent that people acquire actions (*kasb*), see al-Ghazālī, *Al-Ghazali,* 141–46.

49. McGinnis, "Occasionalism, Natural Causation, and Science in al-Ghazālī," 462–63.

50. Griffel, *Al-Ghazālī's Philosophical Theology,* 236–41.

51. Compare with Halevi's comment on the nature of the *Tahāfut al-Falāsifa:* "His project was never to present a unified theological front, free of incoherence. It is interesting not for his personal beliefs but for the manner in which he set up theological against philosophical belief. If this perspective leaves us in the dark about Ghazālī's belief, it nevertheless elucidates the nature of the text." "Theologian's Doubts," 38. See also Perler and Rudolph, *Occasionalismus,* 106.

52. On Averroes as a sympathetic exponent of al-Ghazālī, see Griffel, "Relationship between Averroes and al-Ghazālī."

53. For Ibn al-[c]Arabī's views on causality I have referred to Ṭālibī's *Ārā' Abī Bakr Ibn al-[c]Arabī al-Kalāmiyya,* 1:176–83.

54. See Ibn al-[c]Arabī's *Aḥkām al-Qu'rān,* 3:1082; *[c]Āriḍat al-Aḥwadhī bi-Sharḥ Ṣaḥīḥ al-Tirmidhī,* 7:234–35.

55. Bernard, "La critique de la notion de nature," 63.

56. On Mu[c]tazilī understandings of natures and how they played a role in causality, see ibid., 64–71; and Wolfson, *Philosophy of the Kalam,* 560–77.

57. Bernard, "La critique de la notion de nature," 75–78.

58. For an example of a careful argument that natural phenomena such as rain are effective intermediary causes, see Morrison, "Portrayal of Nature."

59. The best analysis of causality in the work of Averroes is supplied by Kogan, *Averroes and the Metaphysics of Causation.*

60. Griffel, "Relationship between Averroes and al-Ghazālī."

61. Urvoy, *Averroès,* 35, 43, 57. The Arabic text of his commentary on Plato is unfortunately lost, perhaps due to a lack of interest on the part of later generations (152).

62. Urvoy suggests that the condemnation of Averroes and several others may have been an attempt on the part of some Mālikī scholars to reassert the influence they had enjoyed under the Almoravids. Later biographers, with the exception of the eighth/fourteenth-century judge al-Bunnāhī (until recently known as al-Nubāhī), saw Averroes's fall from power as undeserved. Ibid., 179–87.

63. Ibid., 52, 138–39.

64. Griffel, "Ibn Tumart's Rational Proof," 753–64.

65. Kogan, *Averroes and the Metaphysics of Causation,* 45, 48. See also Gómez Nogales, "Teoria de la causalidad," 126–27.

66. The translation is that of Yusuf Ali, modified to reflect Averroes's understanding of the verse. I am drawing here on the analysis of de Libera in his introduction to Averroes, *Averroès,* 31. For the relevant Arabic of the *Faṣl al-Maqāl,* see 121–22. For a comparison of Averroes's understanding of Sura 3:7 with that of other exegetes, see Wild, "Self-Referentiality of the Qur'ān."

67. Kogan, *Averroes and the Metaphysics of Causation,* 162–63.

68. Ibid., 52. Compare with the Arabic text and French translation in Averroes, *Averroès,* 164–67.

69. On the self-conception of philosophers in Andalusī society, see Stroumsa, "Philosopher-King or Philosopher-Courtier?"

70. See Winter's comment in his introduction to *Cambridge Companion to Classical Islamic Theology,* 5.

71. For a reading of twentieth-century Arab intellectuals interpreting the significance of the al-Ghazālī-Averroes debate on causality, see von Kügelen, *Averroes und die Arabische moderne,* 360–85.

Arabic Primary Sources (Including Translations)

Abū Dāwūd. *Sunan Abī Dāwūd.* Beirut: Dār al-Jīl, 1991.

Averroes (Ibn Rushd). *Averroès: Discours decisive.* Edited and translated by Marc Geoffroy, with an introduction by Alain de Libera. Paris: Flammarion, 1996.

Al-ᶜAynī, Ibn Mūsā Badr al-Dīn. *ᶜUmdat al-Qārī fī Sharḥ al-Bukhārī.* 11 vols. Istanbul: Dār al-Ṭibā'a al-'Āmira, 1890.

Al-Bājī, Abū Walīd. *Al-Muntaqā: Sharḥ Muwaṭṭa' Mālik.* 9 vols. Beirut: Dār al-Kutub al-ᶜIlmiyya, 1999.

Al-Banānī, Muḥammad b. al-Ḥasan. *Risāla fī-l-Ṭaᶜn wa-l-Ṭawāᶜīn.* Al-Khizāna al-ᶜĀmma, Rabat, no. d1854, folios 44–48.

Al-Baṣrī, Abū al-Ḥusayn. *Kitāb al-Muᶜtamad.* 2 vols. Damascus: Al-Maᶜhad al-ᶜIlmī al-Faransī li-l-Dirasāt al-ᶜArabiyya, 1965.

Al-Bukhārī, Muḥammad b. Ismāᶜīl. *Ṣaḥīḥ.* 7 vols. Beirut: Dār Ibn Kathīr, 1990.

Al-Burzulī. *Fatāwā al-Burzulī.* 7 vols. Beirut: Dar al-Maghrib al-Islāmī, 2002.

Al-Dhahabī. *Al-Ṭibb al-Nabawī.* Cairo: Sharikat Maktabat wa-Maṭbaᶜat Muṣṭafā al-Bābī al-Ḥalabī, 1961.

Al-Fīlālī (al-Filālī), Muḥammad b. Abī al-Qāsim. *Risāla fī-man Ḥalla bi-Arḍihim Ṭāᶜūn.* Al-Khizāna al-ᶜĀmma, Rabat, no. d2251, pages 49–79.

Al-Gharisī, al-ᶜArabī al-Mashrafi. *Aqwāl al-Maṭāᶜīn fī al-Ṭaᶜn wa-l-Ṭawāᶜīn.* Al-Khizāna al-Mālikiyya, Rabat, no. 2054, folios 1–131.

Al-Ghazālī. *Al-Ghazali: Faith in Divine Unity and Trust in Divine Providence.* Translated by David B. Burrell. Louisville: Fons Vitae, 2001.

Al-Ḥalīmī, Ibn al-Ḥasan. *Kitāb al-Minhāj fī Shuᶜab al-Īmān.* 3 vols. Beirut: Dār al-Fikr, 1979.

Ḥamdān Khoja. *Itḥāf al-Munṣifīn wa-l-Udabā' fī al-Iḥtirāz ᶜan al-Wabā'.* Algiers: Al-Sharika al-Waṭaniyya li-l-Nashr wa-l-Tawzīᶜ, 1968.

———. *Le miroir.* Paris: Sindbad, 1985.

Ibn ᶜAbd al-Barr. *Al-Istidhkār.* 9 vols. Beirut: Dār al-Kutub al-ᶜIlmiyya, 2000.

———. *Al-Tamhīd li-mā fī-l-Muwaṭṭa' min al-Maᶜānī wa-l-Asānīd.* Edited by Suᶜād Aḥmad Aᶜrāb. 26 vols. Tetouan: Wizārat al-Awqāf wa-l-Shu'un al-Islāmiyya, 1967–92.

Ibn Abī Jamra, ᶜAbd Allāh. *Bahjat al-Nufūs.* 2 vols. Beirut: Dar al-ᶜIlm li-l-Malayīn, 1997.

Ibn ᶜAlī Junūn, Muḥammad b. al-Madanī. *Kalām al-A'imma ᶜalā Ḥadīth lā ᶜAdwā.* Al-Khizāna al-ᶜAmma, Rabat, no. d640 (791), pages 46–110.

Ibn Abī Zayd. *Al-Risāla.* Beirut: Dār al-Kutub al-ᶜIlmiyya, 2005.

Ibn Aḥmad al-Ḥājj, Muḥammad. *Mas'ala fī Ḥukm al-ᶜAdwā.* Al-Khizāna al-Mālikiyya, Rabat, Az 12,369, folios 79–95.

Ibn ᶜAjība, Aḥmad. *Sulūk al-Durar fī Dhikr al-Qaḍā' wa-l-Qadar.* Al-Khizāna al-ᶜAmma, Rabat, no. d2589, pages 1–22.

Ibn al-ᶜArabī al-Andalusī, Abū Bakr. *Aḥkām al-Qu'rān.* 3 vols. Cairo: 'Īsá al-Bābī al-Ḥalabī, 1968.

———. *ᶜĀriḍat al-Aḥwadhī bi-Sharḥ Ṣaḥīḥ al-Tirmidhī.* 13 vols. Beirut: Dār al-Kutub al-ᶜIlmiyya, 1980–92.

———. *Al-Qabas fī Sharḥ Muwaṭṭa' b. Anas.* 3 vols. Beirut: Dār al-Gharb al-Islamī, 1992.

Ibn ᶜĀṣim al-Gharnāṭī, Abū Yahyā Muḥammad. *Jannat al-Riḍā fī-l-taslīm li-mā qaddara Allāh wa qaḍā.* 3 vols. Amman: Dār al-Bashīr, 1989.

Ibn al-Athīr. *Jāmiᶜ al-Uṣūl min Aḥādīth al-Rasūl.* 2nd ed. 11 vols. Beirut: Dār al-Fikr, 1985.

Ibn Baṭṭāl, ᶜAlī b. Khalaf. *Sharḥ Ṣaḥīḥ al-Bukhārī.* 10 vols. Riyad: Maktabat al-Rushd, 2000.

Ibn Fūrak. *Bayān Mushkil al-Aḥādīth.* Edited and translated by Raimund Köbert. Rome: Pontificium Institutum Biblicum, 1941.

Ibn Ḥabīb, ᶜAbd al-Malik. *Kitāb al-Wāḍīḥa: Fragmentos extraídos del* Muntajab al-aḥkām *de Ibn Abī Zamanīn (m. 399/1008).* Edited and translated by María Arcas Campoy. Madrid: CSIC, 2002.

———. *Mujtaṣar fī l-Ṭibb.* Edited and translated by Camilo Álvarez de Morales and Fernando Girón Irueste. Madrid: CSIC, 1992.

Ibn Ḥajar al-ᶜAsqalānī. *Badhl al-Māᶜūn fī Faḍl al-Ṭāᶜūn.* 1411. Reprint, Riyad: Dār al-'Āṣima, 1990.

———. *Fatḥ al-Bārī bi-Sharḥ Ṣaḥīḥ al-Bukhārī.* 28 vols. Cairo: Maktabat al-Kullīyāt al-Azharīyah, 1978.

———. *Inbā' al-Ghumr fī Abnā' al-ᶜUmr.* 3 vols. Cairo: Lajnat Iḥyā' al-Turāth al-Islāmī, 1972.

Ibn al-Ḥājj. *Madkhal al-Sharᶜ al-Sharīf.* 4 vols. Cairo: Dār al-Fikr, 1981.

Ibn Ḥanbal, Aḥmad. *Musnad.* 10 vols. Beirut: Dār al-Fikr, 1991.

Ibn al-Jawzī. *Kitāb al-Quṣṣāṣ wa-l-Mudhakkirīn.* Edited and translated by Merlin Swartz. Beirut: Dār al-Mashriq, 1971.

———. *Talbīs Iblīs.* Cairo: Idārat al-Ṭibāᶜa al-Munīriyya, 1966.

Ibn Juzayy, Abū al-Qāsim Muḥammad b. Aḥmad. *Al-Qawānīn al-Fiqhiyya.* Tunis: Al-Dār al-ᶜArabiyya li-l-Kitāb, 1982.

Ibn Kathīr. *Tafsīr al-Qur'ān al-ᶜAẓīm.* 4 vols. Beirut: Al-Maktaba al-ᶜAṣriyya, 1998.

Ibn Khaldūn. *The Introduction to History: The Muqaddimah.* Translated by Franz Rosenthal. Abridged and edited by N. A. Dawood. Princeton, NJ: Princeton University Press, 1969.

———. *Muqaddima.* Beirut: Dār al-Fikr, 1998.

Ibn al-Khaṭīb, Lisān al-Dīn. "Ibnulkhatîbs Bericht über die Pest." In *Sitzungsberichte der königlichen bayerischen Akademie der Wissenschaften zu München,* edited and translated by M. J. Müller, 2:1–34. Munich: J. G. Weiss, 1863.

———. *Al-Iḥāṭa.* 4 vols. Cairo: Maktabat al-Khānjī, 2001.

Ibn Khātima. "Die Schrift von Abi Jaᶜfar Ahmed ibn ᶜAli ibn Mohammed ibn ᶜAli ibn Khatimah aus Almeriah ueber die Pest." Translated by Taha Dinanah. *Archiv für Geschichte der Medizin* 19 (1927): 27–81.

Ibn Lūqā, Qustā. *Abhandlung über die Ansteckung von Quṣṭā Ibn Lūqā*. Translated by Hartmut Fändrich. Stuttgart: Deutsche Morgenländische Gesellschaft, 1987.

———. *Quṣṭā Ibn Lūqā's Medical Regime for the Pilgrims to Mecca: The Risāla fī tadbīr safar al-ḥajj*. Edited by Gerrit Bos. Leiden: Brill, 1992.

Ibn Māja. *Sunan*. 2 vols. Beirut: Dār Iḥyā' al-Turāth al-^{c}Arabī, 1975.

Ibn Manẓūr. *Lisān al-^{c}Arab*. 18 vols. Beirut: Dār Iḥyā' al-Turāth al-^{c}Arabī, 1996.

Ibn Mubārak al-Sijilmāsī al-Lamṭī, Aḥmad. *Jawāb ^{c}amman ḥalla bi-bilādihim ṭā^{c}ūn*. Al-Khizāna al-^{c}Amma, Rabat, no. 2716 (D 1348), folios 125–28.

Ibn Mūsā, ^{c}Iyāḍ. *Ikmāl al-Mu^{c}lim bi-fawā'id Muslim*. 9 vols. Manṣūra: Dār al-Wafā', 1998.

———. *Tartīb al-Madārik*. 4 vols. Beirut, 1968.

Ibn al-Nafīs. *Al-Mūjaz fī l-Ṭibb*. Cairo: Wizārat al-Awqāf, 2001.

Ibn Qayyim al-Jawziyya. *Madārij al-Sālikīn*. 3 vols. N.p., 1955.

———. *Medicine of the Prophet*. Translated by Penelope Johnstone. Cambridge: Islamic Texts Society, 1998.

———. *Miftāḥ Dār al-Sa^{c}āda*. 3 vols. 'Aqrabiyya: Dār Ibn ^{c}Affān, 1996.

———. *Al-Ṭibb al-Nabawī*. Beirut: Al-Maktaba al-^{c}Aṣriyya, 2002.

Ibn Qutayba. *Ta'wīl Mukhtalif al-Ḥadīth*. Beirut: Al-Maktaba al-^{c}Aṣriyya, 2003.

———. *^{c}Uyūn al-Akhbār*. 4 vols. Cairo, 1925.

Ibn Rushd al-Jadd. *Al-Bayān wa-l-Taḥṣīl*. 20 vols. Beirut: Dār al-Gharb al-Islāmī, 1988.

———. *Masā'il Abī al-Walīd Ibn Rushd*. 2 vols. Casablanca: Dār al-Afāq al-Jadīda, 1992.

———. *Al-Muqaddimāt al-Mumahhadāt*. 2 vols. Beirut: Dar al-Kutub al-^{c}Ilmiyya, 2002.

Ibn Sa^{c}d. *Al-Ṭabaqāt al-Kubrā*. 9 vols. Beirut: N.p., 1968.

Ibn al-Ṣalāḥ. *An Introduction to the Science of the Ḥadīth*. Edited and translated by Eerik Dickinson. Reading, England: Garnet, 2006.

———. *^{c}Ulūm al-Ḥadīth*. Damascus: Dār al-Fikr, 1998.

Ibn Sīnā. *Al-Qānūn fī-l-Ṭibb*. 11 vols. Beirut: Nūblīs, 1999.

Ibn Taymiyya. *Al-Fatāwā al-Kubrā*. 6 vols. Beirut: Dār al-Ma^{c}rifa, 1987.

Ibn Waḍḍāḥ al-Qurṭubī, Muḥammad. *Kitāb al-Bida^{c}*. Edited and translated by Maribel Fierro. Madrid: CSIC, 1988.

Al-Khaṭṭābī, Muḥammad. *A^{c}lām al-Sunan fī Sharḥ Ṣaḥīḥ al-Bukhārī*. 2 vols. Rabat: ^{c}Ukaẓ, 1980.

Al-Kattānī, *Salwat al-anfās*, Casablanca, 2004.

Al-Kirmānī, Muḥammad b. Yūsuf b. ^{c}Abd Allāh. *Al-Kawākib al-Darārī fī Sharḥ Ṣaḥīḥ al-Bukhārī*. 25 vols. Cairo: Al-Matba^{c}a al-Bahīyya al-Miṣriyya, 1933–39.

Mālik b. Anas. *Al-Muwaṭṭā'*. Beirut: Dār al-Gharb al-Islāmī, 1994.

Al-Maqqarī. *Azhār al-Riyāḍ*. 5 vols. Cairo: Maṭba'at Lajnat al-Ta'līf wa-al-Tarjamah wa-al-Nashr, 1939.

Al-Mawwāq, Muḥammad, and Muḥammad al-Raṣṣā^{c}. *Al-Ajwiba al-Tūnisiyya ^{c}alā al-Asila al-Gharnāṭiyya*. Beirut: Dār al-Madār al-Islāmī, 2007.

Al-Māzarī, Ibn 'Umar. *Al-Mu^{c}lim bi-fawā'id Muslim*. 3 vols. Beirut: Dār al-Gharb al-Islāmī, 1992.

Al-Miknāsī, Muḥammad b. ^{c}Uthmān. *Al-Iksīr fī Fikāk al-Asīr*. Rabat: Al-Markaz al-Jāma^{c}ī li-l-Baḥth al-^{c}Ilmī, 1965.

Muslim b. al-Ḥajjāj. *Ṣaḥīḥ Muslim*. 5 vols. Cairo: Dār al-Ḥadīth, 1991.

Al-Nasā'ī, Aḥmad ibn Shu'ayb. *Kitāb al-Sunan al-Kubrā.* 6 vols. Beirut: Dar al-Kutub al-'Ilmiyya, 1991.

Al-Nawawī, Muḥyī al-Dīn Abū Zakariyyā. *Sharḥ Ṣaḥīḥ Muslim.* 18 vols. Cairo: Al-Maṭba'a al-Miṣriyya bi-l-Azhar, 1929–30.

Al-Qasṭallānī, Aḥmad b. Muḥammad. *Irshād al-Sārī li-Sharḥ Ṣaḥīḥ al-Bukhārī.* 10 vols. Cairo: Maktabat al-Muthannā, 1887. Reprint, Baghdad, 1971.

Al-Qurṭubī, Ahmad Ibn ᶜUmar. *Al-Mufhim li-mā Ashkala min Talkhīṣ Kitāb Muslim.* 7 vols. Beirut: Dār Ibn Kathīr, 1996.

Al-Qurṭubī, Muḥammad b. Aḥmad. *Al-Jāmiᶜ li-Aḥkām al-Qur'ān.* 21 vols. Cairo: Dār al-Ḥadīth, 1996.

———. *Tafsir al-Qurtubi.* Vol. 1. Translated by Aisha Bewley. London: Dar al-Taqwa, 2003.

Al-Rahūnī, Muḥammad b. Ahmad. *Jawāb fī Āḥkām al-Ṭāᶜūn.* Al-Khizāna al-ᶜĀmma, Rabat, no. d2251, pages 1–48.

Al-Rāzī, Muḥammad b. Zakariyyā. *Al-Ḥāwī fī l-Ṭibb.* 23 vols. in 8. Beirut: Dār al-Kutub al-ᶜIlmiyya, 2002.

Al-Sakūnī, Abū ᶜAlī ᶜUmar. *ᶜUyūn al-Munāẓarāt.* Edited by Saᶜd Ghrab. Tunis: University of Tunis, 1976.

Al-Ṣanᶜānī, ᶜAbd al-Razzāq. *Al-Muṣannaf.* 12 vols. Beirut: Dār al-Kutub al-ᶜIlmiyya, 2000.

Al-Sanūsī, Abū ᶜAbd Allāh Muḥammad b. Yūsuf. *Khayr al-Bariyya min Ghāmiḍ Asrār al-Ṣināᶜa al-Ṭibbiyya.* Edited by Hayā Muḥammad al-Dawsarī and ᶜAbd al-Qādir Aḥmad ᶜAbd al-Qādir. Kuwait: Dār Ibn al-Nadīm, 1999.

———. *Les prolégomènes théologiques de Senoussi.* Edited and translated by J. D. Luciani. Algiers: Imprimérie Orientale Pierre Fontana, 1908.

———. *Sharḥ al-Muqaddimāt.* Edited by Yūsuf Ahnāna. N.p., 1990.

Al-Shāṭibī. *Al-Iᶜtiṣām.* Beirut: Al-Maktaba al-ᶜAṣriyya, 2002.

———. *Al-Muwāfaqāt.* 4 vols. in 2. Beirut: Dār al-Maᶜrifa, 2000.

Al-Shawkānī, Muḥammad. *Fatḥ al-Qadīr.* 5 vols. Beirut: Dār Iḥyā' al-Turāth al-ᶜArabī, 1998.

———. Itḥāf al-Mahara bi-l-Kalām ᶜalā Ḥadīth lā ᶜAdwā wa lā Ṭiyara. Great Library of Sanaᶜa, No. 137. Reprinted in Al-Fatḥ al-Rabbānī, 4:1941–63 (Sanaᶜa: Maktabat al-Jil al-Jadid, 2002).

Al-Subkī, Tāj al-Dīn. *Ṭabaqāt al-Shāfiᶜiyya.* 6 vols. Cairo: Al-Maṭba'ah al-Ḥusaynīya, 1906.

Al-Sūsī, Abū ᶜAbd Allāh Muḥammad al-Shabbī al-Ḥāmidī. *Rāḥat al-Insān fī Ṭibb al-Abdān.* In *Histoire de la medicine au Maroc,* edited by Akhmisse Mustapha, 211–16. Casablanca: Maṭbaᶜa al-Dār al-Bayḍā', 1991.

Al-Ṭabarī, Ibn Sahl b. Rabbān. *Firdaws al-Ḥikma fī l-Ṭibb.* Beirut: Dār al-Kutub al-ᶜIlmiyya, 2002.

Al-Tayālisī, Abu Dāwūd. *Musnad Abī Dāwūd al-Ṭayālisī.* Hyderabad, 1903. Reprint, Beirut: Dār al-Tawfīq, n.d.

Al-Tinbuktī, Aḥmad Bābā. *Nayl al-Ibtihāj.* Tripoli: Manshurāt Kulliyat al-Daᶜwa al-Islāmiya, 1989.

Al-Tirmidhī. *Al-Jāmiᶜ al-Ṣaḥīḥ.* 5 vols. 1965. Reprint, Beirut: Dār al-Fikr, 1983.

Al-Ubbī, Muḥammad b. Khalīfa al-Washtānī. *Ikmāl Ikmāl al-Muᶜlim.* 9 vols. Beirut: Dār al-Kutub al-ᶜIlmiyya, 1994.

Al-Wansharīsī. *Mi^c^yār.* 13 vols. Rabat: Dār al-Gharb al-Islāmī, 1990.

Al-Wazzānī, Abū 'Īsā Sīdī al-Mahdī. *Al-Mi^c^yār al-Jadīd al-Jāmi^c^ al-Mu^c^rib ^c^an Fatāwa al-Muta'akhkhirīn min ^c^Ulamā' al-Maghrib.* 4 vols. Rabat: Wizārat al-Awqāf, 1996.

Yaqūṭ. *Mu^c^jam al-Buldān.* 5 vols. Beirut: Dar al-Kutub al-^c^Ilmiyya, 1955.

Al-Yūsī, al-Ḥasan. *Al-Muḥāḍarāt.* Rabat: Dār al-Maghrib, 1976.

Al-Zayyānī. *Al-Turjamāna al-Kubra.* Rabat: Dār Nashr al-Ma^c^rifa, 1991.

Al-Zurqānī, Muḥammad. *Sharḥ al-Zurqānī ^c^alā Muwaṭṭa' al-Imām Mālik.* 4 vols. Beirut: Dār al-Kutub al-^c^Ilmiyya, 1990.

Latin, Medieval Castilian, and Medieval Valencian Primary Sources (Including Translations)

Alfonso El Sabio. *General estoria.* Edited by Antonio G. Solalinde. Madrid: J. Molina, 1930.

———. *Primera crónica general de España.* Edited by Ramón Menéndez Pidal. 2 vols. Madrid: Editorial Gredos, 1955.

———. *Las siete partidas.* Salamanca, 1555.

Alfonso of Cordoba. "Epistola et regimen Alphontii Cordubensis de pestilentia." *Archive für Geschichte der Medizin* 3 (1910): 223–26.

Alonso of Chirino. *Menor daño de la medicina de Alonso de Chirino.* Edited by Maria Teresa Herrera. Salamanca: Universidad de Salamanca, 1973.

Ambrosiaster. *In epistolam B. Pauli ad Corinthios primam.* In *Patrologia Latina,* 17.209A–210A.

Aquinas, Thomas. *Summa theologiae.* 61 vols. New York: Blackfriars, 1964–81.

Beato of Liebana. *Obras completas de Beato de Liebana.* Edited and translated by Joaquín González Echegaray, Alberto Del Campo, and Leslie G. Freeman. Madrid: Biblioteca de Autores Cristianos, 1995.

Cyprian, Saint. *Liber de habitu Virginum.* In *Patrologia Latina,* 4.455B–457A.

———. *Liber de lapsis.* In *Patrologia Latina,* 4.492A.

Elipando of Toledo. *Obras de Elipando de Toledo: Texto, traducción y notas.* Edited by Gonzalo del Cerro Calderón and José Palacios Royán. Toledo: Diputación Provincial de Toledo, 2002.

El Tostado, Alfonso Fernández de Madrigal. *Las çinco figuratas paradoxas.* Edited by Carmen Parrilla. Alcalá Henares: Universidad de Alcalá, 1998.

Enrique de Villena. *Obras completas.* Edited by Pedro Cátedra. 3 vols. Madrid: Biblioteca Castro, 1994.

Ferrer, Vincent. *Sermons.* Edited by Josep Sanchis Sivera and Gret Schib. 6 vols. Barcelona: Barcino, 1932–88.

Flavius Josephus. *Antigüedades Judías.* Edited by José Vara Donado. 2 vols. Madrid: Akal, 1997.

Haymo Halberstatensis. *In divi Pauli epistolas exposito.* In *Patrolgia Latina,* 117.536B–537A.

Hervé de Bourg Dieu. *Commentaria in epistolas divi Pauli.* In *Patrolgia Latina,* 181.859C–860B.

Isidore of Seville. *Etimologías.* Edited by José Oroz Reta and Manuel-A. Marcos Casquero. Madrid: Editorial Católica, 1982.

———. *Las historias de los godos, vandalos y suevos de Isidoro de Sevilla.* Translated by Cristóbal Rodríguez Alonso. León, Spain: Centro de Estudios e Investigación "San Isidro," 1975.

———. *The Letters of St. Isidore of Seville.* 2nd ed. Translated by Gordon Ford. Amsterdam: A. M. Hakkert, 1970.

Jacme d'Agramont. "Regiment de preservació a epidimia o pestilència e mortaldats." Translated by M. L. Duran-Raynals and C.-E. A. Winslow. *Bulletin of the History of Medicine* 23 (1949): 57–89.

———. *Regiment de preservació de pestilència.* Edited by Jon Arrizabalaga, Luis García Ballester, and Joan Veny. Barcelona: Enciclopèdia Catalana, 1998.

Jerome, Saint. *Commentariorum in epistolam ad Galatas libri tres.* In *Patrologia Latina,* 26.402D–403B.

Lluis d'Alcanyiz. "Lluis d'Alcanyiz: Regiment preservatiu e curatiu de la pestilencia." *Butlletí de la Biblioteca de Catalunya* 7 (1923–27): 25–57.

Rabanus Maurus. *Enarrationem in epistolas Beati Pauli.* In *Patrologia Latina,* 112.51D–52A.

Richard of St. Victor. *Declarationes nonnularum difficultatum scripturae.* In *Patrologia Latina,* 196.258B–260B.

Rupert of Deutz. *Libro de divinis officiis.* In *Patrologia Latina,* 170.48C–51D.

Sermons de quaresma. Edited by M. Sanchs Guarner. 2 vols. Valencia: Albatross Edicions, 1973.

Un sermonario Castellano medieval: El Ms. 1854 de la Biblioteca Universitaria de Salamanca. Edited by Manuel Ambrosio Sánchez Sánchez. 2 vols. Salamanca: Universidad de Salamanca, 1999.

Velasco de Taranta, Licenciado Fores, Fernando Álvarez, and Diego Álvarez Chanca. *Tratados de la peste.* Edited by María Nieves Sánchez. Madrid: Arco/Libros, 1993.

Secondary Sources

Abdel Haleem, M. A. S. *The Qur'an.* New York: Oxford University Press, 2004.

Aberth, John. *The Black Death: The Great Mortality of 1348–1350.* Boston: Bedford/St. Martins, 2005.

Abou El Fadl, Khaled. *Speaking in God's Name.* Oxford: Oneworld, 2001.

Ackerknecht, Erwin. "Anticontagionism between 1821 and 1867." *Bulletin of the History of Medicine* 22 (1948): 562–93.

Alexander, R. McN. "The Evolution of the Basilisk." *Greece and Rome* 10 (1963): 170–81.

Almazan, Vincent. "L'exemplum chez Vincent Ferrer." *Romanische Forschungen* 73 (1967): 288–332.

Alon, Ilai. "Al-Ghazālī on Causality." *Journal of the American Oriental Society* 100 (1981): 397–405.

Amasuno Sárraga, Marcelino V. *La peste en la Corona de Castilla durante la segunda mitad del siglo XIV.* Salamanca: Junta de Castilla y Léon, 1996.

Amster, Ellen. "The Many Deaths of Dr. Emile Mauchamp: Medicine, Technology, and Popular Politics in Pre-protectorate Morocco, 1877–1912." *International Journal of Middle East Studies* 36 (2004): 409–28.

Antuña, Melchor M. "Abenjátima de Almería y su tratado de la peste." *Religión y cultura* 4 (1928): 68–90.

Arié, Rachel. "Un opuscule Grenadin sur la peste noire de 1348: La *"naṣīḥa"* de Muḥammad al-Saqūrī." *Boletín de la Asociación Española de Orientalistas* 3 (1967): 189–99.

Arjona Castro, Antonio. "Las epidemias de peste bubónica en Andalucía en el siglo XIV." *Boletín de la Real Academia de Córdoba de Ciencias, Bellas Artes y Nobles Artes* 56 (1985): 49–58.

Arrizabalaga, Jon. "Facing the Black Death: Perceptions and Reactions of University Medical Practitioners." In *Practical Medicine from Salerno to the Black Death,* edited by L. García-Ballester, R. French, J. Arrizabalaga, and A. Cunningham, 237–88. Cambridge: Cambridge University Press, 1994.

———. "Problematizing Retrospective Diagnosis in the History of Disease." *Asclepio* 54 (2002): 51–70.

Arrizabalaga, Jon, John Henderson, and Roger French. *The Great Pox: The French Disease in Renaissance Europe.* New Haven, CT: Yale University Press, 1997.

Asín Palacios, Miguel. "Un Faqîh Siciliano, contradictor de al Ġazzâlî: Abû 'Abd Allâh de Mâzara." In *Centenario della nascita di Michele Amari,* edited by Giuseppe Salvo Cozzo, 2:216–44. Palermo: N.p., 1910.

Augustine. *Christian Instruction.* Translated by John J. Gavigan. New York: Cima, 1947.

Baer, Yitzhak. *A History of the Jews in Christian Spain.* 2 vols. Philadelphia: Jewish Publication Society of America, 1961–66.

Bashford, Alison, and Clair Hooker, eds. *Contagion: Historical and Cultural Studies.* London: Routledge, 2001.

Basset, Paul. "The Use of History in the Chronicon of Isidore of Seville." *History and Theory* 15 (1976): 278–92.

Al-Bazzāz, Muḥammad al-Amīn. *Tārīkh al-Awbi'a wa-l-Majāʿat bi-l-Maghrib fī-l-Qarnayn al-Thāmin wa-l-Tāsiʿ ʿAshara.* Rabat: Manshūrāt Kulliyāt al-Adab, 1992.

———. "Al-Ṭāʿūn al-Aswad bi-l-Maghrib fī-l-Qarn 14 Milādī." *Majallat Kulliyat al-Ādāb wa-l-ʿUlūm al-Insāniyya bi-l-Rabāṭ* 16 (1991): 109–22.

Beaujouan, Guy. "Philippe Éléphant: Mathématique, alchimie, éthique." In *Science médiévale d'Espagne et d'alentour.* Burlington VT: Variorum, 1992.

Benedictow, Ole J. *The Black Death, 1346–1353: The Complete History.* Woodbridge, UK: Boydell Press, 2004.

Bernard, Marie. "La critique de la notion de nature (*ṭabʿ*) par le kalam." *Studia Islamica* 51 (1980): 59–107.

Berque, Jacques. *Al-Yousi: Problèmes de la culture Marocaine au XVIIIème siècle.* Paris: Mouton, 1958.

Bischoff, Bernhard. "Die europäische Verbreitung der Werke Isidors von Sevilla." In *Mittelalterliche Studien: Ausgewählte Aufsätze zur Schriftkunde und Literaturgeschichte,* 2 vols. 1: 171–94. Stuttgart: Hiersemann, 1966–67.

Blankinship, Khaled. "The Early Creed." In *The Cambridge Companion to Classical Islamic Theology,* edited by Tim Winter, 33–55. Cambridge: Cambridge University Press, 2008.

Booth, Wayne. "Metaphor as Rhetoric: The Problem of Evaluation." In *On Metaphor,* edited by Sheldon Sacks, 47–70. Chicago: University of Chicago Press, 1979.

Borsch, Stuart J. *The Black Death in Egypt and England: A Comparative Study.* Austin: University of Texas Press, 2005.

Bos, Gerrit. "The Black Death in Hebrew Literature: Treatise on Pestilential Fever (Composed by an Anonymous Author). Edition of the Hebrew text with English Translation and Glossary." *European Journal of Jewish Studies* (forthcoming).

———. "R. Moshe Narboni: Philosopher and Physician, a Critical Analysis of *Sefer Oraḥ Ḥayyim'*." *Medieval Encounters* 1–2 (1995): 219–51.

Bos, Gerrit, and Guido Mensching. "The Black Death in Hebrew Literature: Abraham Ben Solomon's Tractatulus de pestilentia; edition of the Hebrew Text and English Translation (with Supplement on the Romance Terminology by Guido Mensching)." *Jewish Studies Quarterly* (forthcoming).

Brody, Saul. *The Disease of the Soul: Leprosy in Medieval Literature.* Ithaca, NY: Cornell University Press, 1974.

Brown, Jonathan. *The Canonization of al-Bukhārī and Muslim.* Leiden: Brill, 2007.

Brown, Michael. "From Foetid Air to Filth: The Cultural Transformation of British Epidemiological Thought, ca. 1780–1848." *Bulletin of the History of Medicine* 82 (2008): 515–44.

Buhindi, Muṣṭafā. *Akthara Abū Hurayra: Dirāsa Taḥlīliyya Naqdiyya.* 2nd ed. Casablanca: N.p., 2003.

Bulaqṭīb, al-Ḥussein. *Jawā'iḥ wa Awbi'at Maghrib ᶜAhd al-Muwaḥḥidīn.* Casablanca: Manshurāt al-Zaman, 2001.

Bürgel, J. Christoph. "Secular and Religious Features of Medieval Arabic Medicine." In *Asian Medical Systems: A Comparative Survey,* edited by Charles Leslie, 44–62. Berkeley: University of California Press, 1976.

Burns, Robert. "Alfonso X of Castile, the Learned: 'Stupor Mundi'." In *Emperor of Culture,* edited by Robert Burns, 1–13. Philadelphia: University of Pennsylvania Press, 1990.

Burton, John. *An Introduction to the Hadith.* Edinburgh: Edinburgh University Press, 1994.

Calero Secall, María Isabel. "La peste en Málaga, según el malagueño al-Nubāhī." In *Homenaje al Profesor Jacinto Bosch Vilá,* 1:57–71. Granada: Universidad de Granada, 1991.

———. "El proceso de Ibn al-Jaṭīb." *Al-Qanṭara* 22 (2001): 421–61.

Callaghan, Joseph. "Image and Reality: The King Creates His Kingdom." In *Emperor of Culture,* edited by Robert Burns, 14–32. Philadelphia: University of Pennsylvania Press, 1990.

Campbell, Anna Montgomery. *The Black Death and Men of Learning.* 1931. Reprint, New York: AMS Press, 1966.

Cañizares-Esguerra, Jorge. "Iberian Science in the Renaissance: Ignored How Much Longer?" *Perspectives on Science* 12 (2004): 86–124.

Cantor, Norman. *In the Wake of the Plague: The Black Death and the World It Made.* New York: Free Press, 2001.

Carmichael, Ann. "Contagion Theory and Contagion Practice in Fifteenth-Century Milan." *Renaissance Quarterly* 44 (1991): 213–56.

Carter, K. Codell. *The Rise of Causal Concepts of Disease: Case Histories.* Burlington, VT: Ashgate, 2003.

Castrillo Márquez, Rafaela. "Yaḥya b. Hudhayl, iniciador de Ibn al-Jaṭīb en el conocimiento de la ciencia medica." *Al-Qanṭara* 7 (1986): 13–18.

Cátedra, Pedro. "La predicación Castellana de San Vicente Ferrer." *Boletín de la Real Academia de Buenas Letras de Barcelona* 39 (1983–84): 235–309.

———. *Los sermones atribuidos a Pedro Marín.* Salamanca: Universidad de Salamanca, 1990.

———. *Los sermones en romance del Manuscrito 40 (Siglo XV) de la Real Colegiata de San Isidoro de León.* Salamanca: Seminario Estudios Medievales y Renacentistas, 2002.

———. *Sermón, sociedad y literatura en la edad media: San Vicente Ferrer en Castilia (1411–12).* Valladolid: Junta de Castilla y León, 1994.

Cavadini, John C. *The Last Christology of the West: Adoptionism in Spain and Gaul, 785–820.* Philadelphia: University of Pennsylvania Press, 1993.

Chase, Melissa. "Fevers, Poisons, and Apostemes: Authority and Experience in Montpellier Plague Treatises." In *Science and Technology in Medieval Society,* edited by Pamela Long, 153–69. New York: New York Academy of Sciences, 1985.

Citrome, William. "Medicine as Metaphor in the Middle English *Cleannesse.*" *Chaucer Review* 35 (2001): 260–80.

Cohen, Ted. "Metaphor and the Cultivation of Intimacy." In *On Metaphor,* edited by Sheldon Sacks, 1–10. Chicago: University of Chicago Press, 1979.

Cohn, Samuel, Jr. *The Black Death Transformed: Disease and Culture in Early Renaissance Europe.* New York: Oxford University Press, 2003.

———. *Cultures of Plague: Medical Thinking at the End of the Renaissance.* Oxford: Oxford University Press, 2010.

Congourdeau, Marie-Hélène, and Mohamed Melhaoui. "La perception de la peste en pays chrétien byzantine et musulman." *Revue des Études Byzantines* 59 (2001): 95–124.

Conrad, Lawrence. "Arabic Plague Chronologies and Treatises: Social and Historical Factors in the Formation of a Literary Genre." *Studia Islamica* 54 (1981): 51–95.

———. "A Ninth-Century Muslim Scholar's Discussion of Contagion." In *Contagion: Perspectives from Pre-modern Societies,* edited by Lawrence Conrad and Dominik Wujastyk, 163–77. Burlington, VT: Ashgate, 2000.

———. "ᶜUmar at Sargh: The Evolution of an Umayyad Tradition on Flight from the Plague." In *Story-Telling in the Framework of Non-fictional Arabic Literature,* edited by Stefan Leder, 488–528. Wiesbaden: Harrassowitz, 1998.

Conrad, Lawrence, and Dominik Wujastyk, eds. *Contagion: Perspectives from Pre-modern Societies.* Burlington, VT: Ashgate, 2000.

Cooter, Roger. "Anticontagionism and History's Medical Record." In *The Problem of Medical Knowledge: Examining the Social Construction of Medicine,* edited by Peter Wright and Andrew Treacher, 87–108. Edinburgh: Edinburgh University Press, 1982.

Corominas, Joan, and José A. Pascual. *Diccionario crítico etimológico Castellano y Hispánico.* Madrid: Gredos, 1980.

Courtenay, William J. "The Critique on Natural Causality in the Mutakallimun and Nominalism." *Harvard Theological Review* 66 (1973): 77–94.

Crosby, Alfred. *The Columbian Exchange: Biological and Cultural Consequences of 1492.* Westport, CT: Greenwood, 1972.

Cunningham, Andrew. "Transforming Plague: The Laboratory and the Identity of Infectious Disease." In *The Laboratory Revolution in Medicine,* edited by Andrew

Cunningham and Perry Williams, 209–44. Cambridge: Cambridge University Press, 1992.

Cunningham, Andrew, and Ole Peter Grell. *The Four Horsemen of the Apocalypse: Religion, War, Famine, and Death in Reformation Europe.* Cambridge: Cambridge University Press, 2000.

Dallal, Ahmad. "Ghazali and the Perils of Interpretation." *Journal of the American Oriental Society* 122 (2002): 773–87.

Dandash, ᶜIsmat ᶜAbd Allāh al-Laṭīf. "Mawqif al-Murābiṭīn min ᶜIlm al-Kalām wa-l-Falsafa." In *Aḍwā' Jadīda ᶜalā'l-Murābiṭīn,* 83–97. Beirut: Dār al-Gharb al-Islāmī, 1991.

Davis, Cynthia J. "Contagion as Metaphor." *American Literary History* 14 (2002): 828–36.

De Epalza, Mikel. "Félix de Urgel: Influencias Islámicas encubiertas de Judaísmo." *Acta Historica et Archaeologica Mediaevalia* 22.2 (1999–2001): 31–66.

De Garganta, José M., and Vicente Forcada. *Biografía y Escritos de San Vicente Ferrer.* Madrid: Editorial Católica, 1956.

De la Granja, F. "La maqama de la peste del Alfaqui ᶜUmar de Málaga." *Al-Andalus* 23 (1953): 107–25.

Demaitre, Luke. "Medieval Notions of Cancer: Malignancy and Metaphor." *Bulletin of the History of Medicine* 72.4 (1998): 609–37.

De Santiago Simón, Emilio. "Un opúsculo inédito de Ibn al-Jaṭīb sobre sufismo." In *Homenaje al Profesor José María Fórneas Besteiro,* 2:1243–53. Granada: Universidad de Granada, 1994.

Deyermond, Alan. "The Sermon and Its Uses in Medieval Castilian Literature." *La Coronica* 8.2 (1980): 127–46.

Diamond, Jared. *Guns, Germs, and Steel.* New York: Norton, 1997.

Díaz y Díaz, Manuel C. "Isidoro en la edad media Hispana." In *De Isidoro al siglo XI,* 141–201. Barcelona: Ediciones El Albir, 1976.

Dickinson, Eerik. "Ibn al-Ṣalāḥ al-Shahrazūrī and the Isnād." *Journal of the American Oriental Society* 122 (2002): 481–505.

Dols, Michael. *The Black Death in the Middle East.* Princeton, NJ: Princeton University Press, 1977.

———. "The Comparative Communal Responses to the Black Death in Muslim and Christian Societies." *Viator* 5 (1974): 269–87.

———. "Ibn al-Wardī's *Risālah al-naba' ᶜan al-waba',* a Translation of a Major Source for the History of the Black Death in the Middle East." In *Near Eastern Numismatics, Iconography, Epigraphy, and History: Studies in Honor of George C. Miles,* edited by Dickran K. Kouymijan, 443–55. Beirut: American University of Beirut, 1974.

———. "The Leper in Islamic Society." *Speculum* 58 (1983): 891–916.

———. "Al-Manbijī's 'Report of the Plague': A Treatise on the Plague of 764–65/1362–4 in the Middle East." In *The Black Death: The Impact of the Fourteenth-Century Plague,* edited by Daniel Williman, 65–75. Binghamton, NY: Center for Medieval and Early Renaissance Studies, State University of New York, 1982.

———. *Medieval Islamic Medicine: Ibn Riḍwān's Treatise "On the Prevention of Bodily Ills in Egypt."* Berkeley: University of California Press, 1984.

———. "Syriac into Arabic: The Transmission of Greek Medicine." Aram 1 (1989): 45–52.

Duart, Thérèse-Anne. "Al-Ghazālī's Conception of the Agent in the *Tahāfut* and the *Iqtiṣād.*" In *Arabic Theology, Arabic Philosophy,* edited by James E. Montgomery, 425–40. Leuven: Peeters, 2006.

Dumont, Jean. *A New Voyage to the Levant: Containing an Account of the Most Remarkable Curiosities.* 3rd ed. London, 1702.

Dutton, Yasin. *Original Islam: Malik and the* madhhab *of Madina.* New York: Routledge, 2007.

Elgood, Cyril. "Tibb-ul-Nabbi or Medicine of the Prophet." *Osiris* 14 (1962): 33–192.

Ernst, Carl. *Words of Ecstasy in Sufism.* Albany: State University of New York Press, 1985.

Fadel, Mohammad. "The Social Logic of *Taqlīd* and the Rise of the *Mukhtaṣar.*" *Islamic Law and Society* 3 (1996): 193–233.

Fahd, Toufic. *La divination arabe.* Paris: sindbad, 1987.

Fermart, José. "Contribución al estudio de la medicina árabe española: El almeriense Aben Jatima." *Actualidad Médica* 44 (1958): 499–513, 566–80.

Fernández Félix, Ana. *Cuestiones legales del Islam temprano: La* ᶜUtbiyya *y el proceso de formación de la sociedad Islámica Andalusi.* Madrid: CSIC, 2003.

Fierro, Maribel. "The Introduction of ḥadīt in al-Andalus." *Der Islam* 66 (1989): 68–93.

———. "El principio mālikī *sadd al-dharāᶜī* en el *Kitāb al-ḥawādith wa'l-bidaᶜ* de Abū Bakr al-Ṭurtūshī." *Al-Qanṭara* 2 (1981): 69–87.

———. "Proto-Malikis, Malikis, and Reformed Malikis in al-Andalus." In *The Islamic School of Law: Evolution, Devolution, and Progress,* edited by Peri Bearman, Rudolph Peters, and Frank Vogel, 57–76. Boston: Harvard University Press, 2005.

Firey, Abigail. "*The Letter of the Law:* Carolingian Exegetes and the Old Testament." In *With Reverence for the Word: Medieval Scriptural Exegesis in Judaism, Christianity, and Islam,* edited by Jane McAuliffe, Barry Walfish, and Joseph Goering, 204–24. Oxford: Oxford University Press, 2003.

Fletcher, Richard. *Moorish Spain.* Berkeley: University of California Press, 1992.

Floriano, Antonio. "San Vicente Ferrer y las Aljamas Turolenses." *Boletín de la Real Academia de la Historia* 84 (1924): 551–80.

Foucault, Michel. *The Order of Things.* 1966. Reprint, New York: Vintage Books, 1994.

Frank, R. M. "Al-Asᶜarī's Conception of the Nature and Role of Speculative Reasoning in Theology." In *Proceedings of the VIth Congress of Arabic and Islamic Studies,* edited by Frithiof Rundgren, 136–54. Leiden: Brill, 1975.

———. "The Structure of Created Causality according to al-Asᶜarî: An Analysis of the *Kitâb al-Luma'.*" *Studia Islamica* 25 (1966): 13–77.

Gallagher, Nancy. *Egypt's Other Wars: Epidemics and the Politics of Public Health.* Syracuse, NY: Syracuse University Press, 1990.

———. *Medicine and Power in Tunisia, 1780–1900.* Cambridge: Cambridge University Press, 1983.

García Ballester, Luis. "Nuevos valores y neuvas estrategías en medicina." In *Historia de la ciencia y de la técnica en la Corona de Castilla,* edited by Luis García Ballester, 630–708. Salamanca: Junta de Castilla y León, 2002.

Garden, Kenneth. "Al-Ghazālī's Contested Revival: *Iḥyā' ᶜUlūm al-Dīn* and Its Critics in Khurasan and the Maghrib." Ph.D. diss., University of Chicago, 2005.

Gascón Vera, Elena. "La quema de los libros de don Enrique de Villena: Una maniobra política y antisemítica." *Bulletin of Hispanic Studies* 56 (1979): 317–24.
Gasse, Rosanne. "The Practice of Medicine in *Piers Plowman*." *Chaucer Review* 39 (2004): 177–97.
Geissinger, Aisha. "The Exegetical Traditions of ᶜĀ'isha: Notes on Their Impact and Significance." *Journal of Qur'anic Studies* 6 (2004): 1–20.
Gerli, E. Michael. "Social Crisis and Conversion: Apostasy and Inquisition in the Chronicles of Fernando del Pulgar and Andrés Bernáldez." *Hispanic Review* (2002): 147–67.
Ghrab, Saᶜd. *Ibn ᶜArafa et le Malikisme en Ifriqiya au VIII*ᵉ */ XIV*ᵉ siècles. 2 vols. Tunis: Faculté des lettres de La Manouba, 1992–96.
———. "Manzilat al-ᶜAql ᶜInd Ibn ᶜArafa." In *Ibn ᶜArafa wa-l-Manzaᶜ al-ᶜAqlī,* 12–25. Tunis: Al-Dār at-Tūnisīya li-l-Nashr, 1993.
Gigandet, Suzanne. "Trois *maqālāt* au sujet des épidémies de peste en Andalousie et au Maghreb." *Arabica* 48 (2001): 401–7.
———. "Trois *maqālāt* sur la prevention des épidémies." *Arabica* 52 (2005): 254–93.
Gilbert-Santamaría, Donald. "Historicizing Vergil: Translation and Exegesis in Villena's *Eneida*." *Hispanic Review* 73 (2005): 409–30.
Gimaret, Daniel. *Théories de l'acte humain en théologie musulmane.* Paris: J. Vrin, 1980.
Gómez Nogales, Salvador. "Teoria de la causalidad en el Tahāfut de Averroes." In *Actas: Primer Congreso de Estudios Arabes e Islamicos,* 115–28. Madrid: Comite Permanente del Congreso de Estudios Arabes e Islamicos, 1964.
Goñi Gaztambide, José. "El tratado "De superstitionibus" de Martín de Andosilla." *Cuadernos de etnología y etnografía de Navarra* 9 (1971): 249–322.
Goodman, Lenn. "Did al-Ghazālī Deny Causality?" *Studia Islamica* 47 (1978): 83–120.
Grell, Ole Peter. "Conflicting Duties: Plague and the Obligations of Early Modern Physicians towards Patients and Commonwealth in England and the Netherlands." In *Doctors and Ethics: The Earlier Historical Setting of Professional Ethics,* edited by A. Wear, J. Geyer-Kordesch, and R. French, 131–52. Amsterdam: Rodopi, 1993.
Griffel, Frank. *Al-Ghazālī's Philosophical Theology.* New York: Oxford University Press, 2009.
———. "Ibn Tumart's Rational Proof for God's Existence and Unity, and His Connection to the Nizamiyya *Madrasa* in Baghdad." In *Los almohades: Problemas y perspectivas,* edited by Patrice Cressier, Maribel Fierro, and Luis Molina, 2:753–812. Madrid: CSIC / Casa de Velásquez, 2005.
———. "The Relationship between Averroes and al-Ghazālī: As It Presents Itself in Averroes' Early Writing, Especially in His Commentary on al-Ghazālī's *Al-Mustaṣfā*." In *Medieval Philosophy and the Classical Tradition in Islam, Judaism, and Christianity,* edited by John Inglis, 51–63. Richmond, Surrey, England: Curzon, 2002.
Grigsby, Byron. "'The Doctour Maketh This Descriptioun': The Moral and Social Meanings of Leprosy and Bubonic Plague in Literary, Theological, and Medical Texts of the English Middle Ages and Renaissance." Ph.D. diss., Loyola University, 2000.
Grmek, Mirko. "Le concept d'infection dans l'antiquité et au moyen âge: Les anciennes measures sociales contre les maladies contagieuses et la fondation de la pre-

mière quarantaine à Dubrovnik (1377).” *Rad Jugoslavenske akademije znanosti i umjetnosti* 384 (1980): 9–54.
Guadalajara Medina, José. “La edad del Antichristo y el año del fin del mundo, según Fray Vicente Ferrer.” In *Pensamiento Medieval Hispano,* edited by José María Soto Rábanos, 1:321–42. Madrid: CSIC, 1998.
Gutas, Dimitri. *Greek Thought, Arabic Culture.* New York: Routledge, 1998.
Halevi, Leor. “The Theologian's Doubts: Natural Philosophy and the Skeptical Games of Ghazālī.” *Journal of the History of Ideas* (2002): 19–39.
Hallaq, Wael. *A History of Islamic Legal Theories.* Cambridge: Cambridge University Press, 1997.
———. *Law and Legal Theory in Classical and Medieval Islam.* Aldershot, England: Variorum, 1995.
———. “Murder in Cordoba: *Ijtihād, Iftā'* and the Evolution of Substantive Law in Medieval Islam.” *Acta Orientalia* 55 (1994): 55–83.
Hamlin, Christopher. “Predisposing Causes and Public Health in Early Nineteenth-Century Medical Thought.” *Society for the Social History of Medicine* 5 (1992): 43–70.
Hanlon, David. “Islam and Stereotypical Discourse in Medieval Castile and Leon.” *Journal of Medieval and Early Modern Studies* 30 (2002): 479–504.
Hanska, Jussi. *Strategies of Sanity and Survival: Religious Responses to Natural Disasters in the Middle Ages.* Helsinki: Finnish Literature Society, 2002.
Hanson, R. P. C. *The Search for the Christian Doctrine of God: The Arian Controversy, 318–381.* Edinburgh: T. & T. Clark, 1988.
Hawting, G. R. *The Idea of Idolatry and the Emergence of Islam: From Polemic to History.* Cambridge: Cambridge University Press, 1999.
Himmich, Bensalem. *The Polymath.* Translated by Roger Allen. Cairo: American University of Cairo Press, 2001.
Al-Hintati, Najmeddine. “Taṭawwur Mawqif ᶜUlamā' al-Mālikiyya bi-Ifrīqiya min al-Ḥawḍ fī-l-Masā'il al-Kalāmiyya wa Tabannī-him li-l-ᶜAqīda al-Ashᶜariyya.” *Revue de l'Institut des Belles Lettres Arabes* 55 (1992): 297–322.
Honerkamp, Kenneth. “Al-Ḥasan ibn Masᶜūd al-Yūsī.” In *Essays in Arabic Literary Biography, 1350–1850,* edited by Joseph Lowry and Devin Stewart, 410–19. Wiesbaden: Harrassowitz, 2009.
Horden, Peregrine. “Disease, Dragons, and Saints: The Management of Epidemics in the Dark Ages.” In *Epidemics and Ideas: Essays on the Historical Perception of Pestilence,* edited by Terence Ranger and Paul Slack, 45–76. Cambridge: Cambridge University Press, 1992.
Horden, Peregrine, and Nicholas Purcell. *The Corrupting Sea: A Study of Mediterranean History.* Oxford: Blackwell, 2000.
Horrox, Rosemary. *The Black Death.* Manchester: Manchester University Press, 1994.
Ibrahim, Yasir. “The Spirit of Islamic Law and Modern Religious Reform: *Maqāṣid al-sharīᶜa* in Muḥammad ᶜAbduh and Rashīd Riḍā's Legal Thought.” Ph.D. diss., Princeton University, 2003.
Idris, H. R. “Essai sur la diffusion de l'aš'arisme en Ifriqiya.” *Les Cahiers de Tunisie* 1 (1953): 126–40.
ᶜInān, Muḥammad. *Lisān al-Dīn ibn al-Khaṭīb: Ḥayātuhu wa-Turāthuhu al-Fikrī.* Cairo: Maktabat al-Khānjī, 1968.

Jacquart, Danielle, and Claude Thomasset. *Sexuality and Medicine in the Middle Ages.* Princeton, NJ: Princeton University Press, 1988.

Jarcho, Saul. *The Concept of Contagion: In Medicine, Literature, and Religion.* Malabar, FL: Krieger, 2000.

Al-Jīdī, ᶜUmar. *Al-Tashrīᶜ al-Islāmī.* Rabat: Manshūrāt ᶜUkāẓ, 1987.

Juynboll, G. H. A. *The Authenticity of the Tradition Literature.* Leiden: Brill, 1969.

Al-Kaḥḥāla, ᶜUmar. *Muᶜjam al-Mu'allifīn.* 4 vols. Beirut: Mu'assasat al-Risāla, 1993.

Kamali, Mohammad Hashim. *Principles of Islamic Jurisprudence.* Cambridge: Cambridge University Press, 1991.

Karmi, Ghada. "Al-Tibb al-Nabawi: The Prophet's Medicine." In *Technology, Tradition and Survival: Aspects of Material Culture in the Middle East and Central Asia,* edited by Richard Tapper and Keith McLachlan, 51–63. London: Frank Cass, 2002.

Katz, Jonathan G. *Murder in Marrakesh: Émile Mauchamp and the French Colonial Adventure.* Bloomington: Indiana University Press, 2006.

Al-Khaṭṭābī, Muḥammad al-ᶜArabī. *Al-Ṭibb wa-l-Aṭibbā' fī-l-Andalus al-Islāmiyya.* 2 vols. Beirut: Dār al-Gharb al-Islāmī, 1988.

Al-Khaṭṭābī, Muḥammad al-ᶜIzzī. *Fahāris al-Khizāna al-Ḥasaniyya bi-l-Qaṣr al-Mālikī.* 6 vols. Rabat, 1983.

Kister, M. J. "Call Yourself by Graceful Names. . . ." In *Society and Religion from Jāhiliyya to Islam,* 12:3–25. Aldershot, England: Variorum, 1990.

Klairmont, Alison. "The Problem of the Plague: New Challenges to Healing in Sixteenth-Century France." *Proceedings of the Annual Meeting of the Western Society for French History* 5 (1977): 119–27.

Kogan, Barry. *Averroes and the Metaphysics of Causation.* Albany: State University of New York Press, 1985.

Kohlberg, Etan. "Medieval Muslim Views on Martyrdom." *Mededelingen van de Koninklijke Nederlandse Akademie van Wetenschappen* 60 (1997): 5–31.

Kugle, Scott. *Rebel between Spirit and Law.* Bloomington: Indiana University Press, 2006.

Kuhnke, LaVerne. *Lives at Risk: Public Health in Nineteenth Century Egypt.* Berkeley: University of California Press, 1990.

Kukkonen, Taneli. "Plenitude, Possibility, and the Limits of Reason: A Medieval Arabic Debate on the Metaphysics of Nature." *Journal of the History of Ideas* 38 (2000): 539–68.

Kuramustafa, Ahmet. *Sufism: The Formative Period.* Berkeley: University of California Press, 2007.

———. "Suicide." In *Encyclopedia of the Qur'ān,* edited by Jane McAuliffe, 5:159–62. Leiden: Brill, 2006.

Lagardère, Vincent. *Histoire et société en occident musulman au Moyen Age: Analyse du Miᶜyār d'al-Wansharīsī.* Madrid: Consejo Superior de Investigaciones Científicas, 1995.

———. "Une théologie dogmatique de la frontière en al-Andalus aux XIᵉ et XIIᵉ siècles: L'Ashᶜarisme." *Anaquel de Estudios Árabes* 5 (1994): 71–98.

Lane, Edward. *Arabic-English Lexicon.* London, 1863.

Latham, J. D. "The Content of the *Laḥn al-ᶜAwāmm* (MS. 2229, al-Maktaba al-ᶜAbdaliyya al-Zaytūniyya, Tunis) of Abū ᶜAlī ᶜUmar b. Muḥammad b. Khalīl al-Sakūnī al-Išbīlī." In *Actas: Primer Congreso de Estudios Arabes e Islamicos,* 293–307. Madrid: Comite Permanente del Congreso de Estudios Arabes e Islamicos, 1964.

Leibniz, G. W. *Theodicy: Essays on the Goodness of God, the Freedom of Man, and the Origin of Evil.* Translated by E. M. Huggard. London: Routledge, 1951.

Lévi-Provençal, E. *Les historiens des chorfas.* 1922. Reprint, Casablanca: Editions Afrique Orient, 1991.

Lewis, Gilbert. "A Lesson from Leviticus: Leprosy." *Man* 22 (1987): 593–612.

Lieber, Elinor. "Old Testament 'Leprosy,' Contagion, and Sin." In *Contagion: Perspectives from Pre-modern Societies,* edited by Lawrence Conrad and Dominik Wujastyk, 99–136. Burlington, VT: Ashgate, 2000.

Lienhard, Joseph. "The Christian Reception of the Pentateuch: Patristic Commentaries on the Books of Moses." *Journal of Early Christian Studies* 10 (2002): 373–88.

Lindberg, David C. "Alhazen's Theory of Vision and Its Reception in the West." *Isis* 58 (1967): 321–41.

———. "Alkindi's Critique of Euclid's Theory of Vision." *Isis* 62 (1971): 469–89.

Lirola Delgado, Jorge. "Ibn al-Khaṭīb." In *Biblioteca de al-Andalus,* edited by Jorge Lirola, 3:643–98. Almería, Spain: Fundación Ibn Tufayl, 2004.

Lirola Delgado, Jorge, and I. Garijo Galán. "Ibn al-Jātima." In *Biblioteca de al-Andalus,* edited by Jorge Lirola, 3:698–708. Almería, Spain: Fundación Ibn Tufayl, 2004.

Lirola Delgado, Pilar, Ildefonso Garijo Galán, and Jorge Lirola Delgado. "Efectos de la epidemia de peste negra de 1348–9 en la cuidad de Almería." *Revista del Instituto Egipcio de Estudios Islámicos en Madrid* 32 (2000): 173–204.

Little, Donald. "Did Ibn Taymiyya Have a Screw Loose?" *Studia Islamica* 41 (1976): 93–111.

Lössl, Josef. "Julian of Aeclanum on Pain." *Journal of Early Christian Studies* 10 (2002): 203–43.

Low, Michael Christopher. "Empire of the Hajj: Pilgrims, Plagues, and Pan-Islam under British Surveillance, 1865–1908." *International Journal of Middle East Studies* 40 (2008): 269–90.

Luther, Martin. "Whether One May Flee from a Deadly Plague." In *Luther's Works: Devotional Writings 2,* edited by Gustav Wiencke, 43:113–38. St. Louis: Concordia Philadelphia, 1968.

Madelung, Wilfred. "The Spread of Māturīdism and the Turks." Reprinted in *Religious Schools and Sects in Medieval Islam,* 109–68. London: Variorum, 1985.

Al-Madgharī, ᶜAbd al-Kabīr al-ᶜAlawī. *Al-Faqīh Abū ᶜAlī al-Yūsī: Namūdhaj min al-Fikr al-Maghribi fī Fajr al-Dawla al-ᶜAlawiyya.* Rabat: Wizārat al-Awqāf, 1989.

Al-Maghrāwī, Muḥammad. "Taṭawwur al-Madhhab al-Ashᶜarī bi'l-Maghrib al-Aqṣā ilā Ḥudūd al-ᶜAṣr al-Murābiṭī." In *Al-Tārīkh wa-l-Fiqh: A'māl muhdā ilā al-marḥūm Muḥammad al-Manūnī,* edited by Muḥammad Ḥajjī, 133–53. Rabat, n.d.

Makdisi, George. "Ashᶜarī and the Ashᶜarites in Islamic Religious History (Part 1)." *Studia Islamica* 17 (1962): 37–81.

———. "Ashᶜarī and the Ashᶜarites in Islamic Religious History (Part 2)." *Studia Islamica* 18 (1963): 19–39.

Makhlūf, Muḥammad. *Shajrat al-Nūr al-Zakiyya.* Beirut: Dār al-Kitāb al-ᶜArabī, 1930.

Mansell, Darrel. "Metaphor as Matter." *Language and Literature* 15 (1992): 109–20.

Al-Manṣūrī, Mabrūk. "Al-Ashᶜariyya fī Bilād al-Maghrib ilā Nihāyat al-Qarn al-Sādis al-Hijrī al-Thānī ᶜAshar Mīlādī wa-Mafhūm al-Adwār al-Ḥaḍariyya." *Revue de l'Institut des Belles Lettres Arabes* 192 (2002–3): 71–98.

Marmura, Michael E. "Al-Ghazālī on Bodily Resurrection and Causality in the Tahafut and the Iqtisad." *Aligarh Journal of Islamic Thought* 1 (1989): 46–75.

———. "Al-Ghazālī's Second Causal Theory in the 17th Discussion of His Tahāfut." In *Islamic Philosophy and Mysticism,* edited by Parviz Morewedge, 85–112. Delmar: Caravan Books, 1981.

Marriott, Edward. *Plague: A Story of Science, Rivalry, and the Scourge That Won't Go Away.* New York: Metropolitan Books, 2002.

Martin, Thomas F. "Paul the Patient: *Christus Medicus* and the *"Stimulus Carnis"* (2 *Cor.* 12:7): A Consideration of Augustine's Medicinal Christology." *Augustinian Studies* 32 (2001): 219–56.

Masud, Muhammad Khalid. *Shatibi's Philosophy of Islamic Law.* New Delhi: Kitab Bhaven, 1997.

Mazzoli-Guintard, Christine. "Notes sur une minorité d'al-Andalus: Les lépreux." In *Homenaje al Profesor Carlos Posac Mon,* 319–25. 2 vols. Ceuta, Spain: Instituto de Estudios Ceutíes, 1998.

McGinnis, Jon. "Occasionalism, Natural Causation, and Science in al-Ghazālī." In *Arabic Theology, Arabic Philosophy; From the Many to the One: Essays in Celebration of Richard M. Frank,* edited by James E. Montgomery, 441–63. Leuven: Peeters, 2006.

McNeill, W. H. *Plagues and Peoples.* New York: Doubleday, 1976.

McWilliam, J. "The Context of Spanish Adoptionism: A Review." In *Conversion and Continuity: Indigenous Christian Communities in Islamic Lands, Eighth to Eighteenth Centuries,* edited by Michael Gervers and Ramzi Jibran Bikhazi, 75–88. Toronto: Pontifical Institute of Mediaeval Studies, 1990.

Melchert, Christopher. "The Piety of the Hadith Folk." *International Journal of Middle East Studies* 32 (2002): 425–39.

Mellor, D. H. *The Facts of Causation.* New York: Routledge, 1995.

Menocal, María Rosa. *The Ornament of the World: How Muslims, Jews, and Christians Created a Culture of Tolerance in Medieval Spain.* New York: Little, Brown, 2002.

Mernissi, Fatima. *Women and Islam.* New Delhi: Kali for Women, 1993.

Meyerhof, Max. "The 'Book of Treasure,' an Early Arabic Treatise on Medicine." *Isis* 14 (1930): 55–76.

Miguel-Prendes, Sol. "Enrique de Villena: Circa 1382–1384–15 December 1434." In *Castilian Writers: 1400–1500,* edited by Frank Domínguez and George D. Greenia, 266–76. Detroit: Gale Group, 2004.

Millán, Cristina A. "Tres opúsculos inéditos sobre la peste en un manuscrito magrebí." *Anaquel de Estudios Árabes* 3 (1992): 183–88.

Molina López, Emilio. *Ibn al-Jatib.* Granada: Editorial Comares, 2001.

———. "La obra histórica de Ibn Jātima de Almería: Los datos geográfico-históricos." *Al-Qanṭara* 10 (1989): 151–73.

Morales Delgado, A. "Abū Yaḥyā Ibn ᶜĀṣim." In *Enciclopedia de al-Andalus,* edited by Jorge Lirola Delgado and José Miguel Puerta Vílchez, 1:495–502. Granada: Fundación El Legado Andalusí, 2005.

Morrison, Robert G. "The Portrayal of Nature in a Medieval Qur'an Commentary." *Studia Islamica* 94 (2002): 115–37.
Moulin, Anne Marie. "The Construction of Disease Transmission in Nineteenth-Century Egypt and the Dialectics of Modernity." In *The Development of Modern Medicine in Non-Western Countries: Historical Perspectives,* edited by Hormoz Ebrahimnejad, 42–58. New York: Routledge, 2009.
Munson Henry, Jr. *Religion and Power in Morocco.* New Haven, CT: Yale University Press, 1993.
Mustapha, Akhmisse. *Histoire de la medicine au Maroc.* Casablanca: Maṭba' al-Dār al-Bayḍa, 1991.
Nagel, Tilman. *The History of Islamic Theology.* Princeton, NJ: Princeton University Press, 2000.
———. "Ibn al-ᶜArabī und das Asch'aritentum." In *Gottes ist der Orient, Gottes ist der Okzident: Festschrift für Abdoljavad Falaturi zum 65. Geburtstag,* edited by Udo Tworuschka, 206–45. Cologne: Böhlau Verlag, 1991.
Nirenberg, David. *Communities of Violence.* Princeton, NJ: Princeton University Press, 1996.
———. "Enmity and Assimilation: Jews, Christians, and Converts in Medieval Spain." *Common Knowledge* 9 (2003): 137–55.
Noordegraaf, Leo. "Calvinism and the Plague in the Seventeenth-Century Dutch Republic." In *Curing and Insuring: Essays on Illness in Past Times,* edited by J. M. W. Binneveld, Rudolf Dekker, and Hans Binneveld, 21–31. Hilversum, Netherlands: Uitgeverij Verloren, 1993.
Nutton, Vivian. "Did the Greeks Have a Word for It? Contagion and Contagion Theory in Classical Antiquity." In *Contagion: Perspectives from Pre-modern Societies,* edited by Lawrence Conrad and Dominik Wujastyk, 137–62. Burlington, VT: Ashgate, 2000.
———. "The Reception of Fracastoro's Theory of Contagion: The Seed That Fell among Thorns?" *Osiris* 6 (1990): 196–234.
———. "The Seeds of Disease: An Explanation of Contagion and Infection from the Greeks to the Renaissance." *Medical History* 27 (1983): 1–34.
Olshewsky, Thomas M. "The Classical Roots of Hume's Skepticism." *Journal of the History of Ideas* 52.2 (1991): 269–87.
Opwis, Felitia. "*Maṣlaḥa* in Contemporary Islamic Legal Theory." *Islamic Law and Society* 12 (2005): 182–223.
Ormsby, Eric L. *Ghazali: The Revival of Islam.* Oxford: Oneworld, 2008.
———. *Theodicy in Islamic Thought: The Dispute over al-Ghazālī's "Best of All Possible Worlds."* Princeton, NJ: Princeton University Press, 1984.
Osswald, Rainer. "Spanien unter den Almoraviden: Die *Fatāwā* des Ibn Rushd als Quelle zur Wirtschafts- und Sozialgeschichte." *Die Welt des Orients* 24 (1993): 127–45.
Ourāb, Muṣṭafā. *Al-Muᶜtaqadāt al-Siḥriyya fī-l-Maghrib.* Rabat: Dār al-Nashr al-Maghribiyya, 2003.
Palazzotto, Dominick. "The Black Death and Medicine: A Report and Analysis of the Tractates Written between 1348 and 1350." Ph.D. diss., University of Kansas, 1973.
Palmer, Richard. "The Church, Leprosy, and Plague in Medieval and Early Mod-

ern Europe." In *The Church and Healing,* edited by W. J. Sheils, 79–99. Oxford: Blackwell, 1981.
Panzac, Daniel. *La peste dans l'empire Ottoman: 1700–1850.* Leuven: Editions Peeters, 1985.
———. *Quarantaines et lazarets: L'Europe et la peste d'Orient.* Aix-en Provence: Edisud, 1986.
———. "Tanzimat et santé publique: Les débuts du conseil sanitaire de l'empire Ottoman." In *Population et santé dans l'empire ottoman (XVIIIe–XXe siècles),* 77–85. Istanbul: Les éditions Isis, 1996. Originally published in *150. Yılında Tanzimat,* edited by H. D. Yıldız, 325–33. (Ankara: Türk Tarih Kurumu, 1992).
Patrides, C. A. *The Grand Design of God.* London: Routledge, 1972.
Paul, Jim. "Medicine and Imperialism in Morocco." *Middle East Research and Information Project* 60 (1977): 3–12.
Pelling, Margaret. "The Meaning of Contagion: Reproduction, Medicine, and Metaphor." In *Contagion: Historical and Cultural Studies,* edited by Alison Bashford and Clair Hooker, 15–39. London: Routledge, 2001.
Perarnau, Josep. "Els quatre sermons de Sant Vicent Ferrer." *Arxiu de Textos Catalans Antics* 15 (1996): 109–340.
Perho, Irmeli. *The Prophet's Medicine—A Creation of the Muslim Traditionalist Scholars.* Helsinki: University of Helsinki, 1995.
Perler, Dominik, and Ulrich Rudolph. *Occasionalimus: Theorien der Kausalität im arabisch-islamischen und im europäischen Denken.* Göttingen: Vandenhoeck & Ruprecht, 2000.
Phillips, William D., Jr. "*Peste negra:* The Fourteenth-Century Plague Epidemics in Iberia." In *On the Social Origins of Medieval Institutions: Essays in Honor of Joseph F. O'Callaghan,* edited by Donald J. Kagay and Theresa M. Vann, 47–62. Leiden: Brill, 1998.
Pormann, Peter E., and Emilie Savage-Smith. *Medieval Islamic Medicine.* Washington, DC: Georgetown University Press, 2007.
Powers, David. *Law, Society, and Culture in the Maghrib, 1300–1500.* Cambridge: Cambridge University Press, 2002.
Al-Qijīrī, Muḥammad. "Al-Āfāt wa-l-Kawārith al-Ṭabīʿiyya bi-l-Maghrib bayna al-Qarnayn 11 wa 15." Master's thesis, Tetouan University, 1990.
Rahman, Sayeed. "The Legal and Theological Thought of Ibn Abī Zayd al-Qayrawānī." Ph.D. diss., Yale University, 2009.
Reilly, Bernard. *The Medieval Spains.* Cambridge: Cambridge University Press, 1993.
Reinert, Benedikt. *Die Lehre vom* tawakkul *in der klassischen Sufik.* Berlin: Walter de Gruyter, 1968.
Reinhardt, Klaus. "Nicolás Eymerich, OP (d. 1399), inquisidor y exegeta: Edición de dos textos selectos de su *Postilla literalis super evangelia.*" In *Pensamiento medieval Hispano,* edited by José María Soto Rábanos, 2:1215–36. Madrid: CSIC, 1998.
Renaud, H. P. J. "Un nouveau document marocain: Sur la peste de 1799." *Hespéris* 5 (1925): 83–90.
———. "La peste de 1799: D'après des documents inédits." *Hespéris* 1 (1921): 160–82.
———. "La peste de 1818: D'après des documents inédits." *Hespéris* 3 (1923): 13–35.
———. "Les "pestes" des XVe et XVIe siècles, principalement d'après des sources

portugaises." *Melanges d'études luso-marocaines dédiés à la mémoire de David Lopes et Pierre de Cenival* 6 (1945): 363–89.

———. "Les pestes du milieu du XVIIIe siècle." *Hespéris* 26 (1939): 293–319.

Rico, Francisco. *Alfonso el Sabio y la "General estoria."* 1972. Reprint, Barcelona: Ariel, 1984.

Rofail Farag, F. "The Muslims' Medical Achievements." *Arabica* 25.3 (1978): 292–309.

Ruben, Miri. *Corpus Christi.* Cambridge: Cambridge University Press, 1991.

Rudolph, Ulrich. "Christliche Theologie und vorsokratische Lehren in der *Turba Philosophorum.*" *Oriens* 32 (1990): 97–123.

Ruiz, Teofilo F. *Spanish Society: 1400–1600.* Essex, England: Longman, 2001.

Sabra, A. I. "The Appropriation and Subsequent Naturalization of Greek Science in Medieval Islam: A Preliminary Statement." *History of Science* 25 (1987): 223–43.

———. "Ibn al-Haytham's Revolutionary Project in Optics: The Achievement and the Obstacle." In *The Enterprise of Science in Islam: New Perspectives,* edited by Jan P. Hodgendijk and Abdelhamid I. Sabra, 85–118. Boston: MIT Press, 2003.

———. "Science and Philosophy in Medieval Islamic Theology: The Evidence of the Fourteenth Century." *Zeitschrift für Geschichte der Arabisch-Islamischen Wissenschaften* 9 (1994): 1–42.

Safran, Janina. "Identity and Differentiation in Ninth-Century al-Andalus." *Speculum* 76 (2001): 573–98.

Al-Ṣaghīr, ᶜAbd al-Majīd. "Al-Buᶜd al-Siyāsī fī Naqd al-Qāḍī Ibn al-ᶜArabī li-Taṣawwuf al-Ghazālī." In *Abū Ḥāmid al-Ghazālī: dirāsāt fī fikri-hi wa ᶜaṣri-hi wa tā'thīr-ihi,* 173–93. Rabat: Jāmi'at Muḥammad al-Khāmis, 1988.

———. "Mulāḥaẓāt ḥawl rudūd fiᶜl baᶜḍ mufakkirī al-maghrib al-ᶜarabī tujāh mushkilat al-wabā' wa-l-ḥijr al-ṣiḥḥī fī-l-qarnayn 18 wa 19." *Majallat Dār al-Niyāba* 2 (1984): 47–51.

Ṣālāḥ al-ᶜAlī, ᶜAbd al-Munᶜim. *Dafāᶜ ᶜan Abī Hurayra.* Beirut: Dār al-Sharq, 1971.

Saliba, George. "Writing the History of Arabic Astronomy: Problems and Differing Perspectives." *Journal of the American Oriental Society* 116 (1996): 709–18.

Salmón, Fernando, and Montserrat Cabré. "Fascinating Women: The Evil Eye in Medical Scholasticism." In *Medicine from the Black Death to the French Disease,* edited by R. French, J. Arrizabalaga, A. Cunningham, and L. García-Ballester, 53–84. Burlington, VT: Ashgate, 1998.

Sánchez-Albornoz, Claudio. *Historia de España: El Reino Astur-Leonés (722–1037): Sociedad, economía, gobierno, cultura y vida.* Madrid: Espasa-Calpe, 1980.

Savage-Smith, Emilie. "Gleanings from an Arabist's Workshop: Current Trends in the Study of Medieval Islamic Science and Medicine." *Isis* 79 (1988): 246–66.

———. "Medicine." In *Encyclopedia of the History of Arabic Science,* edited by Roshdi Rashed, 3:903–62. London: Routledge, 1996, 3 vols.

Schmidtke, Sabine. "Neuere Forschungen zur *Muᶜtazila.*" *Arabica* 45 (1998): 379–408.

Serrano Ruano, Delfina. "Los Almorávides y la teología Ashᶜarí: Contestación o legitimación de una disciplina marginal?" In *Identidades Marginales,* edited by Cristina de la Puente, 461–516. Madrid: CSIC, 2003.

———. "Por qué llamaron los almohades antropomorfistas a los almorávides?" In *Los almohades: Problemas y perspectives,* edited by Patrice Cressier, Maribel Fierro, and Luis Molina, 2:815–52. Madrid: CSIC, 2005.

———. "Why Did the Scholars of al-Andalus Distrust al-Ghazālī? Ibn Rushd al-Jadd's *Fatwā* on *Awliyā' Allāh.*" *Der Islam* 83 (2006): 137–56.

Sezgin, Fuat. *Geschichte des Arabischen Schrifttums* (*GAS*). 9 vols. Leiden: Brill, 1967–84.

Sharpe, William. "Isidore of Seville: The Medical Writings; An English Translation with an Introduction and Commentary." *Transactions of the American Philosophical Society* 54.2 (1964): 1–75.

Singer, Dorothea. "Some Plague Tractates." *Proceedings of the Royal Society of Medicine* 9 (1916): 159–211.

Smalley, Beryl. *Studies in Medieval Thought and Learning.* London: Hambledon, 1981.

Soifer, Maya. "Beyond Convivencia: Critical Reflections on the Historiography of Interfaith Relations in Christian Spain." *Journal of Medieval Iberian Studies* 1 (2009): 19–35.

Sontag, Susan. *AIDS and Its Metaphors.* New York: Farrar, Straus and Giroux, 1988.

———. *Illness as Metaphor.* 1978. Reprint, New York: Farrar, Straus and Giroux, 1988.

Stearns, Justin. "Considering the Maliki madhhab in Nasrid Granada: Two Significantly Different Views (Review of Dutton and Lohlker)." *Al-Qanṭara* 30 (2009): 664–70.

———. "Contagion in Theology and Law: Ethical Considerations in the Writings of Two 14th Century Scholars of Naṣrid Granada." *Islamic Law and Society* 14 (2007): 109–29.

———. "New Directions in the Study of Religious Responses to the Black Death." *History Compass* 7 (2009): 1–13.

———. "Representing and Remembering al-Andalus: Some Historical Considerations regarding the End of Time and the Making of Nostalgia." *Medieval Encounters* 15 (2009): 355–74.

Strohmaier, Gotthard. "Die Ansteckung als theologisches und als medizinisches Problem." *Oriente Moderno* 19 (2000): 631–45.

Stroumsa, Sarah. "Philosopher-King or Philosopher-Courtier? Theory and Reality in the *falāsifa's* Place in Islamic Society." In *Identidades Marginales,* edited by Cristina de la Puente, 433–59. Madrid: CSIC, 2003.

Sublet, Jaqueline. "La peste prise aux rêts de la jurisprudence: Le traité d'Ibn Ḥajar al-ᶜAsqalānī sur la peste." *Studia Islamica* 33 (1971): 141–49.

Sudhoff, Karl. "Ein Pestregimen aus dem Anfange des 15 Jahrhunderts." *Archive für Geschichte der Medizin* 3 (1910): 407–8.

———. "Pestschriften aus den ersten 150 Jahren nach der Epidemie des 'schwarzen Todes' 1348." *Archive für Geschichte der Medizin* 4 (1911): 191–222, 389–424; 5 (1912): 36–87, 332–96; 6 (1913): 313–79; 7 (1913): 57–114; 8 (1915): 175–215, 236–89; 9 (1916): 53–78, 119–67; 11 (1918): 44–92; 17 (1925): 241–91.

Ṭālibī, ᶜAmmār. *Ārā' Abī Bakr ibn al-'Arabī al-kalāmiyya.* Algiers: Al-Sharikah al-Waṭanīyah, 1974.

Temimi, A. "L'activité de Hamdan Khudja à Paris et à Istambul pour la question Algérienne." *Revue d'Histoire Maghrebine* 7-8 (1977): 234–43.

———. "Sidi Hamdan Bin Othman Khudja (1773–1842?)." *Revue d'Histoire Maghrebine* 25–26 (1982): 85–87.

Temkin, Owsei. "An Historical Analysis of the Concept of Infection." In *The Double*

Face of Janus, 456–71. 1953. Reprint, Baltimore: Johns Hopkins University Press, 1977.

Tokatly, Vardit. "The *Aʿlām al-Ḥadīth* of al-Khaṭṭābī." *Studia Islamica* 92 (2001): 53–91.

Tolan, John. *Saracens: Islam in the Medieval European Imagination.* New York: Columbia University Press, 2002.

Torres-Alcalá, Antonio. *Don Enrique de Villena: Un mago al dintel del renacimiento.* Madrid: Studia Humanitas, 1983.

Touati, François-Olivier. "Contagion and Leprosy: Myth, Ideas, and Evolution in Medieval Minds and Societies." In *Contagion: Perspectives from Pre-modern Societies,* edited by Lawrence Conrad and Dominik Wujastyk, 179–201. Burlington, VT: Ashgate, 2000.

———. *Maladie et societé au Moyen Age: La lepre, les lépreux et les léproseries dans la province ecclésiastique de Sens jusqu'au milieu du XIVe siècle.* Paris: De Boeck Université, 1998.

Travaglia, Pinella. *Magic, Causality, and Intentionality: The Doctrine of Rays in al-Kindi.* Florence: Edizioni del Galluzzo, 1999.

Travis, Peter. "Chaucer's Heliotropes and the Poetics of Metaphor." *Speculum* 72 (1997): 399–427.

Twigg, Graham. *The Black Death: A Biological Reappraisal.* New York: Schocken Books, 1984.

Ubieto Arteta, Antonio. "Cronología des desarrolló de la peste negra en la peninsula Iberica." *Cuadernos de Historia* 5 (1975): 47–66.

Ullmann, Manfred. *Islamic Medicine.* Edinburgh: Edinburgh University Press, 1978.

———. *Die Medizin im Islam.* Leiden: Brill, 1970.

Urvoy, Dominique. *Averroès: Les ambitions d'un intellectuel musulman.* Manchecourt France: Flammarion, 2001.

———. "Les conséquances christologiques de la confrontation islamo-chrétienne en Espagne au VIII siècle." In *The Formation of al-Andalus, Part 2,* edited by Maribel Fierro and Julio Samsó, 37–48. Brookfield, VT: Aldershot, 1998.

———. *Pensers d'al-Andalus: La vie intellectuelle á Cordoue et Seville au temps des empires berberes.* Toulouse: Presses Universitaires du Mirail, 1990.

Van Arsdall, Anne. "Reading Medieval Medical Texts with an Open Mind." In *Textual Healing: Essays on Medieval and Early Modern Medicine,* edited by Elizabeth Lane Furdell, 9–29. Leiden: Brill, 2005.

Van Ess, Josef. *Der Fehlschritt des Gelehrten.* Heidelberg: C. Winter, 2001.

———. "Ein unbekanntes Fragment des Naẓẓām." In *Der Orient in der Forschung,* edited by Wilhelm Hoenerbach, 170–201. Wiesbaden: Harrassowitz, 1967.

Vásquez de Benito, Concepción. "La materia médica de Ibn al-Jaṭīb." *Boletín de la Asociación Española de Orientalistas* 15 (1979): 139–50.

Von Kügelen, Anke. *Averroes und die Arabische Moderne: Ansätze zu einer Neubegründung des Rationalismus im Islam.* Leiden: Brill, 1994.

Wensinck, A. *Concordance et indices de la tradition musulmane.* 8 vols. Leiden: Brill, 1992.

Wesseling, Klaus-Gunther. "Rupert von Deutz." In *Biographisch-bibliographisches Kirchenlexikon,* edited by Traugott Bautz, 8:1021–31. Herzberg: Otto Harrassowitz, 1994.

Wild, Stefan. "The Self-Referentiality of the Qur'ān: Sura 3:7 as an Exegetical Challenge." In *With Reverence for the Word: Medieval Scriptural Exegesis in Judaism, Christianity, and Islam,* edited by Jane McAuliffe, Barry Walfish, and Joseph Goerin, 422–36. Oxford: Oxford University Press, 2003.

Winter, Tim, ed. *The Cambridge Companion to Classical Islamic Theology.* Cambridge: Cambridge University Press, 2008.

Wolf, Kenneth. *Christian Martyrs in Muslim Spain.* Cambridge: Cambridge University Press, 1988.

———. "Muḥammad as Antichrist in Ninth-Century Córdoba." In *Christians, Muslims, and Jews in Medieval and Early Modern Spain,* edited by Mark Mayerson and Edward English, 3–19. Notre Dame, IN: University of Notre Dame Press, 1999.

Wolfson, Harry Austryn. *The Philosophy of the Kalam.* Cambridge, MA: Harvard University Press, 1976.

Worboys, Michael. "Review of *The Rise of Causal Concepts of Disease.*" *Bulletin of the History of Medicine* 79 (2005): 832–33.

———. *Spreading Germs: Disease Theories and Medical Practice in Britain, 1865–1900.* Cambridge: Cambridge University Press, 2000.

Wray, Shona Kelly. "Boccaccio and the Doctors: Medicine and Compassion in the Face of Plague." *Journal of Medieval History* 30 (2004): 301–22.

York, William Henry. "Experience and Theory in Medical Practice during the Later Middle Ages: Valesco de Tarenta (fl. 1382–1426) at the Court of Foix." Ph.D. diss., Johns Hopkins University, 2003.

Yver, Georges. "Si Hamdan ben Othman Khodja." *Revue Africaine* 57 (1913): 96–138.

Ziriklī, *al-Aᶜlām.* Beirut: Dār al-ᶜIlm li-l-Milāyīn, 1989.

Zomeño, Amalía. "Ibn Lubb." In *Biblioteca de al-Andalus,* edited by Jorge Lirola, 4:24–8. Almería: Fundación Ibn Tufayl, 2006.

Zuckerman, Arnold. "Plague and Contagionism in Eighteenth-Century England: The Role of Richard Mead." *Bulletin of the History of Medicine* 78 (2004): 273–308.